MEASURING DIFFERENCE,
NUMBERING NORMAL

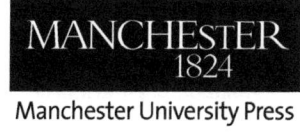

Manchester University Press

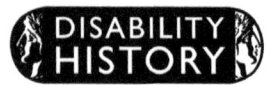

Series editors
Dr Julie Anderson, Professor Walton O. Schalick, III

This series published by Manchester University Press responds to the growing interest in disability as a discipline worthy of historical research. The series has a broad international historical remit, encompassing issues that include class, race, gender, age, war, medical treatment, professionalisation, environments, work, institutions and cultural and social aspects of disablement including representations of disabled people in literature, film, art and the media.

Already published

Deafness, community and culture in Britain: leisure and cohesion, 1945–1995
Martin Atherton

Disability in industrial Britain: a cultural and literary history of impairment in the coal industry, 1880–1948
Kirsti Bohata, Alexandra Jones, Mike Mantin and Steven Thompson

Disability and the Victorians: attitudes, interventions, legacies
Iain Hutchison, Martin Atherton and Jaipreet Virdi (eds)

Rethinking modern prostheses in Anglo-American commodity cultures, 1820–1939
Claire L. Jones (ed.)

Destigmatising mental illness? Professional politics and public education in Britain, 1870–1970
Vicky Long

Intellectual disability: a conceptual history, 1200–1900
Patrick McDonagh, C. F. Goodey and Tim Stainton (eds)

Fools and idiots? Intellectual disability in the Middle Ages
Irina Metzler

Framing the moron: the social construction of feeble-mindedness in the American eugenics era
Gerald V. O'Brien

Recycling the disabled: army, medicine, and modernity in WWI Germany
Heather R. Perry

Shell-shocked British Army veterans in Ireland, 1918–39: a difficult homecoming
Michael Robinson

Eradicating deafness? Genetics, pathology, and diversity in twentieth-century America
Marion Andrea Schmidt

Disability in the Industrial Revolution: physical impairment in British coalmining, 1780–1880
David M. Turner and Daniel Blackie

Worth saving: disabled children during the Second World War
Sue Wheatcroft

MEASURING DIFFERENCE, NUMBERING NORMAL

SETTING THE STANDARDS FOR DISABILITY IN THE INTERWAR PERIOD

Coreen McGuire

Manchester University Press

Copyright © Coreen McGuire 2020

The right of Coreen McGuire to be identified as the author of this work has been asserted by her in accordance with the Copyright, Designs and Patents Act 1988.

An electronic version of this book is also available under a Creative Commons (CC-BY) licence, which permits distribution and reproduction provided the author(s) and Manchester University Press are fully cited and any changes are acknowledged. Details of the licence can be viewed at https://creativecommons.org/licenses/by/4.0/

Published by Manchester University Press
Altrincham Street, Manchester M1 7JA
www.manchesteruniversitypress.co.uk

British Library Cataloguing-in-Publication Data
A catalogue record for this book is available from the British Library

ISBN 978 1 5261 4317 4 hardback
ISBN 978 1 5261 4316 7 open access

First published 2020

The publisher has no responsibility for the persistence or accuracy of URLs for any external or third-party internet websites referred to in this book, and does not guarantee that any content on such websites is, or will remain, accurate or appropriate.

Typeset by Newgen Publishing UK

Contents

List of figures		vii
Series editors' foreword		x
Acknowledgements		x
Acknowledgements of previously published material		xiii
Note on terminology		xiv
1	Numbering normal	1
2	Measuring disability	36
3	The artificial ear and the disability data gap	65
4	The audiometer and the medicalisation of hearing loss	105
5	The spirometer and the normal subjects	140
6	The respirator and the mechanisation of normal breathing	174
7	Measuring ourselves	202
Bibliography		210
Index		228

This volume is dedicated with much love and respect to my mother, Yvonne Margaret McGuire (née Hogshaw)

Figures

3.1 'How to pass and receive a telephone call', in 'Guidance for Subscribers on How to Articulate and Pronounce Vowels and Consonants, and Phrases to Use When Speaking on the Telephone', October 1923. British Telecom Archives, London, TCB 325/EHA 197 — 71

3.2 The artificial ear, Post Office Research Station, Dollis Hill. Records created and used by the Post Office telegraph and telephone service 1854–1969. British Telecom Archives, London, TCB 473/P 3513 — 78

3.3 Advertising booklet, 'A Telephone for Deaf Subscribers', 1936. British Telecom Archives, London, TCB 318/PH 632 — 84

3.4 'Telephone Service for the Deaf', 1938. British Telecom Archives, London, TCB 318/PH 632 — 89

3.5 'Suggestion that a flat mouthpiece, instead of the normal cupped one, should be provided to facilitate the use of a telephone in conjunction with a deaf aid worn on the chest'. Letter from W. S. Clark to Telephone Headquarters, 20 March 1954. British Telecom Archives, London, TCB 2/172, folder 'Telephones for Deaf People' — 93

4.1 Audiometer. Image and object courtesy of Thackray Medical Museum, Leeds — 112

4.2 Engineer's drawing of the hearing aid adaptor. The Services Division, letter dated September 1947, in 'Special Apparatus Fitted on Telephone Exchange Lines Rented by Deaf Subscribers'. British Telecom Archives, London, TCB 2/172 — 127

4.3 The Medresco hearing aid telephone adapter, in 'Special Apparatus Fitted on Telephone Exchange Lines Rented by Deaf Subscribers'. British Telecom Archives, London, TCB 2/172 — 130

5.1 Lowne spirometer, 1904. Image and object courtesy of the Thackray Medical Museum, Leeds — 143

5.2 Map of the south Wales coalfield marking the positions of the sixteen collieries of the MRC chronic pulmonary disease inquiry, 1942. *Chronic Pulmonary Disease in South Wales Coalminers: Report by the Committee* (Medical Research Council Special Report Series No. 243) (London: His Majesty's Stationery Office, 1942). The National Archives, London, FD 41243, p. 11 — 161

6.1 Drinker respirator and Drinker–Collins respirator. *'Breathing Machines' and Their Use in Treatment: Report of the Respirators (Poliomyelitis) Committee* (Medical Research Council Special Report Series No. 237) (London: His Majesty's Stationery Office, 1939), plate 1 — 186

6.2 Bragg–Paul pulsator and Burstall jacket respirator. *'Breathing Machines' and Their Use in Treatment: Report of the Respirators (Poliomyelitis) Committee* (Medical Research Council Special Report Series No. 237) (London: His Majesty's Stationery Office, 1939), plate 3 — 189

Series editors' foreword

You know a subject has achieved maturity when a book series is dedicated to it. In the case of disability, while it has co-existed with human beings for centuries the study of disability's history is still quite young.

In setting up this series, we chose to encourage multi-methodologic history rather than a purely traditional historical approach, as researchers in disability history come from a wide variety of disciplinary backgrounds. Equally 'disability' history is a diverse topic which benefits from a variety of approaches in order to appreciate its multi-dimensional characteristics.

A test for the team of authors and editors who bring you this series is typical of most series, but disability also brings other consequential challenges. At this time disability is highly contested as a social category in both developing and developed contexts. Inclusion, philosophy, money, education, visibility, sexuality, identity and exclusion are but a handful of the social categories in play. With this degree of politicisation, language is necessarily a cardinal focus.

In an effort to support the plurality of historical voices, the editors have elected to give fair rein to language. Language is historically contingent, and can appear offensive to our contemporary sensitivities. The authors and editors believe that the use of terminology that accurately reflects the historical period of any book in the series will assist readers in their understanding of the history of disability in time and place.

Finally, disability offers the cultural, social and intellectual historian a new 'take' on the world we know. We see disability history as one of a few nascent fields with the potential to reposition our understanding of the flow of cultures, society, institutions, ideas and lived experience. Conceptualisations of 'society' since the early modern period have heavily stressed principles of autonomy, rationality and the subjectivity of the individual agent. Consequently we are frequently oblivious to the historical contingency of the present with respect to those elements. Disability disturbs those foundational features of 'the modern.' Studying disability history helps us resituate our policies, our beliefs and our experiences.

Julie Anderson
Walton O. Schalick, III

Acknowledgements

This book is about failed attempts to measure things that cannot really be quantified, and so, accordingly, I will now attempt to sum up the overwhelming contributions of the individuals and institutions that helped me write it.

First, I want to thank all the disabled people featured in this book, who fought back against attempts to categorise the diverse and innovative experiences of their lives.

The materials for half of this book derive from research I undertook at the University of Leeds with support from BT Archives. I am grateful to BT Archives and the AHRC for funding this research, and to David Hay for sharing his knowledge of the Post Office and allowing me to reproduce images from BT Archives. I am especially appreciative of the support of Professor Graeme Gooday for his incisive intellectual commentary on my work and his generous friendship over the past six years. His book, *The Morals of Measurement*, has been central to the development of my thinking about surrogate measurements and their use in healthcare. I am appreciative of the contributions of the scholarly community of The Centre for History and Philosophy of Science at Leeds between 2013 and 2016. I am thankful for the enduring friendships formed during that time with Alice Haigh, Rebecca Bowd, Anne Hanley, Kiara White, Gemma Almond and Nick Marsh. I have also gained immeasurably from the scholarship and friendship of Emily Herring, Jade Fletcher, Alice Murphy and Laura Sellers who have all read chapter drafts, encouraged me to keep writing when I was worried about the process and encouraged me to keep drinking when on girls' nights out.

The other half of this book was written in the Department of Philosophy at the University of Bristol. My research there was made possible through the support of the Wellcome Trust and I am very grateful that their generosity has allowed this book to be open access. I thank all the staff and students who helped shape my scholarship between 2017 and 2019. I am especially appreciative of the cross-disciplinary engagement, reading and encouragement of my work from friends and colleagues: Ana-Maria Crețu, Karim Thébault, Jason Konek, and Robert Chapman. Thanks also to my office-mates Joshua Habgood-Coote, Sean Gryb and Johannes Stern. I miss our coffees and our climate-challenged office!

I am indebted to all the members of the Life of Breath team at Durham University and Bristol. Being a part of this project with its amazing group of interdisciplinary scholars has changed the way I think about history, and convinced me that one of the best ways we can think about the past is in relation to how we can shape the present. Thanks to all the team and especially to Kate Binnie, Alice Malpass, Tina Williams, James Dodd and Jane Macnaughton. Thank you to Havi Carel for hiring me on the project. Before I started working with Havi, I expressed my hope to a mutual colleague that she would be nice, and they responded, 'Nice? She's far too intelligent and interesting to be described as nice!' I have since appreciated the truth of this descriptor, and have sincerely appreciated Havi's intellectual power, her unpredictability and especially her luminous prose. But in fact, she has been very nice to me, and I appreciate the many and various kindnesses that she has extended to me over the last two years. I have also benefited from the wisdom and efficiency of our project manager Jordan Collver who designed the image used on the cover of this book. The Life of Breath Project also allowed me to invite Lundy Braun to Bristol to give a brilliant lecture on 'race correction in medicine' in the summer of 2018. Braun's *Breathing Race into the Machine* is the most exciting history of medicine book I have ever read and has hugely influenced my thinking.

As well as individuals, this book was made possible by institutions, and I am grateful to the National Archives and its staff (especially Paul Johnson) and all the archivists at the wonderful South Wales Miners' Library. I have been lucky enough to work closely with the incredible object collections at the Thackray Medical Museum and I appreciate the help with sourcing and reproducing the images in this book given by Alan Humphries and Louise Crossley. Further thanks to the Action on Hearing Loss Library, principally to librarian extraordinaire Dominic Stiles. Thanks also to the Consortium for History of Science, Technology and Medicine and all those who contributed to the 'Measuring Aurality' group. I greatly appreciated the feedback Mara Mills gave me on Chapter 4, which dovetails most closely with her brilliant scholarship on telephony in the US context. This group was organised by Jaipreet Virdi, who I owe huge thanks to for her help with this book and her generous encouragement throughout the last six years. I first met Jai at a conference in Leeds in 2013, and this encounter totally changed my sense of how a historian could be. Her vision, scholarship, humour and grace are unparalleled. Manchester University Press has been a wonderful place to publish a first book. I particularly appreciate the professionalism and kindness of Emma Brennan, Julie Anderson, Jen Mellor and Paul Clarke. Thanks also to those involved in the production process, especially Christopher Feeney and Helen Flitton. I am very grateful to the anonymous reviewer for their astute observations and encouraging remarks on earlier drafts. If you confirm your identity, I would love to buy you a cake.

My family have been a constant source of love, support and encouragement throughout my life. It is too big to really commend all its members to paper, but I want to convey special thanks to the Crawford family, especially my Gran and Grandad (Maureen and David Crawford) and the McGuire family, especially my Grannie Anne (Anne McGuire). Thanks also to Tracey Barr, and Anthony, Maria, George and Claudia Pace. My Uncle Ernie (Pace) and Uncle Billy (Barr) passed away before seeing this book but were both instrumental in facilitating its completion. Thank you to my incredible brother Michael, who I love, and am unutterably proud of, and my (almost) sister Camilla. Not technically a sister either, but much more than a best friend, thank you to Victoria Brown. And to my Mum and Dad, Yvonne and Ewan McGuire – thank you for everything. Everything I am or will ever be is owed to you both. I love you very much.

And with love, I come at last to my husband. I am so happy to be part of your family, and want to thank Ian, Janet, Gaz, Amy, Neil, Sophie and Daphne Bellis, Uncle Rob and the Cater family for their warm support throughout the last four years. Richard, I could never attempt to measure (directly or indirectly) the infinite amount of love we have. However, I know you will want me to at least try. So, thank you for bearing with me while I wrote this. For reading and editing my entire first draft, listening to me and helping me, for probably helping me a bit too much with the bibliography, for cooking and cleaning so I could work, for making me laugh always, for everything. We are both aware of the vastness of history and our relatively small space in it, yet I cannot be made to believe that any other two people could ever have been as happy as we are right now.

Acknowledgements of previously published material

Chapter 3, 'The artificial ear and the disability data gap', is derived in part from an article published in *History and Technology* on 3 September 2019 © 2019 The Author(s), available online: https://doi.org/10.1080/07341512.2019.1652435 I would like to extend my thanks to editors Gabriele Balbi, Christiana Berth, Amy Slaton and Tiago Saraiva, as well as publishers Taylor & Francis for allowing me to reproduce this material.

Thank you to Clare Jones for giving me permission to reframe some of the material for my Chapter 3 section on 'Case studies: individual users versus institutional innovations', which was originally published as: McGuire, C., 'Inventing Amplified Telephony: The Co-Creation of Aural Technology and Disability', in C. Jones (ed.), *Rethinking Modern Prostheses in Anglo-American Commodity Cultures, 1820–1939* (Manchester: Manchester University Press, 2017), pp. 70–90.

Thank you to Havi Carel, Adam Cureton, David Wasserman and Oxford University Press for giving me permission to reframe the material in the Chapter 4 section 'Putting the user in the picture' and in the Chapter 6 section 'The Bragg-Paul Pulsator', some portions of which were originally published as: McGuire, C., and Carel, H., 'The Visible and the Invisible: Disability, Assistive Technology, and Stigma', in D. T. Wasserman and A. Cureton (eds), *The Oxford Handbook of Philosophy and Disability* (Oxford: Oxford University Press, 2019), pp. 598–615.

Chapter 5, 'The spirometer and the normal subjects', is derived in part from an article published in the *British Journal of the History of Science*. I would like to extend my thanks to Trish Hatton and editors Charlotte Sleigh and Amanda Rees for allowing me to reproduce this material. McGuire, C. '"X- Rays Don't Tell Lies": The Medical Research Council and the Measurement of Respiratory Disability 1936-1945', *British Journal for the History of Science*, 52:3 (2019), 447–465.

Finally, parts of Chapter 6, 'The respirator and the mechanisation of normal breathing', have been developed alongside my co-authors Jaipreet Virdi and Jenny Hutton and will feature in the forthcoming edited collection *Patient Voices in Britain, 1840–1948: Historical and Policy Perspectives*, published by Manchester University Press. I am very grateful to Jaipreet and Jenny for their permission to use this work and also extend my gratitude to editors Anne Hanley and Jessica Meyer.

The roles of all these editors in helping me to originally refine this material is much appreciated and their influence has helped to shape the ideas and content of this book in its entirety.

Note on terminology

I have used the word 'disabled' in this book in relation to hearing loss, with full awareness that many deaf people do not consider themselves disabled. I have avoided referring to people 'with disabilities' in order to emphasise, in line with the social model of disability, that people are disabled as a result of the workings of society. Disablement is often contingent on temporality, spaces, cultures and contexts. In this book, I demonstrate the way in which people have also been disabled by technology and measurement systems. Therefore, while I use the word disabled, I am fully aware that it does not reflect the experiences of most people with hearing loss, or the Deaf. In this context and in this book, the word Deaf is capitalised in order to indicate the way that the term is being used to represent the members and views of a group identified by culture and community rather than through their medical status. The Post Office often referred to 'Deaf Subscribers' and a 'Deaf Telephone Service', and I have reproduced primary sources verbatim. However, it is important to note that in those instances, the capitalisation of Deaf indicates the historically accurate title but is not indicative of the cultural identity now attached to the Deaf.

1

NUMBERING NORMAL

Waking up different

In 1998, thousands of men and women in the United States woke up and found themselves changed. These individuals may have felt the same as they did the day before. They may have got out of bed, showered, made breakfast and driven to work as if it were any other day. Yet overnight they had become overweight. Some had become obese, others morbidly so. Still more had moved from the underweight category to become 'normal'. What kind of drastic vicissitudes had been realised to change so many bodies so rapidly? A sudden increase in nocturnal sleep-related eating disorders? Icing sugar falling like snow from the night sky? No: the National Institutes of Health (NIH) had changed the way the way that it measured Body Mass Index (BMI).

Previously the United States had classified men with a BMI of 27.8 or above and women with a BMI of 27.3 or above as overweight. However, in 1998 it shifted the measurement down to 25, to fall in line with the World Health Organization's (WHO) standardised classification system and to allow for easier calculability.[1] In one fell swoop thousands more people in the US were obese. The media responded with panicked commentary about the obesity epidemic, without mentioning the artificial inflation of these new statistics. But why would they? It is perfectly natural to trust in the classification systems of scientists. Yet this example demonstrates that the thresholds of normalcy that we rely on for the classification of health are more fluid that we might imagine. In this book I argue that our bodies have been changed by measurement technology. Our capabilities and parameters have been defined so that we – you – shift from states of normalcy to disability at the whim of mercurial thresholds.

Disability history fascinates because it forces us to ask questions about our universal lived experience and how we ascribe meaning and significance to certain attributes and values. What should we be capable of?

What matters to us? Would these things have mattered in the same way to those living a hundred or so years ago? Does this change anything about how we feel? Such questions are, of course, subject to diversity of experience. Yet the need to standardise and objectify levels of disability using measurement technologies is often in opposition with individual variance. Measuring normalcy has never been simple. The choice of certain measurement systems was influenced by the relative difficulty or ease of their implementation. Subsequently, these chosen measurement classifications have had a crucial impact on our concept of disability, and I show here that these processes were perpetuated and perfected in the interwar years in Britain. This book thus provides a new perspective on the relationship between the measurement and understanding of disability.

The central thesis of this book is that health measurements are given artificial authority if they are particularly amenable to calculability and easy measurement. Furthermore, the selection of people we have chosen to measure as standard is subject to discrimination and bias as we prioritise the measurement of easily recognisable groups. This, I contend, has led to biased data sets that have conflicted with individual perceptions of health, especially in cases of invisible but experiential disability. The real-world consequences of this are highlighted in cases of invisible disability that have been contested, for instance in compensation procedures. Difficulties around diagnosis are compounded by invisible experiences, and so measurement tools are used to make the invisible visible. However, problems often coalesce around felt experiences that do not lend themselves to easy quantification. Dissonance between objective measurement and subjective experience is therefore a recurring theme, resounding in each chapter of this book. Measurement technologies were a crucial component of the drive to quantify bodily norms and grade sensorial symptoms and are thus an important but unrecognised area for the historical investigation of disability.

The historical technologies I am primarily concerned with here relate to the measurement of hearing and breathing. However, I am not providing a history of the modern fields of audiometry or spirometry.[2] Rather, I aim to reveal the data gaps in these fields. In the book *Invisible Women: Exposing Data Bias in a World Designed for Men*, feminist activist Caroline Criado Perez coined the phrase 'Henry Higgins Effect', to describe the data gap that leads to technologies designed as neutral really only being suitable for the neutral *male*.[3] Examples of this are legion, ranging from mildly inconvenient to dangerous (offices too cold, phones too large, loads too heavy), to fatal (ineffective drugs, unrecognised symptoms, fatal car accidents). Why is this happening? To take the example of fatal car accidents, Perez explains that:

Men are more likely than women to be involved in a car crash, which means they dominate the numbers of those seriously injured in car accidents. But when a woman is involved in a car crash, she is 47% more likely to be seriously injured than a man, and 71% more likely to be moderately injured, even when researchers control for factors such as height, weight, seat-belt usage, and crash intensity. She is also 17% more likely to die. And it's all to do with how the car is designed – and for whom.[4]

These dire statistics are reflective of the fact that women's (on average) shorter torsos and legs mean that they sit further forward while driving; a 'wilful deviation from the norm' which corresponds to increased internal injuries in front-facing collisions.[5] Using only data related to men's bodies means that the average is biased towards a male driver. However, it is often only this data that is available and this, of course, is related to ease of measurement. Specifically, the fact that women are regarded as more expensive and difficult to measure, primarily due to the perceived unpredictability of hormonal fluctuations.[6] Perez explains, 'Female bodies (both the human and animal variety) are, it is argued, too complex, too variable, too costly to be tested on.'[7] And yet, Perez's central argument – that we need more research on sex differences to take women's bodies and experiences into account – shows a startling degree of historical naivety about the reasons why we have in the past chosen to measure certain bodies and not others. It is the project of this book to outline the complex historical circumstances and contingencies which have led to the prioritisation of particular measurements of particular kinds. In doing so, I reveal the political expediencies often hidden in the construction of measurement instruments and explicate the potential negative consequences of essentialising social groups as distinct kinds to be categorised for measurement. As Steven Epstein has pointed out, 'Recent reformers assume that a medical insistence on difference necessarily advances the interest of historically disadvantaged groups; but the old medical theories of group difference had just the opposite effect, reinforcing oppression and helping them to consolidate the very disadvantages that we now hope to overturn.'[8] Angela Saini has also warned of the 'ugly and dangerous history' of research into sex differences.[9] Moreover, measuring only the '70 kg white man' as a representative average has further, entirely unexplored implications for the understanding of disability.

Disability data gaps can be similarly distorting of normal capabilities. Such omissions are evident in the data sets used in the nascent field of audiometry during the interwar period. Data sets which excluded those with imperfect hearing meant that the average threshold, which represented normalcy, was distorted. Thus, the line of normalcy was artificially high, and the range of those categorised as deaf was too broad. As we will see in Chapter 3, this was because these data sets came from telephone companies who needed a minimum efficiency standard for their male customer base. Economic imperatives generated these data, not medical considerations. And, as scientist Dr Phyllis Margaret Tookey Kerridge (1901–1940) pointed out as early as 1937 while using these standards to measure hearing in a medical context, it was an assumption that hearing was universal, with no variation within the normal between groups, such as children.[10]

Within spirometric studies the situation was more complex. The idea that we are all breathing the same air in the same way was problematised from the beginning of spirometry. Data sets were specifically constructed around appropriate reference classes. I use the term reference classes throughout this book to refer to the categories of difference such as race, sex, age, weight, height and class which are variously employed to both produce of knowledge about our health *and* to validate our social classification systems. For example, sociologist Janet Shim illuminates the fact that the epidemiology of heart disease 'both emerges out of and contributes to systems of social classification by race, class, sex, and gender'.[11]

However, the selection of these groups or reference classes was contested and variable throughout the twentieth century. Indeed, the selection of easily recognisable groups promoted the idea of normalcy within certain *social* groups. This had drastic consequences in impeding the availability of occupational compensation for respiratory disability. Conversely but perhaps equally tragically, the failure to use such reference classes for apparently *biological* groups (such as women) meant that our understanding of what it meant for women to breathe normally was also misrepresented. The historical use of these reference classes, as we will see in Chapter 2, has been variously linked with the social determination that certain bodies were superior or inferior, which has consequently impacted on our understanding of disability.

Disability everywhere and nowhere

Historian Lennard Davis has argued that the anthropometric measurements and systematic setting of the 'normal' body's limits that took place in the nineteenth century led to significant and enduring changes to our understanding of disability. As the rise of eugenics-based statistics worked to create a standard of 'normalcy', increased measurement and statistical analysis created a symbiotic relationship between what could be defined as the 'normal' body and the 'disabled' body.[12] As this book will demonstrate, such strict dichotomies were challenged by individuals who disputed their status as normal or disabled, especially in compensation disputes. Davis focused especially on deafness to argue that 'the problem is the way that normalcy is constructed to create the "problem" of the disabled body'.[13] Davis's work highlights what has become an important part of disability history. That is, acknowledgement of the fact that the construction of normalcy and deviance from normalcy (disability) is dependent on the time, place and context in which the judgement is made. Although this book takes a similar theoretical stance to Davis, it differs in its focus on the interwar years in Britain and in its critical emphasis on measurement technologies. While Davis drew attention to the power of statistics, I extend his argument to argue that technological instruments have been underestimated as crucial tools for developing our conceptualisation of disability.

For instance, the complex connection between deafness and sound technologies continued in interwar Britain, I argue, when the telephone became a tool for identifying and categorising hearing loss. The telephone's power in interwar Britain was linked to the fact that between 1912 and 1981, the British Post Office had control over a nationalised telephone system. Bell's Telephone Company was the first independent telephone company and Alexander Graham Bell (1847–1922) fought zealously to retain his right over the telephone patent, making himself a fortune in the process.[14] However, eventually Thomas Edison's (1847–1931) competing telephony company forced Bell to co-create the Bell and Edison telephone company and the Edison Gower-Bell Telephone Company of Europe, which extended one long arm of its monopoly into Britain with the National Telephone Company (the NTC). Therefore the Bell and Edison conglomerate controlled most of telephony in Britain. That is until the 1880 ruling on the 1869 Telegraph Act mandated a nationalised service, which was summarily instated in 1911. The 1869 Telegraph Act had granted the UK government a complete monopoly over all communications and it was confirmed in 1880 that this Act included telephony even though the telephone had not been invented when the Act was first conceived.[15]

The telephone in interwar Britain was an important tool in both the identification and categorisation of individual hearing loss, and the ability to hear normally was both defined and moderated by the telephone. Linkage between telephony and hearing has long been noted by historians of sound and science, and Post Office engineers in the interwar period had considerable expertise in both telecommunications and hearing assistive devices. Telephone technology thus contributed to increased quantification of the human body and the interwar shift towards mechanised practical measures of hearing.

Using machines in this way led to what Daston and Galison term 'mechanical objectivity'. In their framing, technologies such as photography led to distrust in human visual perception due to expectation of perception; so it was feared that scientists were irrevocably biased by their expectations and that only machines could be trusted to be objective and honest.[16] They point out that by the late nineteenth century, mechanical objectivity was installed as the guiding ideal of scientific representation across a range of disciplines, including medicine.[17] For instance, in Chapter 4 we will see that the mechanised standards of hearing set up by the telephone system enabled the quantitative measurement of hearing through the audiometer. This circumvented the need to rely on the subjective assessment of personal hearing loss and allowed for the graphical inscription of individual deviation from 'normal hearing' – a term which I contest and problematise in Chapter 3 and Chapter 4. Indeed, the claim that audiometers provide a trustworthy representation is highly contentious: hearing is facilitated by the whole body and the way we access speech is dependent on a variety of factors, including accent, speech, facial expression and lip-reading. Communication is a two-way street, after all. Indeed, historical analysis of the long and difficult process of training machines to hear speech clarifies the fact that hearing is more complex than a simple mechanical process, 'spectrographic data had to be further quantified and expressed mathematically in order for a machine to "objectively" discern patterns that were apparent to the "subjective scale" of the ear or eye'.[18] As Chapter 4 outlines, claiming to be able to measure hearing was largely a matter of technocratic control which was often at odds with the experience of those subjected to such measures.

Patient reporting of symptoms was thus downgraded in a way memorably described by Jewson as resulting in 'the disappearance of the sick man'.[19] While Jewson's original analysis related primarily to the social changes that attended the shift from bedside medicine to hospital medicine, he also argued that the technical apparatus used in 'laboratory medicine' at the end of the nineteenth century further objectified the body of the patient.[20] Daniel Goldberg has maintained that this naturalistic epistemic framework is best described as 'somaticism' – a focus on materially identified body pathologies endorsed by the ideology of mechanical objectivity.[21]

In this book, I extend these analyses to the interwar years in Britain, and argue that at that point, measurement instrumentation became a crucial component of the process of measuring disability and numbering normalcy. Tools like the audiometer and the spirometer defined disability as measurable pathology within the epistemic framework of mechanical objectivity, which linked instruments with impersonality, and thus with truth.[22] The subsequent pursuit of standardisation reflected an attitudinal shift in the twentieth century that meant many no longer considered individual perception to be sufficiently accurate, or to be an appropriate channel for measurement. Since instrument users had to trust the maker, materials and theory embodied in the device, this meant trust was not automatically assumed; often, users artificially privileged preferred values by using easily measurable (surrogate) parameters to achieve practical ends.[23] Trust was embedded in machinery and preferred to the kind of knowledge that could be generated by the individual human body.

The natural sciences' embrace of mechanical objectivity during the interwar years occurred alongside a crucial change in the tone of wider ideological thinking about society in Britain. While industrialising Victorian Britain was characterised by broad social and cultural confidence in empire and industry, the interwar years featured growing pessimism and fears of British decline and degeneration, alongside the apparent rise 'of the survival of the unfittest'.[24] The 1904 Committee on Physical Deterioration was set up to explore how realistic these fears were and, while it found no evidence of overall decline, it did posit that poor food choices could be one of 'the causes to which degenerative tendencies might be assigned'.[25] Such statements, which presented degeneration as evident and apparent, added to the growing public rhetoric of deterioration.[26] Its expression was funnelled, increasingly, through the conduit of eugenics – the pursuit of the exceptional man initiated by Francis Galton (1822–1911).

The eugenics paradigm rested on a social determination of idealised bodies positioned in opposition to the abnormal. I argue in Chapter 5 that the historical use of reference classes in spirometery was linked with and supportive of this framework. Spirometry was originally designed in the late nineteenth century to quantify the volume of air that an individual could exhale as 'vital capacity'. At this point, the spirometer presented vital capacity as lung capacity and its usage was often extrapolated into the measurement of normal breathing. Yet using this measure as representative of health or even levels of breathlessness was immediately problematic.

Normal breathing was never for all; rather, the spirometer was employed to enhance the differences between us. Spirometric data sets were specifically constructed around groups, which promoted the idea of normalcy within certain *social* groups (such as coal miners). This had drastic consequences in impeding the availability of occupational compensation for respiratory disability.

In Chapter 3 and Chapter 5 I show that technologies such as the spirometer and audiometer led to increased quantification of the human body and a shift towards more mechanistic perception which intensified the need to assign equivocal values to scale applicable measures of normal hearing and normal respiratory function. The impetus behind the reduction of these multidimensional sensorial qualities stemmed from powerful bureaucratic forces for which classification was especially important, namely, the British Post Office and the Medical Research Council (MRC), and I detail the importance of these two bodies to British society during the interwar years and explain the drive behind their standardisation of normalcy. In these chapters I make visible the invisible workings of these technologies, and in Chapter 4 and Chapter 6 I detail their consequences for individual bodies by exploring how standard thresholds of normalcy impacted on assistive technologies such as hearing aids and respiratory prostheses.

Scholars including Ian Hacking, Ted Porter and Stephen Jay Gould have all linked eugenic thinking to the expansion and veneration of measurable, numerical data. I situate their arguments within the historical context of the nineteenth century in the next section of this chapter. However, at this point, I simply point out that for all their insight, it is puzzling that such scholars did not recognise the relevance that their analysis had on the categorisation of disability. With the exception of the work of the aforementioned Lennard Davis, these classic texts linking the rise of standardised classification systems to eugenics do not make the leap to connect biometrics to disability.

Disability is everywhere and nowhere in these texts. And, as disability historian Douglas Baynton points out, disability is everywhere in history. As he puts it, 'there are no histories in which a disability analysis would be out of place and many that are diminished by its absence'.[27] Indeed, Baynton elucidates the fact that the concept of disability was integral to eugenic thought and practically expressed in the United States through anti-immigration laws that were designed broadly to safeguard against abnormal individuals entering society.[28] Such concerns were allied to the twentieth-century culture of industrialisation and efficiency, 'a culture that was increasingly intolerant and afraid of difference'.[29] Twentieth-century standardisation of medical practices took place against a background of standardisation which extended into the home and the office.

> The industrialist Frederick Winslow Taylor's attempts to standardize all aspects of the workplace, including the workers, the need to develop standard sizes for the ready-to-wear clothing industry, and the emerging field of life insurance and the apparent link between height, weight, and health all contributed to a growing tendency to see the human body in terms of statistical averages established through rigorous scientific investigation.[30]

The body of the patient, too, became conceptualised within this universal standardisation framework and the increased intolerance of difference resulted in an analogous standardisation of disability. As Baynton's immigration example demonstrates, disability is a particularly important grouping to study because it allows us to consider how it functions as a key defining social category *alongside* the categories of race, class and gender.[31] It also reinforces historian Catherine Kudlick's compelling insight that when we are studying disability we are in fact studying power.[32] Such power is often attached to numerical data.

Why was the Post Office involved in standardising normalcy thresholds? To understand its role in our story, we need to go back to the late nineteenth century, and the beginning of telephony.[33]

In 1874, Scottish-American inventor and teacher of the deaf Alexander Graham Bell managed to procure a dissected human ear 'fresh' from a recently deceased cadaver. He attached this to a needle and was thus able to transcribe sound waves onto smoked glass.[34] This was one of the experiments that eventually led to the 'invention' of the telephone, which was patented by Bell in 1876. Bell's obsession with deafness, his desire to cure it, or to at least make speech visible so that lip-reading and forced speech could give the appearance of a cure, is well known. His mother was deaf, and his father and grandfather were both elocutionists. Bell's visible speech (a kind of physiological alphabet used for oral instruction) was the invention of his grandfather, Alexander Melville Bell.[35] And, like his father and grandfather, Alexander initially worked as an elocutionist. He moved to Canada in 1870, and then to Boston in 1871 to take up work as a teacher of the deaf.[36] It was there that he met Mabel, the student that he would eventually marry. The neurologist Oliver Sacks memorably described Bell's life-long obsession with curing deafness as 'half-terrible, half-promethean'-like in its fury and vigour.[37] This fury had far-reaching effects. Multiple scholars have demonstrated the extent to which Bell's promotion of oralism helped to enact it as the only suitable method for teaching the deaf following the infamous 1880 Milan Conference which forbade sign language and forced generations of deaf children to undergo unsuitable and cruel education practices.[38] Oralism was further motivated by Christian ideology which emphasised that citizens must be able to speak to claim the right to abode in the kingdom of heaven.[39] One had to be able to speak to affirm one's faith, and (under Roman law) to claim property, which meant that oralism was heavily promoted by aristocratic families where interbreeding had caused hereditary deafness that subsequently threatened their ability to retain their lands and property.[40] As Douglas Baynton notes, simply 'to be human was to speak'.[41] The practice of oralism used various breathing techniques to make the voice visible and then audible. The spirometer was thus used in the nineteenth century in deaf education as well as in medical researches into respiration.[42] Deafness echoes through technologies as varied as shorthand, multiple telegraphy, oralism, speech therapy and, above all, telephony.[43]

The Post Office brought telephony under its control through its unique position as an office of state that also had to function as a profitable business. Stephen Tallents, the public relations guru who spearheaded the Post Office's major rebranding campaign during the 1930s, articulated the conflict of interest between profit and the state that was integral to the Post Office in the interwar years:

> The Post Office of today is a combination between great business corporation and a government department. As such its publicity ... must be organised to combine, with such modifications as its special position demands, the well-tried methods of commercial advertising and the wholly unexplored and almost wholly unpractised methods of government publicity. That combination breeds certain advantages and certain difficulties.[44]

As a result of what Tallents termed its 'special position' within the government, the Post Office developed amplified telephone technology according to its changing relationship with the Treasury, whose priorities regarding welfare were simultaneously in flux. The certain advantages alluded to by Tallents included the total control that the Post Office had over the telephone network. But this state backing also meant that it was required to work under the demands and financial constraints of the Treasury and act as an arm of the wider government. For this reason, the state and the newly enfranchised public expected the Post Office to provide telephones that could be used by people with some hearing loss. Amplified telephony was thus developed alongside the embryonic welfare state.

Writing history based around the activities of the Post Office is challenging because of its institutional set-up. The interwar structure of the Post Office business model complicates and conceals the agency directing amplified telephone development. Until the Bridgeman Report was instigated by the wider government in 1932, the Post Office Telecommunications Department was run on the same lines as its predecessor, the National Telephone Company. However, the rapid growth of its telephone network put pressure on the larger Post Office operation. This pressure was exaggerated by the fact that any problems related to engineering had to be referred to the Engineer-in-Chief in London and this meant that any changes to equipment became extremely complicated. This also led to internal disputes, as historian Campbell-Smith has explained: 'Local telephone operations were run from day to day by twenty-eight "District Managers", ... who were not entirely comfortable being subordinated to colleagues with no technical training whatever.'[45] In practice, this meant that all complaints about the efficacy of the amplified telephones and planned changes to their design were filtered through the London

Office at St Martin's Le Grand via the Engineer-in-Chief's research station at Dollis Hill. It is thus sometimes difficult to recover agency in the direction of telephone improvements, as individual actions were immersed in extensive bureaucracy. The Telecommunications Department of the Post Office exemplifies an office hidden behind its role as a cog driving the larger Post Office 'Government Machine', with its role in providing a telephone for people with hearing loss 'marked by opaqueness and discretion'.[46]

Like the British Post Office, the MRC was part of the government but remained apart from it. As discussed earlier in this chapter, the interwar years were permeated by pessimistic ideas about degeneration and featured a succession of governmental social surveys, largely targeted at children and the working classes. Researchers worrying about 'physical efficiency' designed studies on nutrition and minimal calorie intake, which prominently featured attempts to objectively calculate individual physical needs.[47] Interrelated with such health concerns were economic worries, especially since the 1911 National Insurance Act had begun providing disability benefits and free medical treatment for insured workers.[48] The Act gave special provision for the treatment of tuberculosis for both the insured and their dependants, partly to ensure that Britain kept up with Germany, who were the major threat invoked in relation to 'national efficiency'.[49]

Crucially, *research* into tuberculosis was also included in the 1911 proviso, and by exploiting this research clause the Departmental Committee on Tuberculosis was able to morph into the broader Medical Research Committee. The outbreak of war in 1914 severely curtailed the planned tuberculosis research. However, the department's contributions to medical science throughout the war were afterwards deemed essential by the War Office. These contributions were especially directed towards the compilation, sorting and classification of medical statistics. The MRC combined the medical and surgical statistics of military hospitals in an enterprise of 'formidable' import.[50]

Therefore, in 1919 the Medical Research Committee was re-designated as the Medical Research Council.[51] The fact that it was directly responsible only to the Privy Council meant that the MRC was endowed with significant freedom in its organisation and investigations into a variety of medical and biological researches. This research diversity meant that during the interwar years, the council was split into numerous sub-sections which were usually represented by committees, research boards or advisory boards with specific focal points.[52] Wider interwar concerns about 'National Efficiency' were allied with the MRC's drive for standardisation, especially of anthropometric measurements. The war had highlighted the need for fixed, standardised measurements in the medical sciences, and the MRC believed that Britain was falling behind other countries, becoming subject to other standards rather than setting them. In Austoker and Bryder's terms: 'Standardization thus assumed not just scientific or medical but also economic and political significance.'[53]

In Chapter 5 I make the argument that the MRC's focus on medical statistics impeded recognition of the risk of coal-dust to miners' lungs. Yet ironically, the MRC's focus on medical statistics in the twentieth century overwhelmingly aligned with its increased recognition of the social determinants of health. For instance, after the Second World War the industrial health research board of the MRC sponsored a wide-scale survey on the occupation factors implicated in ulcers.[54] Many of the clinicians working for the MRC in the interwar years and after were politically left-wing, and emphasised the impact that social deprivation, malnutrition and living conditions had on health.[55] MRC researchers like Richard Doll (1912–2005) and Archie Cochrane (1909–1988) were not only cognisant of the environmental causes of illness, they instituted practices in medical statistics and epidemiology (such as the randomised control trial) to reveal them and force the instigation of public health measures. Concurrently, the randomised control trial helped to usher in an era of measured quantification directed towards the simultaneous standardisation of medical practice and the patient.[56]

Measurement matters

The idea that numerical measurable data has privileged (and powerful) epistemological significance is sometimes referred to as the 'Curse of Kelvin', because of a remark he made to the Institute of Civil Engineers in 1883: 'I often say that when you can measure what you are speaking about, and express it in numbers, you know something about it; but when you cannot measure it, when you cannot express it in numbers, your knowledge is of a meagre and unsatisfactory kind.'[57] Kelvin's implicit suggestion was taken to mean that ease of measurement should therefore be prioritised over theoretical accuracy. That is, what cannot be easily measured can be at best dismissed, and at worst denied. The problem with this has been most thoughtfully articulated by Graeme Gooday in his classic study of the measurement of electricity, in which he writes:

> If privileged significance is attached only to that which is easily measurable. Then those people who cherish what cannot easily be thus quantified are likely to experience injustice or at least marginalization. Less extreme, but of great significance to this volume, is that such unfortunates may find their positions all too easily devalued by quantitative experts as deficient in (numerical) evidential support or even as grounded on mere speculation or delusion.[58]

Gooday follows this preface remark with a thorough study of the intersections between measurement, trust and instrumentation in the context of nineteenth-century electrical technologies. Part of his argument rests on the claim that because the human body was no longer trusted as a reliable vector of knowledge, individual testimony was subsumed through the use of reliable laboratory instruments.[59] *Measuring Difference, Numbering Normal* extends this argument to the arena of healthcare in the twentieth century to explore how personal testimony about the body has been commodified, then devalued by standardised measurement technologies and indirect measurements.

There are two kinds of measurement: direct and indirect. Direct measurements are primary values that are measured directly through a system or tool. Examples include measurements of weight, height, size, temperature, time, capacity and so forth. However, indirect measurements make inferences from another parameter, usually when direct measures are unavailable or unobservable. Gooday has termed such indirect measures 'proxy' or 'surrogate' measures. As the section below will discuss in detail, head size, IQ and life insurance are all examples of proxy measurements.

An above-mentioned example of such artificial privileging of measurement in healthcare is the Body Mass Index scale, which was originally invented by Adolphe Quetelet (1796–1874). Quetelet was a mathematician and astronomer who introduced statistical methods to the social sciences.[60] He did pioneering work in what we would now term cross-sectional-style studies of human growth, and developed 'the Quetelet index', a formula that estimated whether a person was healthy by dividing their weight by height in metres squared. This method of measuring health was dubbed the 'Body Mass Index' by Ancel Keys in 1972. But its ancestor the Quetelet Index was developed and used by actuaries and insurers as a strong predictor of health and mortality throughout the nineteenth century.[61] Using this scale, they could make inferences about health based on direct measurements of height and weight. However, in terms of gaining significant information about health, measuring body fat against body mass would be better, but measuring that has been historically far more difficult, time-consuming and expensive. Instead, BMI was used. Ease of measurement should not be underestimated as a powerful reason for choosing one kind of measurement over another. The BMI scale demonstrates how the artificial privileging of measurement is perpetuated. Indeed, for most of his career, Ancel Keys (though he coined the term) railed against its use as a measure of health, although he eventually gave up attempts to institute the more precise but far more difficult measurement of adiposometry (using callipers to measure skinfold fat).[62] I make this point not to decry the usefulness of BMI to clinical studies, but simply to reinforce the point that it is artificially privileged as a simple and cheap indirect measurement.

Easy quantifiable measurements are thus elevated as objective, and yet indirect or proxy measurements are necessarily subjective. For instance, other examples of proxy measures in healthcare include fMRI (functional magnetic resonance imaging or functional MRI), which does not directly measure neuronal activity, but rather measures 'the indirect consequences of neuronal activity'.[63] Changes in neural activity are associated with oxygenated blood, and oxygenated blood has different magnetic susceptibility, so fMRI measures blood oxygen levels as a proxy for neuronal activity. Similarly, in economics, the unemployment rate is used as a proxy for the health of the economy; a notable example of a measure that can be manipulated, for instance by counting zero hours contracts in labour market statistics related to employment. Similarly, GDP (gross domestic product) is used as a proxy for quality of life. Yet GDP is far more subjective than it seems. Measuring GDP is a blended measurement, characterised by judgements about what should be included in its definition. Scholar Marilyn Waring has therefore argued that GDP can distort our economic reality through its perpetuation of patriarchal values.[64] Breastfeeding, for example, is not currently included in Britain's GDP despite the contributions to the economy that it makes based on its health benefits for infants, which results in cost benefits like fewer hospital visits.[65] Its exclusion has had the unfortunate consequence of elevating the contribution of formula milk to the economy, while simultaneously lowering the contributions of breastfeeding mothers and hence contributing to the gender pay gap.[66] GDP is 'not like measuring how high the mountain is'.[67] Proxy measures are therefore more likely to be easily manipulated, more likely to miss key information and more likely to denigrate important information. Their enduring appeal, however, lies in their greater propensity to quantification and scalability.

The problem with numbers on a scale, though, is the potential of distance between them. One apposite example is the decibel scale we use to measure sound, which is logarithmic rather than linear. That is, each value is multiplied by an order of magnitude. Whereas on a linear scale, the variation between one and two is the same as that between seven and eight, on a logarithmic scale, variation between values increases in proportions. This can be problematic when numbers are elevated as markers of objectivity and inappropriately used to represent qualitative research concerned with non-additive units. Jane Macnaughton has identified that 'the important point is that when qualities are arranged in a series and identified with numbers, the use of those numbers to do calculations such as averages or percentages is meaningless, since the relation between points 1 and 2 and between 5 and 6 in the series may be completely different.'[68] Eula Biss has written beautifully of how this lack of meaning manifests in the numerical scales used to measure pain, asking: 'where does pain worth measuring begin? With poison ivy? With a hang nail? With a stubbed toe? A sore throat? A needle prick? A razor cut?'[69] As Joanna Bourke has outlined, the historical imperatives driving the creation of such scales were linked to the drive to bring objectivity to the idiosyncratic experience of pain.[70] Yet many have pointed out that any pain scale rests upon a fixed zero point of no pain, or an average ideal of normalcy. Even scales that dispense with numbers altogether, such as the Wong–Baker scale, are subject to this criticism. As the writer Abby Norman memorably put it in her critique of this scale: 'It has cartoon faces wearing expressions that range from Kurt Vonnegut's "Everything is beautiful and nothing hurts" to Leslie Knope's "Everything hurts and I'm dying".'[71] Individual normalcy is inevitably personal, and interrelated with an individual's experiences, culture, environment and history. Indeed, the idea that normalcy as an average of many can tell us anything meaningful on the individual level may be entirely misguided.

In Georges Canguilhem's classic exploration of nineteenth-century medicine, he critiques the idea that pathology is the same as normal function and only differs quantitatively.[72] Canguilhem makes a crucial distinction between individual normalcy and the normal as an average. That is, what is considered normal as an average of many might not account for the variance of individual functioning. Moreover, Canguilhem questioned the conflation of divergence with abnormality, arguing that 'in order to represent a species we have chosen norms which are in fact constants determined by averages. The normal living being is the one who conforms to these norms. But must we consider every divergence abnormal?'[73] An example used in Cryle and Stephens's genealogy of normalcy vividly illustrates just how the average can work in opposition to individual variance, which I now discuss.[74]

In 1945, two statues were displayed in the American Museum of Natural History in New York.[75] Named Norma and Normman, they were carved from alabaster and were made by a gynaecologist called Robert Dickinson working with the sculptor Abram Belskie to represent the 'perfectly average' American body. A competition was held to 'find Norma' but, although there were thousands of applicants, no one American woman embodied these average measurements. Not even close: as Todd Rose explains, fewer than '40 of the 3,864 contestants were average-size on just five of the nine dimensions' and none of them were close to the average of all the measurement dimensions.[76] The unfortunate American contestants who failed to meet the ideal represented by

Norma were chided for being 'unhealthy and out of shape'.[77] Conversely, when the same finding was made in 1952 in relation to Air Force pilots who did not fit cockpits designed for the 'average man', the discovery led to the development of ergonomic design in cockpits.[78] However, as Rachel Weber has explained, using ergonomic designs based on the anthropometric measurements of men still led to the exclusion of women and shorter-statured men. Even when the ninety-fifth and fifth percentile male dimensions were used as guidelines, 'the gap between a 5th percentile woman and a 95th percentile man can be very large'.[79] And there is more to this story. The fact that Dickinson's statues were carved from alabaster is not the only reason that they looked white. This is in fact because of the data sets that were used to create the averages for the statues. Normman's data came from records of First World War soldiers that had been collected by the eugenics records office, whilst Norma's came from the anthropometric measurements of 15,000 'native white' American women which had been gathered by the Bureau of Home Economics to create a standardised system of sizing for readymade clothes.[80]

Thus, the subjects that we decide to measure as standard have an important influence on our conception of normalcy. Such standardisation can have particularly pernicious effects in healthcare if we equate normalcy with whiteness or maleness. For example, historian Heather Prescott has argued that US college physicians used students to establish paradigm 'standards of normality' across a range of bodily functions, including 'blood pressure, lung capacity, pulse rate, basal metabolism and other physiological processes'.[81] In establishing these standards, any students with any sort of disability was excluded, as were women, as 'researchers also continued to assume that students, particularly white males from the upper middle classes, best represented the normal human population'.[82] This decision, Prescott argued, was politically motivated. Not only were white male students considered ideal specimens to represent humanity, they were also assumed to be the best group to study because they were the 'most valuable to society'.[83]

A similar case of politically motivated measurement occurred in 1994, when a group associated with the WHO met to define normal bone density. In this meeting, young women were chosen to represent the standard of normal bone density. Peter Gotzsche argues that

> the group – completely arbitrarily – defined osteoporosis as present if the bone mineral density was 2.5 standard deviations below that in a young woman, and didn't even stop there, but defined osteopenia as present if the measurement lay between 1.0 and 2.5 standard deviations below. These criteria were intended for epidemiological research but were a bonanza for the drug industry, as they rendered half of all older women 'abnormal'.[84]

Gotzsche suggests that the fact that a drug industry sponsored the meeting was not unrelated to the creation of this standard. And these examples lead us to more substantial questions about how we measure health. How arbitrary are the thresholds we use in healthcare? How much are they influenced by the form and ease of measurement? How has the drive for quantified data shaped our conception of the normal as strictly dichotomous to the abnormal?

Strict dichotomies have also characterised the literature concerning disability and measurement. Disability studies developed as a discipline relatively recently, concurrent with social changes concerning the perception of disability and the work of activists campaigning for greater rights for the disabled, starting around the mid-1980s.[85] It is important to emphasise this grounding in political activism because this has influenced the kinds of histories that have been told about disability, and has oriented the focus of these histories. For example, campaigns for greater rights for the disabled in the US have been linked by historian David Gerber to the impact of the Vietnam War.[86] Thus, veterans were the first major group to instigate the fight for greater recognition of disability rights. Reflecting the strongest aspect of disability activism and political interest, research into disabled veterans has been a major component of disability history.

Understanding the quantification of sensorial symptoms poses a challenge of epistemological as well as historical significance and thus necessitates engagement with philosophical theory as well as relevant medical and disability history. While disability history has received increased scholarly attention in recent years, it has not often engaged with science and technology studies, partly because of politicised concerns about medical technologies functioning as tools of oppression.

As the title suggests, *Measuring Difference, Numbering Normal* instead provides a detailed study of the technological construction of disability by examining how the audiometer and spirometer were used to create numerical proxies for invisible and inarticulable experiences. This is particularly relevant to our understanding of unseen but experiential disability. The audiometer was critical both for providing proof of hearing loss in the industrial/military complex, and for managing the threat posed by 'hysterical' deafness and malingerers. When instrumentation was used in this way and conflicted with an individual's own perception of health, I argue that this created a specific kind of instrument-based epistemic injustice – mechanical epistemic injustice. In Chapter 2 I discuss how these instruments have been used in relation to disability measurement to perpetuate mechanical epistemic injustice. I argue that as well as the distinctive kind of epistemic injustice levelled at the disabled there is further such injustice inherent to the processes of instrument-based confirmation testing that compensation or social support often necessitates.

However, while this book does explore the experience of hearing loss, it does not focus on Deaf history, which has been thoroughly explored by others.[87] Rather, it is concerned with the experiences of the 'deafened'. That is, those who identify as hearing and experience their hearing loss as a loss.[88] Indeed, this book is unique in its specific consideration of late-onset disability, which means the subjects under consideration are unlikely to have identified as disabled. Both hearing loss and breathlessness are associated with ageing and entail negative stereotypes that can be avoided by hiding or rejecting the related assistive technology.[89]

Both hearing and breathing are invisible, and so, too, are hearing loss and breathlessness. This categorisation conflict is highly relevant to the themes of this book. The medical measurements designed to quantify and define hearing loss and breathlessness are often incongruent with extremely diverse and individual conditions and experiences. Indeed, this project is of significance precisely because of the amorphous nature of the phenomena under consideration; that is, the fact that breathing and hearing are singularly difficult to measure and standardise. There are other pertinent commonalities between hearing and breathing. Air is the medium through which we hear. As both noise and air pollution move through space, they resist easy quantification and measurement, making them difficult to regulate. Similarly, hearing and breathing are characterised by extreme diversity in personal experience, which similarly eludes fixed representation. Hearing and breathing are experienced and facilitated by the whole body and our understanding of how these processes work is still somewhat uncertain.[90] As Williams and Carel explain, 'breathlessness is a unique medical symptom and experience that of its essence involves sensation, cognition, and reasoning, none of which are reducible to the other.'[91] To understand multisensorial phenomena, I argue that we need a multidisciplinary approach, blending science and technology studies (STS) approaches with medical history and disability history.

Disability studies is often multidisciplinary; and invites scholars to think about disability not as an isolated, individual medical pathology but instead as a key defining social category on a par with race, class and gender. Disability studies is not concerned with analysing human variation, rather it considers how we *define* categories of variation and make them meaningful.[92] In focusing on these definitional processes, disability studies made use of the influential concept of the social model of disability. The history and development of this concept will be explored in full detail in the following chapter but to put it most simply, the medical model defines disability as located in an individual's pathology, whereas the social model defines disability as resulting from environmental barriers which impact on the individual's ability to live and work. The stark division between the social and medical model of disability has meant that collaboration between science and technology studies and disability studies has been regarded as counterproductive and even inappropriate. The social model presents particular problems for historians because it does not fit with the idea that 'the impaired body is part of the domain of history, culture and meaning, and not – as medicine would have it – an ahistorical, presocial, purely natural object'.[93] Technology and medicalisation have been negatively linked in the minds of many, and likewise associated with the oppression and normalisation of disability by the medical profession. Therefore, certain proponents of disability history define the discipline explicitly in opposition to medical history.[94]

In this research, by contrast, answering what motivations underpinned the development of the spirometer and audiometer necessitates studying technology alongside disability history. Historian Julie Anderson has argued that it is essential to consider medical as well as social developments in disability history to reveal the full lived experience of individuals.[95] Too narrow a focus on the social model of disability risks missing the perspectives and experiences of the users of technology *and their reciprocal impact* on measurement technologies.

Furthermore, while the social model has been incredibly successful in forcing through legislative changes and in creating a radical and effective politics of disability, its theoretical framing has led to conceptual criticism.[96] For example, the social model's separation of body from impairment risks disowning medical approaches to the extent that it implies that 'impairment is not a problem'.[97] The social model therefore risks eliding the importance of the body and its impact on our health. We are becoming increasingly aware that the Cartesian separation of mind and body has prevented us from realising the importance of biography to health.[98] The blurriness of the distinction between mind and body has been repeatedly shown in studies concerned with breathlessness. For instance, neuroimaging studies demonstrate that an individual's past experiences and personal psychology mediate their experience of breathlessness.[99] Both the mind and body process breathlessness, and, relatedly, its severity does not correlate with disease stage.[100] However, prior experiences, expectations and individual psychology do impact on the effect of breathlessness, much like the feeling of pain.[101] Parallels with pain are also notable in studies that show that vicarious dyspnoea (breathlessness) can be induced in empathetic individuals watching others struggling to breathe.[102]

Breathlessness thus offers distinct challenges for those attempting to measure it. The 'Life of Breath' project has been designed to explore this as part of its remit to investigate how the humanities can shed light on the experience of breathing and breathlessness.[103] As such, many of its publications have illuminated the personal and intangible nature of breathing and breathlessness. Moreover, project research has demonstrated that objective measurements have been assumed to correlate with the lived experience of breathlessness, so that 'breathlessness has for the most part been subsumed by objective measurements'.[104] This research represents the increasing awareness of disconnect between the subjective individuality of breathlessness and attempts to mark out a numerical correlation. In fact, the premise of being able to achieve a reliable and valid objective measurement of breathlessness has recently been called into question by physiotherapist David Nicholls, who argues that:

> The importance placed upon achieving a reliable and valid objective measurement of breathlessness is confusing a basic fact. Breathlessness is a unique human phenomenon that can be understood and interpreted only by sufferers. In that sense no amount of objective complexity will ever obtain a true representation of a sufferer's experience.[105]

Thus, two crucial tensions are presented by the usage of standardised frameworks in medicine applied to the more intangible aspects of ourselves (like breathing and hearing) through instrumentation. Firstly, in the correlation between subjective experience and objective measurement; and secondly, in the question of what exactly is being measured through tools like the spirometer.

Now, perhaps more than ever, data sits higher in the hierarchy of medical knowledge than the kinds of knowledge gained from subjectively experienced symptoms and embodied experience. Do my experiences matter as much as the data that I generate? A position that prioritises such data (implicitly or explicitly) suggests that quantifiable numbers are understood as neutral, objective and valid in a way that lived experience is not. Moreover, normalcy and the normative standards embodied in instrumentation have often rendered themselves invisible to both the measurers and the measured.

A normal history

Even our idea of the word 'normal' as the opposite of abnormal or pathological has a long and obscure history. The term originated from geometry as a way of describing the relationship between lines.[106] In what we might term the 'pre-normal' era, alternative words such as orderly, regularly, natural and virtuous were used, but historian Caroline Warman contends that such conceptions of normality were tied: '(a) with measurement and senses of straight or deviating lines (b) moral and sexual behaviour, and thus, with binaries of values which are generalised into morality'.[107] These links between measurement, morality and normalcy were strengthened by the work of Adolphe Quetelet.

As well as developing height and weight tables to study the relationship between them, Quetelet demonstrated that normal distribution could be applied to physical attributes of humans through population studies.[108] So, he applied normal distribution to human qualities. Starting with height, Quetelet showed that when individual characteristics were measured the values tended to cluster around the average, 'the polygon of frequency tends towards a so called "bell-shaped" curve' – in other words, the normal curve.[109] He thus developed the concept of 'the average man', and from this point the average was held up as the ideal – a shift that had significant consequences for our understanding of normalcy. As Neff and Nafus emphasise: 'This conflation of mathematically normal distribution with "normal" as a kind of ideal gives tremendous power to those who decide what to measure.'[110] And, I argue, to those who decide *who* to measure.

Quetelet's ideas were taken forward by Francis Galton, but for Galton, the average man was not ideal, he was mediocre.[111] Using quantitative statistical methods to investigate biological phenomena is closely linked to Francis Galton's researches. Charles Darwin's cousin, Galton believed that anything could be measured, and that measurement was the most important aspect of scientific study.[112] This was reflective of his interest in measuring the exceptional rather than the average in order to facilitate the improvement of races.[113] In 1883 he coined the term eugenics and advocated positive eugenics, that is, the promotion of 'good stock', through regulation of marriage and family size. Because of his interest in heredity, Galton's life work was devoted to accurate precision measurements of human characteristics and functions, based on instrument derived quantitative data. Certain aspects of his work betray his more idiosyncratic and subjective measures. For instance, his beauty map of the United Kingdom involved him ranking the women he met numerically and then putting them on a scale which put women from London on the top and women from the north-east coast of Scotland at the bottom.[114]

Eugenicists like Galton used the power and prestige attached to large amounts of data on head sizes to legitimate their claims about differences between races. As Stephen Jay Gould identified in *The Mismeasure of Man*:

> The second half of the nineteenth century was not only the era of evolution in anthropology. Another trend, equally irresistible, swept through the human sciences – the allure of numbers, the faith that rigorous measurement could guarantee irrefutable precision, and might mark the transition between subjective speculation and a true science as worthy as Newtonian physics.[115]

Gould traces the history of intelligence testing from its inception in France as a way of identifying children that needed more help to its eventual mutation into a trusted measure of absolute intelligence. In doing so, he shows that IQ's design was predicated on the expected knowledge norms of its designers, meaning that users who were not immersed in an Anglo-American worldview were at an immediate disadvantage. Failure to recognise this led to the apparently damming objective claims concerning difference between races, which inevitably positioned white men at the top. Nineteenth-century scientists' elevated positions were thus reflected in the apparently objective hierarchy of nature. Thus, statistics about the human body gained authority in an increasingly eugenic framework which worked to quantify and rationalise the human body. Fear of disability was disguised in 'objective' biometrics such as those proposed by Galton's protégé, Karl Pearson (1857–1936), who set up a large-scale investigation into the racial qualities of Jewish schoolchildren and concluded that 'taken on the average, and regarding both sexes, this alien Jewish population is somewhat inferior physically and mentally to the native population'.[116]

Gould argues that it is this kind of 'science' that Charles Murray and Richard J. Herrnstein restored in *The Bell Curve* in 1994, when they argued for the existence of inherited racial differences in IQ.[117] Their analysis has been notably countered by the existence of 'the Flynn effect', which shows that there were IQ gains through time across all groups during the twentieth century, thus suggesting that it is environmental factors and perhaps specific features of modern living (such as increased leisure time, greater education and exposure to abstract concepts) that impact IQ difference.[118] Yet even before the existence of IQ, craniometrists believed that the shape and size of the head gave clues to reveal an individual's intelligence level by proxy. Head measurers focused on physical measurements of the skull; either on the outside, using ruler and callipers to measure various indices and ratios, or filling the cranium with seed or shot to measure the volume of the brain indirectly.[119] Measuring skulls was popularised earlier in the nineteenth century by US scientist Samuel George Morton. Morton believed that the races could be ranked, and that the existing societal hierarchy was an objective reflection of nature. He could support this by citing the evidence of his rigorous measurements on large amounts of data. In fact, he was famously described as 'the objectivist of his age'.[120]

Gould went to great lengths to refute the science behind the *Bell Curve* thesis, by actively recalculating and re-analysing the statistics used by craniometrist Samuel Morton to decisively demonstrate the subjective and biased nature of Morton's calculations. He thus demonstrated that Morton's data were unreliable and distorted by his preconceived views on the intelligence of the different races. Regardless of their precision, it is notable that these researchers chose arbitrary racial groupings over other possible categories and it is pertinent to question whether this led to increased acceptance of these classifications.

The statistical tools interrelated with these classification systems have been explored by philosopher Ian Hacking, who has argued that the 'avalanche of numbers' following this process was precipitated at a specific point in the nineteenth century, that is, 1820–40.[121] Historian Ted Porter is less specific, but agrees that it was the nineteenth century that featured the initial drive for standardised quantitative measurement units. Porter has analysed how power to monitor, observe and normalise individuals was especially invested in single numbers as representative of truth and objectivity[122] The association between single numbers and objectivity was strengthened in the 'measured world' of the twentieth century, and Porter has demonstrated that by the 1920s, there was a strong association between statistical methods and standardised IQ tests. Porter points out that IQ tests were privileged as a form of measurement in schools not just because of their perceived objectivity, but also because of their convenience and cheapness. And furthermore, as historian Dan Bouk reminds us, these objective measures impacted on individual subjectivities, through 'the power of statistical studies to inform ordinary people's understandings of themselves'.[123]

Such single numbers were used to demonstrate objectivity in the natural sciences, but soon extended into the realm of life insurance, which began 'in Britain in the mid-eighteenth century and became a signature feature of modernity around the world in the nineteenth century'.[124] For example, in economic principles, the value of a life should mean just how much it is worth to the person living it.[125] In practice, it was (and remains) difficult for people to put a quantitative value on their own existence. As a result, the measure used instead is the average lost income on death. Actuaries tried to arrive at a legitimate sum of money that could compensate families for the loss of the main breadwinner rather than attempting to determine a numerical monetary value for the incalculable value of life.[126] This pragmatic move towards cost-benefit logic has had significant consequences to public health, for example in the way that heart disease as the leading cause of death in men in the US was treated as a public health emergency while the fact that heart disease was the leading cause of death in women was ignored. This was because although heart disease killed both sexes at equal rates, it killed men *earlier*, while they were still working.

The assumption, then, that the leading cause of women's death was less of a public health emergency than the leading cause of men's death just because men were more likely to be affected at a younger age was, ultimately, a value judgement, though one consistent with the cost-benefit logic often used in the health-care arena, which emphasises the years of 'productive' life lost to illness. (It also raised the interesting question of how much of the underrepresentation of women in heart disease research was actually a consequence of the tendency to underrepresent the elderly.)[127]

As this book shows, the development of schemes designed to recompense for disability were similarly criticised for their apparently arbitrary scaling of disability levels. In this book, I link the analysis of historians and sociologists from STS focused on measurement and categorisation together with work from disability studies in order to make a radical addition to work on the social construction of disability. In arguing that technological processes have been ignored as important contributors to the classification of disability, I make these processes visible and reveal that seemingly purely technical issues such as how to categorise data thus has an important impact on what we consider to be natural. Kohrman explains that: 'At the close of the last millennium some of the most powerful institutional artefacts of modernity – nation states – came to define, standardize, and medicalize aspects of human existence under and within a relatively new social category; that is, disability.'[128] Large bureaucracies like the MRC and the Post Office exemplify offices of such administrative biopower.

Michel Foucault introduced this influential concept in *The History of Sexuality* in which he argued that, from the seventeenth century, 'there was an explosion of numerous and diverse techniques for achieving the subjugation of bodies and the control of populations, marking the beginning of an era of "biopower"'.[129] Biopower is power over life, constituted of two separate forms.[130] The first is concerned with the body as a machine, and the second pole is concerned with the body of *species*. It is the second form that is explored in this book through the context of early twentieth-century biomedicine. Hacking takes Foucault's concept further, to show that even the *process* of dividing people into categories for statistical analysis means that we need to then name these subdivisions and classify people into certain categories. This can, in turn, lead to the perpetuation of these artificial groupings as if they were real, natural entities. He explains that 'Counting is hungry for categories. Many of the categories we now use to describe people are by-products of the needs of enumeration.'[131]

These newly created body categories exerted powerful influence over their subjects through the prism of medico-legal forces. Historian Lundy Braun's 2014 book, *Breathing Race into the Machine*, vividly illustrated the real-world consequences of these classificatory forces. Braun has shown that the practice of correcting for race in spirometry measurement promoted scientific acceptance of difference between racial groups, without due concern to the racial categories employed to organise this data in the first place, or to the way that social conditions and living conditions affected lung function in these groups.[132] Further examples of biopower in action feature in historian Vanessa Heggie's work on testing sex and gender in sports, which shows that the tests we use to measure sex rely on arbitrary cut-off points which are strongly influenced by our cultural attitudes towards gender.[133] Sex is, of course, very intimate, hidden and embodied and so attempts to standardise its measurement have been fraught and conflicted: 'The story of sex testing, and *histories* of sex testing, in international sport tell us a great deal about social attitudes to gender, and how the co-option of science in sport (however it is resisted by scientists and human rights campaigners) can act to essentialise social categories.'[134] These essentialised social categories are all too often those associated with non-standard bodies. This is a reference class problem, and the threat represented by contested reference classes to the apparent objectivity of normalcy will be explained and further explored in Chapter 2.

In this context, measurement devices offered scientific objectivity but also offered a way to *make the invisible visible*. By this I mean not just invisible disability, but also the intangible characteristic of 'fitness' that concerned eugenicists. Indeed, while British eugenicists are often considered to have been more concerned with class degradation than with racial purity, Dan Stone argues that class and race were intertwined and inseparable in eugenic thought during the interwar period. Although class was central to British eugenics, the idea that 'there were two strands of eugenic thought, a German one emphasising race and a British one stressing class, was promoted, after the Second World War, by the eugenicists themselves'.[135] Moreover the fears of degeneration from 'alien' immigrants were consistently couched in terms that emphasised disability. Just as Baynton has outlined in the US context, so too in the interwar years in the UK the threat of immigration was highlighted in rhetoric connoting disability. Immigrants were described as 'inferior', 'weak', 'feeble-minded', 'unfit' and as a national 'impediment'.[136]

Measurement devices like the spirometer and audiometer were used during the interwar period not just to measure specific health features but rather to divine more generally some intrinsic *quality* of the measured. These devices were perfected in an era that was overwhelmingly concerned with degeneration and disability and ways of measuring these deviant attributes. In this way, these tools endowed such studies with a veneer of scientific objectivity and contributed to essentialist notions about certain group categories.

Resisting categorisation

This book is framed around a comparative study of hearing loss and breathlessness undertaken through examination of the tools that were developed to quantify these experiences in Britain during the interwar period. Structured chronologically and divided into two main sections, the first on hearing and the second on breathing, these parallel case studies allow us to compare first the process of quantifying normal hearing and breathing, and then the impact this measurement had on a range of disability experiences; from wealthy businessmen disputing their levels of deafness and arguing that their phones weren't loud enough, to miners arguing that they deserved compensation for respiratory disability.

Such injustices are especially problematic for the kinds of disability where the experience of it constitutes its essence, and so in Chapter 2, 'Measuring disability', I elucidate the epistemological implications of the historical case studies which follow in Chapters 4 to 6. These begin with hearing and start in Chapter 3, 'The artificial ear and the disability data gap', with an investigation of how the telephone was used as a tool for the categorisation of hearing through the British Post Office's nationalised telephone system. Utilising underused sources from BT Archives, Chapter 3 argues that the Post Office functioned as an arbitrator of both hearing loss and hearing aids and demonstrates that the Post Office's standard of hearing was set by a machine called the artificial ear, which used data from just ten 'normal' male ears, and elevated enduring thresholds of hearing in the fledgling field of audiometry. However, its standardisation of 'normal' hearing and devices to correct 'abnormal' hearing did not always correlate with the needs and experiences of its users. Indeed, the focus of Chapters 4, 'The audiometer and the medicalisation of hearing loss', is on how the standard of normal hearing for telephony use failed to correlate with the experience of people with hearing loss in the interwar years and argues that this led to the eventual failure of the Post Office's hearing assistive technologies. The narrative then shifts back in Chapter 5, 'The spirometer and the normal subjects', to consider processes of standardisation. The MRC's interest in normal functioning is recovered through archival sources from The National Archives, and it weaves through all these chapters, with its focus on objective anthropometric standards situated within the interwar context of heightened awareness of disability and concern about national fitness.

The MRC's remit of mechanical objectivity is thus further developed in the second half of the book, which is concerned with breathing. In Chapter 5 we return to the late nineteenth century with a detailed exploration of the initial uses of spirometric data and the development of relevant reference classes.

To combat the difficulty of measuring breathlessness and the impossibility of making direct measurements of lung capacity, the surrogate measurement of vital capacity was developed and measured with spirometers. However, the attempt to standardise the parameters of normal breathing has been complicated by the drive to *categorise* the social groups that should represent the standard of normal breathing *for* that particular group. Thus, attempts to accurately measure and scale breathing through the spirometer were complicated by the need to first define the measure for normal breathing; there can be no abnormal without an initial definition for the normal. However, recurring questions over whether the parameters of normal breathing were universal or varied between groups marked all such attempts: normal breathing for whom? Embodied knowledge is also central to this chapter, which looks at the MRC's use of spirometry in the 1936–45 investigation of pneumoconiosis in south Wales. The chapter again focuses on the subjects used to set the standards of normalcy. I reveal that the spirometric data sets used a normal standard set by apparently healthy miners rather than a non-mining control group, thus taking its measure of normalcy from a population in which abnormality was already apparent. Spirometer tests were used as a crucial marker of the presence of respiratory disease which could not be made visible through X-rays. Thus, my focus is on the historical attempts to correlate subjective reports of breathlessness with an objective quantifiable measurement as a way to adjudicate, scale and compensate respiratory disability. By examining the history of measuring lung function in British miners, we see that the threshold for normal lung function was taken from a baseline measurement of other miners, rather than a normal comparison group. This meant that miners who felt their respiratory health to be diminished could be dismissed as healthy by apparently objective instruments. Such cases are revealed in trade union records held by the South Wales Miners' Library, Bristol University's Special Collections and Swansea University's Richard Burton Archives. Thus, central to this book is consideration of *disputed* disability in compensation cases focused on hearing loss and breathlessness.

The attempt to create data on such an intimate life experience is characteristic of the tension between embodied knowledge and scientific knowledge. This tension is explored throughout this book but is particularly concentrated in Chapter 6, 'The respirator and the mechanisation of normal breathing', which explores how issues pertaining to the experience of the patient were utilised in the development of resuscitation technologies. Chapter 6 thus moves to a consideration of user involvement in developing early mechanical respirators. The focus both here and in Chapter 3 is on the ways that personal bodily knowledge has been commodified and utilised in assistive technology. Tracing the origins of assistive breathing technologies design, with focus on engagement and co-production with users, allows for exploration of the conflict between assistive technology and lived experience. Rejection of assistive technology seen as stigmatising or inappropriate is an ongoing problem. Such assistive technology represents a twofold problem for users, in that it not only makes an invisible disability visible to the public but also makes the illness more visible to themselves. By exploring how patients have incorporated medical technology into their lives, this chapter will illuminate the dissimilitude between the engineering of assistive technology and the needs and wants of users.

The quantification of the body has resulted in the privileging of mechanical authority over subjective experience for explicitly political ends. The literal process of encoding biostatistics into machines has been used to create standard norms for specific groups of people. Through this process, the classifications used in creating these standards became invisible and appeared as natural divisions, as machines like the spirometer or the audiometer and the data they generated were venerated as objective and authoritative. In making the invisible visible and making the personal visible we are led to situations where objective measures do not correlate with lived experience. When measurement instruments are trusted over testimony in order to deny compensation, the lived experience of the disabled is denied, and it is this that represents mechanical epistemic injustice.

At its heart, this book is about resistance to standardisation and categorisation. It is a story about individual experience and its resistance to easy quantification. By studying historical attempts to measure disability, we can recover the lives and the voices of those individuals who have *not* been easily categorised.

Notes

1 See Nuttall, F. W., 'Body Mass Index: Obesity, BMIT, and Health: A Critical Review', *Nutrition Today*, 50:3 (2015), 117–128, and Gay, R., *Hunger: A Memoir of (My) Body* (London: HarperCollins, 2007).
2 For that, look to Brueggemann, B. J., *Lend Me Your Ear: Rhetorical Constructions of Deafness* (Washington, DC: Gallaudet University Press, 1999) and Berger, K. W., *The Hearing Aid: Its Operation and Development* (Livonia, MI: National Hearing Aid Society, 1970) for the former, and see the introduction to Braun, L., *Breathing Race into the Machine: The Surprising Career of the Spirometer from Plantation to Genetics* (Minneapolis: University of Minnesota Press, 2014) and Spriggs, E. A., 'The History of Spirometry', *British Journal of Diseases of the Chest*, 72 (1978), 165–180, for the latter.
3 This is in reference to a song, 'A Hymn to Him', delivered by the character Professor Henry Higgins in the 1964 film *My Fair Lady* which includes the immortal line

'Why can't a woman be more like a man?'. See Perez, C. C., *Invisible Women: Exposing Data Bias in a World Designed for Men* (London: Chatto & Windus, 2019), pp. 122–123. I love the film and recommend watching it to see Higgins playing with all sorts of technologies related to oralism: tuning forks, universal speech charts, a manometer flame, Edison phonographs and, of course, lots of lovely candlestick-style telephones. (Alexander Melville Bell was mentioned in George Bernard Shaw's original preface to *Pygmalion*, though the inspiration for Higgins is normally identified as Professor Daniel Jones of UCL.)

4 Perez, *Invisible Women*, p. 186.
5 Ibid.
6 Epstein, S., 'Bodily Differences and Collective Identities: The Politics of Gender and Race in Biomedical Research in the United States', *Body and Society* 10:2/3 (2004), 183–203, p. 186.
7 Perez, *Invisible Women*, p. 202. I should note here that Perez advocates for increased sex-disaggregated data and more scientific research on sex differences.
8 Epstein, S., *Inclusion: The Politics of Difference in Medical Research* (Chicago: University of Chicago Press, 2007), p. 33.
9 In her nuanced and historically aware book, Saini reminds us that 'as science enters this new era, scientists need to be careful. Research into sex differences has an ugly and dangerous history'. Saini, A., *Inferior: The True Power of Women and the Science that Shows It* (London: HarperCollins, 2017), p. 64.
10 Such as between adults and children. See Virdi, J., and McGuire, C., 'Phyllis M. Tookey Kerridge and the Science of Audiometric Standardisation in Britain', *British Journal for the History of Science*, 51:1 (2018), 123–146.
11 Shim, J. K., *Heart-Sick: The Politics of Risk, Inequality, and Heart Disease* (New York: New York University Press, 2014).
12 Davis, L. J., *Enforcing Normalcy: Disability, Deafness, and the Body* (London: Verso, 1995), p. 67.
13 Ibid., p. 24.
14 The telephone is often described as the most lucrative patent ever.
15 Campbell-Smith, D., *Masters of the Post: The Authorised History of the Royal Mail* (London: Penguin Books, 2011), p. 193.
16 Daston, L., and Galison, P., *Objectivity* (New York: Zone Books, 2007), p. 34.
17 Ibid., p. 125.
18 Li, X., and Mills, M., 'Vocal Features: From Voice Identification to Speech Recognition by Machine', *Technology and Culture*, 60:2 (2019), p. 151.
19 Jewson, N. F., 'The Disappearance of the Sick Man from Medical Cosmology, 1770–1870', *Sociology*, 10:2 (1976), 225–244.
20 Armstrong, D., 'The Rise of Surveillance Medicine', *Sociology of Health and Illness*, 17:3 (1995), 393–404, p. 395.
21 Goldberg, D. S., 'Pain, Objectivity and History: Understanding Pain Stigma', *Medical Humanities*, 42 (2017), 238–243, p. 240.
22 Daston and Galison, *Objectivity*, p. 125.

23 Gooday, G., *The Morals of Measurement: Accuracy, Irony, and Trust in Late Victorian Electrical Practice* (Cambridge: Cambridge University Press, 2004). p. 68.
24 Stone, D., *Breeding Superman: Nietzsche, Race and Eugenics in Edwardian and Interwar Britain* (Liverpool: Liverpool University Press, 2002), p. 7.
25 Petty, C., 'Primary Research and Public Health: The Prioritization of Nutrition Research in Interwar Britain', in J. Austoker and L. Bryder (eds), *Historical Perspectives on the Role of the MRC: Essays in the History of the Medical Research Council of the United Kingdom and Its Predecessor, the Medical Research Committee, 1913–1953* (Oxford: Oxford University Press, 1989), pp. 83–108, p. 83.
26 Stone, *Breeding Superman*, p. 116.
27 Baynton, D. C., *Defectives in the Land: Disability and Immigration in the Age of Eugenics* (Chicago: Chicago University Press, 2016), p. 2.
28 Ibid.
29 Ibid., p. 4.
30 Prescott, H. M., 'Using the Student Body: College and University Students as Research Subjects in the United States during the Twentieth Century', *Journal of the History of Medicine and Allied Sciences*, 57:1 (2002), 3–38, p. 14.
31 Kudlick, C., 'Disability History: Why We Need Another "Other"', *American Historical Review*, 108:3 (2003), 763–793, p. 764.
32 Ibid., p. 765.
33 For a detailed account of the controversies around Bell's invention and the contenders for the role of inventor of the telephone see Shulman, S., *The Telephone Gambit: Chasing Alexander Graham Bell's Secret* (New York: Norton, 2008).
34 Lane, H., *When the Mind Hears: A History of the Deaf* (New York: Random House, 1984), p. 352. Recently, the Science and Technology Museum of Canada recreated this experiment (opting for 3D printing and silicone rather than human flesh).
35 Brueggemann, *Lend Me Your Ear*, p. 111.
36 Lane, *When the Mind Hears*, p. 345.
37 Sacks, O., *Seeing Voices: A Journey into the World of the Deaf* (Berkeley and Los Angeles: University of California Press, 1989), p. 152 (at n. 162, p. 151).
38 See for example: Gooday, G., and Sayer, K., *Managing the Experience of Hearing Loss in Britain, 1830–1930* (London: Palgrave Macmillan, 2017); Lane, *When the Mind Hears*; and Padden, C. and Humphries, T., *Inside Deaf Culture* (Cambridge, MA: Harvard University Press, 2005).
39 Hutchison, I., 'Oralism: A Sign of the Times? The Contest for Deaf Communication in Education Provision in Late Nineteenth-Century Scotland', *European Review of History*, 14:4 (2007), 481–501, p. 484.
40 Eriksson, P., *The History of Deaf People: A Source Book* (Orebro: Daufr, 1991), p. 18 and p. 28.
41 Baynton, D. C., '"Savages and Deaf Mutes": Evolutionary Theory and the Campaign against Sign Language in the Nineteenth Century', in J. V. van Cleve (ed.), *Deaf History Unveiled* (Washington, DC: Gallaudet University Press, 1993), pp. 92–112, p. 108.

42 See, for example, Behnke, E., and Browne, L., *Voice, Song, and Speech: A Practical Guide for Singers and Speakers* (London: Sampson Low, Marston and Company, 1891).
43 Sterne, J., *The Audible Past: Cultural Origins of Sound Reproduction* (Durham, NC: Duke University Press, 2003), p. 41.
44 Tallents, S., *Post Office Publicity* (Post Office Green Paper No. 8) (London: His Majesty's Stationery Office, 1935), British Telecom Archives, London (BTA), TCB 350/8.
45 Campbell-Smith, *Masters of the Post*, pp. 270–271.
46 Agar, J., *Constant Touch: A Global History of the Mobile Phone* (Cambridge: Icon Books, 2003), p. 395.
47 Glynn, S., and Oxborrow, J., *Interwar Britain: A Social and Economic History* (London: George Allen & Unwin, 1976), p. 24.
48 Bryder, L., 'Tuberculosis and the MRC', in J. Austoker and L. Bryder (eds), *Historical Perspectives on the Role of the MRC: Essays in the History of the Medical Research Council of the United Kingdom and Its Predecessor, the Medical Research Committee, 1913–1953* (Oxford: Oxford University Press, 1989), pp. 1–21, p. 1.
49 Ibid., p. 2.
50 Austoker, J., and Bryder, L., 'The National Institute for Medical Research and Related Activities of the MRC', in J. Austoker and L. Bryder (eds), *Historical Perspectives on the Role of the MRC: Essays in the History of the Medical Research Council of the United Kingdom and Its Predecessor, the Medical Research Committee, 1913–1953* (Oxford: Oxford University Press, 1989), pp. 35–57, p. 50.
51 Bryder, 'Tuberculosis and the MRC', p. 8.
52 Valier, H., and Timmermanns, C., 'Clinical Trials and the Reorganization of Medical Research in Post-Second World War Britain', *Medical History*, 52 (2008), 493–510.
53 Austoker and Bryder, 'The National Institute for Medical Research', p. 53.
54 Keating, C., *Smoking Kills: The Revolutionary Life of Richard Doll* (Oxford: Signal Books, 2014), p. 57.
55 Ibid., p. 17 and p. 62.
56 Epstein, *Inclusion*, p. 48.
57 Kelvin, W. T., 'Electrical Units of Measurement: A Lecture Delivered at the Institution of Civil Engineers on May 3, 1883; Being One of a Series of Six Lectures on "The Practical Applications of Electricity"', *Nature Series: Popular Lectures and Addresses* (London: Macmillan and Co., 1889), p. 73. The Kelvin scale is used to measure absolute temperature. It is useful because it includes no negative numbers, absolute zero is its fixed point.
58 Gooday, *The Morals of Measurement*, Preface, p. 17.
59 Ibid., p. 21 and p. 33.
60 Cryle, P., and Stephens, E., *Normality: A Critical Genealogy* (Chicago: University of Chicago Press).

61 Eknoyan, G., 'Historical Note: Adolphe Quetelet (1796–1874) – The Average Man and the Indices of Obesity', *Nephrology Dialysis Transplantation*, 23:1 (2008), 47–51.
62 Rasmussen, N., 'Downsizing Obesity: On Ancel Keys, the Origins of BMI, and the Neglect of Excess Weight as a Health Hazard in the United States from the 1950s to 1970s', *The History of the Behavioral Sciences*, 55:4 (2019), 299–318.
63 Stokes, M., '"What Does fMRI Measure?" Brain Metrics: How Measuring Brain Biology Can Explain the Phenomena of Mind', *Nature Blog*, 16 May 2019. www.nature.com/scitable/blog/brain-metrics/what_does_fmri_measure/. Accessed May 2019.
64 Waring, M., *If Women Counted: A New Feminist Economics* (London: Macmillan, 1989).
65 The NHS website highlights the fact that breastfeeding reduces the risk of infant infections, which means a reduction in hospital visits. See www.nhs.uk/conditions/pregnancy-and-baby/benefits-breastfeeding/. Accessed July 2019.
66 BBC Radio 4, 'The Real Gender Pay Gap', *Analysis*, 10 June 2019. www.bbc.co.uk/programmes/m0005t3n?fbclid=IwAR1ESVFYDqjKurDDbkxU4eROmOdmPY-3nooXJOl5KqSkldX2Xc8Kcl7XDQtE. Accessed June 2019.
67 Professor Diane Coyle of Manchester University Economics Department, quoted in Perez, *Invisible Women*, pp. 239–240.
68 Macnaughton, J., 'Numbers, Scales, and Qualitative Research', *The Lancet*, 347:9008 (1996), 1099–1100, p. 1099.
69 Biss, E., 'The Pain Scale', in J. E. Sullivan III (ed.), *Ways of Reading: An Anthology for Writers* (Boston and New York: Bedford/St. Martins, 2011), pp. 171–182, p. 178.
70 Bourke, J., *The Story of Pain: From Prayer to Painkillers* (Oxford: Oxford University Press, 2014).
71 Norman, A., *Ask Me about My Uterus* (New York: Nation Books, 2018), Kindle version location 252 of 4573.
72 Canguilhem, G., *The Normal and the Pathological* (Cambridge, MA: Zone Books, 3rd edn, 1991).
73 Ibid., p. 154.
74 Cryle and Stephens, *Normality*.
75 Stephens, E., 'The Object of Normality: The Search for Norma Competition', Queer Objects Symposium Paper, October 2014. www.academia.edu/8893077/The_Object_of_Normality_The_Search_for_Norma_Competition. Accessed May 2019.
76 Rose, T., *The End of Average* (London: Allen Lane, 2016), p. 7.
77 Ibid., p. 8.
78 Weber, R. N., 'Manufacturing Gender in Commercial and Military Cockpit Design', *Science, Technology, and Human Values*, 22:2 (1997), 235–253.
79 Ibid., p. 238.
80 Stephens, 'The Object of Normality'.
81 Prescott, 'Using the Student Body', p. 16.
82 Ibid., p. 30.
83 Ibid., p. 38.

84 Gotzsche, P. C., *Deadly Medicine and Organised Crime: How Big Pharma has Corrupted Healthcare* (London: Radcliffe Publishing, 2013).
85 Partly as a result of this activism, the Americans with Disabilities Act (1990) and the Disability Discrimination Act (1995) in Britain were enacted. See Gerber, D. A., 'Introduction: Finding Disabled Veterans in History', in D. A. Gerber (ed.), *Disabled Veterans in History* (Ann Arbor: University of Michigan Press, 2000), pp. 1–52.
86 Ibid.
87 See: Lane, *When the Mind Hears*; Padden and Humphries, *Inside Deaf Culture*; Sacks, *Seeing Voices*; Eriksson, *The History of Deaf People*; Baynton, ' "Savages and Deaf Mutes" '; and Branson, J., and Miller, D., *Damned for Their Difference: The Cultural Construction of Deaf People as Disabled* (Washington, DC: Gallaudet University Press, 2002).
88 This category was explored for the first time in a recent monograph, Gooday and Sayer, *Managing the Experience of Hearing Loss*.
89 Assistive technology such as hearing aids and ambulatory oxygen. See McGuire, C., and Carel, H., 'The Visible and the Invisible: Disability, Assistive Technology, and Stigma', in D. T. Wasserman and A. Cureton (eds), *The Oxford Handbook of Philosophy and Disability* (Oxford: Oxford University Press, 2019), pp. 598–615.
90 For discussion of the difficulty of distinguishing between somatic and physiological breathlessness see Williams, T., and Carel, H., 'Breathlessness: From Bodily Symptom to Existential Experience', in K. Aho (ed.), *Existential Medicine: Essays on Health and Illness* (London: Rowman & Littlefield, 2018), pp. 145–159, p. 147. For discussion of how individual psychology and past experiences affect neurological processing of breathlessness see Faull, O. K., Hayen, A., and Pattinson, K. T. S., 'Breathlessness and the Body: Neuroimaging Clues for the Inferential Leap', *Cortex*, 95 (2017), 211–221. For personal perspective and more on how we use our whole body to process sounds see Bathurst, B., *Sound: Stories of Hearing Lost and Found* (London: Profile Books, 2017).
91 Williams and Carel, 'Breathlessness', p. 152.
92 Kudlick, 'Disability History', p. 765.
93 Hughes, B., and Paterson, K., 'The Social Model of Disability and the Disappearing Body: Towards a Sociology of Impairment', *Disability and Society*, 12:3 (1997), 324–340, p. 326.
94 For a review of the divergences between medical history and disability history in the USA see Linker, B., 'On the Borderland of Medical and Disability History: A Study of the Fields', *Bulletin of the History of Medicine*, 87:4 (2013), 499–535.
95 For a discussion of the history of the medical and social model of disability see Shakespeare, T., 'The Social Model of Disability', in L. J. Davis (ed.), *The Disability Studies Reader* (London: Routledge, 4th edn, 2013), pp. 214–221. For a discussion of the problems of the social model for historians see Anderson, J., *War, Disability and Rehabilitation in Britain* (Manchester: Manchester University Press, 2011), pp. 5–6.

96 For a comprehensive overview of these criticisms see Shakespeare, T., *Disability Rights and Wrongs Revisited* (London: Routledge, 2nd edn, 2013).
97 This has also made the social model incompatible with disability history focused on prostheses, etc. which one could argue were a very important part of historical actors' lives. Shakespeare, 'The Social Model of Disability', p. 221.
98 Mjolstad, B. P., Kirkengen, A. L., Getz, L., and Hetlevik, I., 'What Do GPs Actually Know about Their Patients as Persons?', *European Journal for Person Centered Healthcare*, 1:1 (2012), 149–160.
99 Faull et al., 'Breathlessness and the Body'.
100 See Booth, S., Chin, C., and Spathis, A., 'The Brain and Breathlessness: Understanding and Disseminating a Palliative Care Approach', *Palliative Medicine*, 29:5 (2015), 396–398, and Spathis, A., Booth, S., Moffat, C., Hurst, R., et al., 'The Breathing, Thinking, Functioning Clinical Model: A Proposal to Facilitate Evidence-Based Breathlessness Management in Chronic Respiratory Illness', *NPJ Primary Care Respiratory Medicine*, 27:1 (2017), 1–6.
101 Faull, O. K., Marlow, L., Finnegan, S. L., and Pattinson, K. T. S., 'Chronic Breathlessness: Re-Thinking the Symptom', *European Respiratory Journal*, 51:1 (2018), 1–5.
102 Herzog, M., Sucec, J., Diest, I. V., Chevinesse, C., et al., 'Observing Dyspnoea in Others Elicits Dyspnoea, Negative Affect and Brain Responses', *European Respiratory Journal*, 51:4 (2018), 1–10.
103 See www.lifeofbreath.org and Macnaughton, J., and Carel, H., 'Breathing and Breathlessness in Clinic and Culture: Using Critical Medical Humanities to Bridge an Epistemic Gap', in A. Whitehead and A. Woods (gen. eds), *The Edinburgh Companion to the Critical Medical Humanities* (Edinburgh: Edinburgh University Press, 2016), pp. 294–309.
104 Carel, H., Macnaughton, J., and Dodd, J., 'Invisible Suffering: Breathlessness in and beyond the Clinic', *The Lancet: Respiratory Medicine*, 3:4 (2015), 278–279, p. 278.
105 Nicholls, D., 'Breathlessness: A Qualitative Model of Meaning', *Physiotherapy*, 86:1 (2000), 23–27, p. 23.
106 Warman, C., 'From Pre-Normal to Abnormal: The Emergence of a Concept in Late Eighteenth Century France', *Psychology & Sexuality*, 1:3 (2010), 200–213, p. 206.
107 Ibid.
108 Eknoyan, 'Historical Note'.
109 Ibid.
110 Neff, G., and Nafus, D., *Self-Tracking* (Cambridge, MA: MIT Press, 2016), p. 39.
111 Eknoyan, 'Historical Note'.
112 Gould, S. J., *The Mismeasure of Man* (New York: Norton, 2nd edn, 1996), p. 107.
113 Braun, *Breathing Race into the Machine*, p. 92.
114 It feels important to note here that I am a woman from the north-east of Scotland and that I thoroughly disagree with this assessment.
115 Gould, *The Mismeasure of Man*, pp. 105–106.

116 Stone, *Breeding Superman*, p. 105.
117 Gould, *The Mismeasure of Man*, p. 31.
118 Flynn, J. R., *What is Intelligence?* (Cambridge: Cambridge University Press, 2007), p. 8.
119 Gould, *The Mismeasure of Man*, p. 23.
120 Lewis, J. E., DeGusta, D., Meyer, M. R., Monge, J. M., et al., 'Correction: The Mismeasure of Science: Stephen Jay Gould versus Samuel George Morton on Skulls and Bias', *PLoS Biology*, 9:7 (2011), 1–6.
121 Hacking, I., 'Biopower and the Avalanche of Printed Numbers', *Humanities in Society*, 5 (1982), 279–295.
122 Porter, T. M., 'Measurement, Objectivity, and Trust', *Measurement: Interdisciplinary Research and Perspectives*, 1:4 (2003), 241–255, p. 246.
123 Bouk, D., *How Our Days Became Numbered: Risk and the Rise of the Statistical Individual* (Chicago: University of Chicago Press, 2015).
124 Ibid., Preface, p. 28.
125 Porter, 'Measurement, Objectivity, and Trust', p. 250.
126 Porter, T. M., 'Objectivity as Standardization: The Rhetoric of Impersonality in Measurement, Statistics, and Cost-Benefit Analysis', in A. Megill (ed.), *Rethinking Objectivity* (Durham, NC and London: Duke University Press, 1994), pp. 197–237, p. 216.
127 Epstein, *Inclusion*, p. 60.
128 Kohrman, M., 'Why Am I Not Disabled? Making State Subjects, Making Statistics in Post-Mao China', *Medical Anthropology Quarterly*, 17:1 (2003), 5–24, p. 6.
129 Foucault, M., *The History of Sexuality: Volume One* (London: Penguin Books, 1976), p. 140.
130 Ibid., p. 139.
131 Hacking, 'Biopower and the Avalanche of Printed Numbers'.
132 Braun, *Breathing Race into the Machine*.
133 Heggie, V., 'Testing Sex and Gender in Sports: Reinventing, Reimagining and Reconstructing Histories', *Endeavour*, 34:4 (2010), 157–163.
134 Ibid., p. 157.
135 Stone, *Breeding Superman*, p. 99.
136 This is the central thesis of Baynton, *Defectives in the Land*. The quoted terminology is from primary sources used in the chapter 'The "Lethal Chamber" in Eugenic Thought', in Stone, *Breeding Superman*, although there is no explicit discussion in Stone's book of disability.

2

MEASURING DISABILITY

The ubiquitous desire for uniqueness

As I write this, I have a clear view over the busy intersection between the main roads dividing the University of Bristol's central campus. The campus scene below is punctuated by constant flashes of brightness. The students that walk past are arrayed in an impressive spectrum of colour: yellow raincoats, lilac Puffa-jackets, red backpacks, floral umbrellas, purple windbreakers, neon blues and pinks offset by fresh white trainers. It is a paean to uniqueness and originality. For many of the vibrant individuals traversing the campus, to be described as normal or average would be akin to an insult. This is not a comment on the student mindset; it is a comment on the average mindset. A recent BBC Radio 4 documentary explained that 85 per cent of us would identify ourselves as above average, a huge increase compared with the 1950s, when only 50 per cent would make such a claim.[1] Many have noted this societal shift – everyone wants to be unique. Yet when it comes to our health, we still strive to remain within the boundaries of normalcy. We might all desire to be uniquely dressed, uniquely intelligent or above average in certain prized areas, but nobody wants above-average cholesterol or abnormal test results. When it comes to our health, we all want to be normal.

This book's central thesis is that health measurements are validated if they are particularly amenable to calculability and easy measurement. In this chapter, I grapple with the epistemological implications of this claim as a contention which relates to two philosophical theses. Although this is a historical book with interdisciplinary influences, this chapter explicitly discusses the philosophical implications of my historical analysis. First, I argue that the naturalist position on disease and disability is undermined by consideration of how statistical normality is technologically constructed. The naturalist position maintains that the threshold level of normal functioning (the line of normalcy) is objective and value-free. However, by examining the data used to create the standards of normalcy, this book demonstrates that these thresholds – fundamental to technologies we use and trust – are often constructed through measurement instruments built with biased data sets. The threshold line of normal functioning that naturalists hold to be objective and value-free is thus also subject to bias and social evaluations. Furthermore, the changing use of appropriate reference classes has further concealed the variability of health within groups, simultaneously masking the social determinants of health that have affected these groups. That is, the judgements that we make concerning our biology are also normative. In sum, by exploring issues of trust in measurement through analysing the bodies used in defining the technical parameters of disability, I argue that the statistical definition of impairment is undermined by its technological construction. In relation to this, I argue that the need for objectivity in adjudicating and measuring disability has led to devaluation of individual experience and reduced understanding of the lifeworld of the disabled person.

Second, I argue that this presents a problem of 'mechanical' epistemic injustice. Measurement tools have been prioritised as authoritative and trusted ahead of individual testimony about personal experiences of health. While there was some acknowledgement of the individual, personal and intangible nature of breathlessness and hearing loss, the processes of testing for confirmation of pathology prioritised instrumental evidence over user voices. This, I argue, is an example of mechanical epistemic injustice. Epistemic injustice connotes the scepticism that greets certain (discriminated) groups' claims to knowledge.[2] In healthcare, this can affect individuals' access to treatment as testimonies about their own bodies and health are placed under extra and unnecessary scrutiny.[3] Such extra scrutiny and disbelief often attend the claims of the disabled, especially when claiming social support such as welfare benefits, which necessitates strict definitions of general disability and normalcy.[4] However, this book does not attempt to theorise about disability generally. My attention is specifically on the historical experiences of adults who (broadly speaking) were unlikely to have identified as disabled. Furthermore, the primary focus here is on invisible but experiential disability as a category. Hearing and breathing are thus united through the processes of making these invisible sensorial experiences visible, which were characterised by a correspondent focus on objectivity and the use of precision measurement tools.

Although invisible, breathlessness and hearing loss are usually presumed to be somatic though in certain instances this is not the case. This kind of heterogeneity – inherent to disability – has long been problematic for philosophers attempting to detail a comprehensive metaphysics of disability. This chapter's consideration of mechanical epistemic injustice therefore holds additional relevance for those interested in mental illness, chronic illness and undiagnosable conditions.

Our understanding of what is normal in healthcare contains complex philosophical baggage. In what follows, I unpack these conceptual trappings. Further, I argue that the historical case studies in this book exemplify how the measurement of normalcy and the tools we use to make these measurements have shaped our understanding and judgements about disability. Illuminating the way that disability has been technologically constructed simultaneously sheds light on our understanding of normal functioning as a threshold and adds to our understandings of what medicine has historically and currently called 'normal'. This builds on philosopher Havi Carel's observation that 'the world of the ill is dependent upon the world of the healthy for its norms; and the world of the healthy is dependent on the world of the ill for the aberration of these norms'.[5] I am concerned with exactly how these aberrations are *constructed by technology* through the creation of measurement standards, and aim to disentangle the processes and materials through which we make reliable and trusted measurements.

In the following section, 'Defining disease', I begin by outlining the main arguments relevant to philosophical attempts to define disease – naturalism and normativism. I bring sustained attention to the reference class problem in the section titled 'By no means average: the reference class problem' and explore the ways in which 'correcting' for attributes like sex, class and race (or not) impacts on the measurement of normalcy. In relation to the scholarship on reference classes, I discuss whether disability could ever be considered as a reference class and ask why it has not been previously considered to be a medically separable identity. When philosophers of medicine have focused on these definitional questions, they have tended to categorise disability under the heading of disease, using disease as an umbrella term which can encompass disability as pathology alongside disease in the narrow sense, as well as wounds and injuries and various other unhealthy conditions. Although taking this position allows us to do useful conceptual work on the metaphysics of disease, such a position has been critiqued by scholars of disability, who argue that disability is by no means necessarily 'a bad thing', an issue that I explore in the section on 'Defining disability'.[6] After considering the ways in which Elizabeth Barnes's recent metaphysics of disability has problematised the concept of normalcy, I go on to argue that defining disability using a naturalistic framework is problematised not only by scholarship from disability studies but also by researches from the field of hedonic psychology. In the section on 'Well-being and disability', I argue that the existence of the disability paradox suggests that the measurement of disability is far more complex than naturalist accounts suggest. Finally, in the section on 'Disability and epistemic injustice', I argue that the move to define disability through technological construction has created a phenomenon I term mechanical epistemic injustice.

Defining disease

Within philosophy of medicine, defining disease has inspired a vast amount of literature which has crystallised around the naturalism versus normativism debate. In this section, I outline these two positions and argue that taking an interdisciplinary approach that encompasses insights from disability studies can allow for a compromise between these two dichotomous positions. Broadly speaking, naturalism holds that health and disease are objective biological facts that should not be influenced by 'our subjective evaluations of a state', while normativists maintain that health and disease are value-laden concepts.[7] Before considering the various arguments against naturalism, we need to spend some time detailing the exact parameters of the naturalist account, which I start to set out below.

Naturalism is committed to the thesis that typical species' efficiency is objective and nonevaluative. Health and disease are hence objective biological facts. Disease is statistically defined biological dysfunction and health is the absence of disease. This is sometimes termed the 'negative conception of health' or the 'species norm account' and it holds that disease is simply an impairment of normal functional ability.[8] A function is normal if it makes 'a statistically typical contribution ... to individual survival and reproduction'.[9] The threshold of normal functional ability is determined by taking the statistical norm as an index of normal functioning. So, for example, we map the variability of human functioning onto a bell curve with cut points divided into units of standard deviation – which represent the positions low, medium, normal and high. If you fall below these thresholds that means you are sufficiently far from normal to be diseased. This is the dominant paradigm in medical practice and this account defines disability as 'a stable intrinsic property of subject S that deviates from the normal functioning of the species to which S belongs'.[10]

Christopher Boorse is the best-known proponent of this view and has advanced it primarily through his development of the bio-statistical theory (BST).[11] Jerome Wakefield's account of disorder as harmful dysfunction is like the BST in that it is naturalistic, that is, it rests on the idea of objective biological dysfunction (independent of value judgements). However, it differs in its conception of function and its inclusion of 'harm' as an essential criterion.[12] However, there is not adequate space in this chapter to fully consider Wakefield's theory, particularly due to its specific focus on mental disorders, which are largely outside the scope of my analysis. It is important to note that in his 2010 chapter on disability Boorse does distinguish between disability and disease by making it clear that disability judgements vary with contextual factors independent of medicine'.[13] For instance, he acknowledges that 'the judgement about whether x is disabled is not always purely medical'.[14] However, his original iteration of the BST is consistently conflated with the medical model or 'common'-sense view. Therefore, I concentrate in the remainder of this chapter on Boorse's primarily proposed BST as representative of the medical model view on disability.

In the BST paradigm, the body (whether it be a human, animal or plant body) is made up of systems and sub-systems. 'System' is a broad term which includes organs, the nervous system and functions/systems of the mind such as memory.[15] All the systems and sub-systems of the body ideally work towards the goal of survival and reproduction, and, for Boorse, normal function is the statistically normal contribution of any given system or subsystem towards this goal. Disease is dysfunction of the system (or sub-system), so disease is an internal state that is an impairment of normal functional ability.[16] The inclusion of 'internal' here is important because it indicates that the aberration from normalcy is not caused by something external. For example, if I was to decide after Scotland winning a football game to celebrate by taking recreational drugs (equally unlikely scenarios) this activity might raise my heart rate. However, my temporary elevated heartrate would not count as disease unless it persisted after the effects of the drugs should have worn off.[17] The advantages of the BST system lies in its practical use for clinical studies and clinicians, its broad and general applicability, its simplicity and apparent objectivity and political neutrality.

But do the dynamic and unpredictable functions of day-to-day normal physiology point towards a serious flaw in Boorse's account? That is, unless the BST is modified to situation-specific cases, it is unable to account for dynamic physiological functions.[18] The philosopher Elselijn Kingma argues that this is a significant problem, pointing out that

> the normal ranges of heart rate and cardiac output are very different on the occasions of sleeping (when both are low), and the less common occasion of strenuous exercise (when both are very high). Normal ranges of insulin production, glucose absorption and glycogen synthesis are very different depending on whether and what a person is eating and/or doing. Therefore, what the normal, healthy, correct or appropriate quantitative normal level for a specific function is depends on the situation or occasion too.[19]

Another criticism of the BST's statistical basis rests on the fact that there are conditions that affect many people (such as athlete's foot) which are statistically normal in the sense that they are widespread, but are nonetheless still considered pathological. The philosopher Rachel Cooper has pointed out the intrinsic difficulty of using the statistical norm as a guide to natural functioning, which 'makes it difficult for Boorse to include near universal diseases, for example dental caries, in his account'.[20] Cooper's work on intellectual disability further demonstrates the extent to which economic concerns impact where the threshold is set on a bell-curve, as she shows how the cut-off point for mild intellectual disability shifted during the twentieth century in response to economic considerations such as the need for labour.[21]

Other philosophers have argued that the naturalistic account overgeneralises because there are many departures from normal functioning that are not considered to be markers of disease or disability. As Amundson has also pointed out, 'Better-than-average function is not usually labelled as abnormal even though it is statistically atypical.'[22] Barnes considers as an exemplar of this point the most successful Olympian of our time – swimmer Michael Phelps.[23] Most people's wingspan is proportionate to their height, but Phelps is 6 ft 4, with a 6 ft 7 wingspan. He has hypermobile joints so his size 14 feet bend 15 per cent more than they should, and his muscles produce less lactic acid than is considered 'normal'. Moreover, Barnes points out that his lanky physique (also known as marfan syndrome) could put him at a higher risk for cardiac problems.[24] This, she argues, means that the traits that allow us to be Olympic swimmers are not necessarily the same ones that promote survival. This conflicts with the naturalist view that considers a function to be normal only if it makes a statistically typical contribution to individual survival and reproduction; but it is surely counterintuitive to consequently argue that Phelps should be classed as disabled. This aspect of the naturalist account might also then consider being gay to be a disability (in the sense that it is not promotive of reproduction) and Barnes succinctly points out that any successful account of disability needs to be able to 'distinguish between being disabled and being gay'.[25] Given this unwelcome consequence of the BST, Barnes argues that in fact the naturalist account is implicitly normative. If we can accept that our definitions of disability are inevitably value-laden, could we define disability in terms of lack of ability?

Barnes would suggest not, as doing so would still result in an inadequate definition of disability. Disability as lack of ability does not hold for several reasons. First, we do not consider the common lack of certain abilities, or certain inabilities, to denote disability.[26] For instance, I cannot touch my toes and never have been able to, a consequence of short hamstrings and my enjoyment of running, perhaps – but I am not considered disabled in virtue of that lack of ability. Second, a condition which means you are debilitated by a higher than usual sensitivity (for example, hyperacusis, which involves greater sensitivity to sound) is arguably an enhanced ability and yet it is still debilitating. Third, many disabilities are characterised by unpredictable and fluctuating capabilities, so that sometimes you can do something, but at other times you cannot; sometimes you can do it, but with assistance or the aid of a prosthetic, or in pain or at a cost to time or personal effort.[27] The example of prosthetic assistance points to another flaw within to the naturalist account, which does not allow for the ways in which technologies (such as tool use and environmental design) change the ways that humans can function. Yet philosopher Ron Amundson believes that this is important: 'A weak person using an atlatl can throw a spear farther than a strong person without one. A weak person can walk faster on pavement than a strong person can walk on a sandy beach.'[28] Consideration of such factors may become more important in the future with the rise of transhumanism.

In summary, the BST has been criticised because of its inability to account for situation-specific functioning, the fact that statistical normalcy does not denote biological normalcy, its tendency to overgeneralise and its failure to successfully define enhanced or fluctuating disabilities. In addition, I argue that another profound criticism against the apparent 'objectivity' of the BST relates to the process of drawing the line of normal species functioning. There are two facets to my criticism. First, the threshold of normalcy presents the ideal as the normal so does not represent true variability among the population. I define this as a 'disability data gap' (see Chapter 3). Second, thresholds of normalcy are influenced by the inclusion of reference classes (see Chapter 5). In the next section I argue that while conventional medical distinctions by their nature must be arbitrary, the arbitrary choice of bodies to present certain classes does denote a significant flaw in the BST.

By no means average: the reference class problem

To briefly reiterate, the naturalist position holds that health is simply the absence of disease and that disease is simply an impairment of normal functional ability. A function is normal if it makes 'a statistically typical contribution … to individual survival and reproduction'.[29] Therefore, the BST defines health as the absence of disease, and disease as the adverse departure from normal species functioning. Health is normal function, where normal function is the statistically typical contribution to survival and reproduction for my *reference class*.[30] That is, 'The threshold for dysfunction is determined statistically, occurring at an arbitrarily chosen minimum level below the mean of the relevant reference class.'[31]

It is this inclusion of reference classes that further complicated the issue. We do not tend to think of normalcy all in one go, rather we think about categories of difference or subgroups of people – reference classes. For instance, a physician considering whether patient Alex's inability to become pregnant is a problem would first need to know whether Alex was male or female and whether they were pre or post menopause. But what other factors do we take into consideration? When, for example, might race matter? Normality is always defined in relation to reference classes – normal function for that age, or sex, or race or species. And how we *define and classify* people into such groups is *inherently* value-laden.

Moreover, Cooper would argue that reference classes like age, sex and race are too broad for the purpose of defining disease and that they need to take into account other factors such as past training, environment, living conditions, as well as many other factors: 'Thus the organisms in a reference class must not only be of the same species, sex and age as the organism under consideration, but must also be of the same race and must have undergone similar training and have lived in the same kind of environment.'[32] That is, if you are a healthy but fairly sedentary person your resting heart rate would likely be slightly higher compared with someone identical to you who has lived a parallel life but pursued a professional athletic career. Similarly, if we took the average liver function of a group of alcoholics and used it to measure normalcy for the individuals therein, many members of this group would be considered normal, although through a broader population comparison they would be deemed pathological. That is, the statistically normal range in these groups would include function levels more broadly considered to indicate disease. There is thus a related (and already acknowledged) need to use separate reference classes for groups with distinct lifestyles (for instance, when measuring vital capacity in groups of smokers) so as to recognise disease that is distinct and unrelated to this lifestyle.

Therefore, the BST only works in reference to 'appropriate' reference classes.[33] But what are the appropriate reference classes? And are appropriate reference classes equally appropriate for all conditions? While it seems intuitive to use categorical reference classes like age, sex and race, Steven Epstein argues that these classifications are based on a somewhat arbitrary supposition of relevance:

> Out of all the ways by which people differ from one another, why should it be assumed that sex and gender, race and ethnicity, and age are the attributes of identity that are most medically meaningful? Why these markers of identity and not others? And are there differences among these types of difference, such that the same policy remedies may not be appropriate for each case?[34]

To use a sporting analogy, we divide competitors into weight classes for boxing, but do not divide high jumpers by height though it seems that this would have relatively similar import on the competition. When using the BMI scale, we correct for age and sex. We make use of reference classes including height, weight, age, sex and race in lung function tests, but we do not use class; and we use of none of these categories in hearing tests. As we will see in the following chapters, this is a result of complex historical processes, with decisions regarding what categories to consider often having more to do with the measurement's development than with any supposedly relevant features of health.

For example, in epidemiological studies of heart disease, correcting for race, sex and class is standard practice. Janet Shim's study of the politics of heart disease illuminates the fact that

> the custom of including racial categories, socioeconomic status, and sex in epidemiologic studies was so taken for granted that in presentations and conversations about their methods, researchers often referred simply to 'controlling for the usual suspects' as a shorthand gloss for the practice.[35]

Shim's account highlights the *blurriness* inherent in defining causation of disease as either biological or environmental. For instance, Shim explains that race in the context of epidemiology studies was not always considered to be of biological significance. Rather, it tended to be used as a proxy for the kinds of cultural differences and related health behaviours (such as diet) which were assumed to be relevant to the development of heart disease.[36] Similarly, class was variously (and contentiously) defined through proxy measures such as income, occupation or education attainment.[37] Conversely, sex (and especially oestrogen in the case of women) was consistently highlighted as being a meaningful *biological* factor relevant to heart disease, while the impact of gender (and its attendant impact on social biases, stresses, pressures and access to resources) was not considered relevant. This is despite the fact that researchers have linked the difference between men's and women's presentation of heart attacks to women's lack of reporting of chest pain due to (gendered) fears about wasting the doctor's time.[38] Shim further describes a lack of interest in the 'emerging literature which asserts that sex and gender are not the clear, biological binaries we have imagined them to be'.[39] Yet this categorical approach risks obscuring the social causes of health inequities. Not only does it ignore the impact of biography and developmental plasticity on health, as Epstein explains, by 'valorizing certain categories of identity, they conceal others from view'.[40]

The work that reference class categorisation systems can do to obscure social causes of disease is an especially significant issue to consider in light of recent researches on allostatic load theory. Allostatic load refers to the concept that long-term stress exposure leaves a marked physiological stamp on the body, evidenced in biomarkers such as shortened telomeres.[41] If, as seems to be the case, groups (such as racial groups) suffer from health inequalities not as a result of any factor related to their race but rather as a result of increased allostatic load caused by long-term stress, then we may need to consider whether using racial reference classes has obscured this social cause of ill health. We might also ask whether, if living under oppression is a significant determinant of health, we should categorise other social groups, for example those of lower socioeconomic status (or the disabled), as a meaningful reference class. This would be a politically charged move, as Epstein makes clear: 'Indeed, if social class were incorporated as a standard classifier, the political effects might be significant: because social class is not seen as a biological category, to call attention to differential health outcomes by class is to call attention to the effects of social inequality on health.'[42] Indeed, such processes of knowledge production have often been promoted explicitly as part of political agendas.

For instance, it is relevant to question whether grouping people into these categories affects the perpetuation of these categories. This is an increasingly relevant concern in the age of big data, which relies on such processes of categorisation. Chow-White and Green have argued that the development of genome technologies has resulted in an attendant acceptance of clear-cut racial boundaries purportedly correspondent to measurable genetic factors. Epstein points out the irony in the fact that since the sequencing of the human genome in 2000 demonstrated the commonality between humans, using racial categories to measure genetic difference has increased:

> Unlike other species, including other primates, humans cannot be disaggregated into clearly defined genetic subspecies – meaning that the eighteenth-and-nineteenth-century racist and imperialist conception of humanity as divided into biologically discrete groups simply has no basis in fact.[43]

Yet Chow-White and Green point out that using racial categories as a surrogate measure in genetics is simply easier – at least for the purposes of the researchers. Moreover, data-driven processes' apparent objectivity masks the way in which 'the decision to group racial data into three large samples of Asian, African, and European requires a complex social calculus for groups at the boundaries.'[44] Similarly, understanding of sex/gender as existing on a spectrum rather than on a binary complicates its previous simple division. The apparent neutrality of big data disguises its ability to categorise and shape the social world and 'this seeming neutrality obfuscates domain assumptions and leaves cultural values and practices of power unexamined.'[45]

Similarly, researchers such as Safiya Noble and Anna Hoffman have recently drawn attention to issues of fairness within algorithmic systems, demonstrating that technologies, like, for example, search engines, can work to architect and perpetuate structural biases.[46] Prejudices, cultures, biases and decisions are thus invisibly embedded in digital products through the categorisation of big data. As well as reflecting inequalities in society, these processes can work to perpetuate them. One of the ways that we can start to recognise and deal with the categorisations that lead to data discrimination is through examining the *historical* classification and categorisation of relevant groups. This is particularly relevant within healthcare classification systems, which often split up the world into useful categories. Classification systems section the world and allow us to put things or people into neat sets of boxes, which then work in the promotion of knowledge production.[47]

My argument here is not just that the variable use of reference classes undermines the naturalist conception of disease, but also that their use may serve to essentialise inappropriate social classes, and through this process conceal causes of health inequality. Classification of entities like race, disease, disability and patients is highly controversial and extremely important, as in the process of being classified they are often fashioned as natural divisions. But when we read studies that purport to demonstrate a biological basis for inequality, it is worth thinking about the underlying motivations for classifying their subjects into different groupings. Medical classifications divide our world into convenient categories, shaping our reality.[48] The process of categorisation and standardisation in knowledge classification systems has often been promoted explicitly as part of political agendas. Yet the objectivity and trust that we associate with numerical classification means that whatever classification schema these standards mark out becomes invisible as it upholds the categories it uses as inevitable, immutable, natural kinds – a process that philosopher Ian Hacking has described as 'Kind making'.[49] To say that a kind is natural is to say that it corresponds to nature's architecture as opposed to human interests. There is much debate, however, over whether things like races, sexes or sex orientations are natural kinds, or if they reflect the classifying interests of humans.

These are accordingly referred to as Social Kinds, and while sex categories have until recently been accepted as being (on average at least) as binary, there are more long-term definitional difficulties associated with racial and ethnic categories. As Amundson puts it: 'We were not carving nature at its joints when we partitioned human variability into races.'[50] Epstein outlines the questions connected with this difficulty in healthcare classifications by asking: 'How many racial and ethnic categories are there? What about people who are multiracial or multi-ethnic?'[51] To clarify, Kingma makes the point that we might be able to make a useful distinction here between ideas and objects. She explains:

> Take, for example, race. We might make a distinction between the object race – that is the existence of groups of people that share some (biological) differences, such as a difference in skin colour or ancestry – and the idea race, that is the practice of using certain physical characteristics to sort people into groups, and to use this classification for various purposes. The idea of race is the idea that sorting people into groups by, for example, skin colour, is a relevant means of classification.[52]

This is the kind of sorting process that has been illuminated by the work of Lundy Braun, who has explained that racialised lung function measurements are rooted in white supremacist ideologies of difference between races.[53] Race correction is literally programmed into the spirometer. It will not work unless you select race by either pushing a button, touching the screen or selecting race on a pull-down menu. It is unclear how the operator is meant to determine their patient's race. Moreover, because this function is 'black boxed', inside the machine as standard, many medics are unaware of how this process impacts on lung capacity measurements. This is just the kind of successful standard that disappears as a result of its success and becomes a ubiquitous and unremarkable aspect of scientific/industrial infrastructure.[54] Yet its apparent irrelevance gives the lie to its significance, as it could affect claims for compensation for occupational disease. For example, if you are black, a lower lung function norm means that you could be deemed ineligible for compensation even with the same degree of lung damage as your white co-worker. This works either through a scaling factor (of up to 15 per cent) or through use of race-specific population standards, usage of which varies between different manufacturers and different regions.[55]

However, it may nonetheless be necessary to use these corrections to ensure we gain accurate information when we assess someone's health for the first time. As a tool for evaluating respiratory health the spirometer is very useful – it is necessary for diagnosis of COPD (complex obstructive pulmonary disease – an umbrella diagnosis of various lung diseases), for example. Moreover, it provides crucial information about the *progression* of an individual's illness over time. Normal reference population values are used for many reasons in medicine, not least because they offer easy and fast ways to assess health. Yet Braun concludes that we must move towards a more intersectional understanding of health inequality, with more consideration for how socioeconomic status affects lung function. She argues that by 'considering race, class, and gender as deeply intertwined and the lungs as sensitive indicators of lived experience, we can ask how global inequality affects respiratory health'.[56]

Health inequalities are interconnected with the use of reference classes. As we will see in Chapter 5, using corrections for social groups as though they were biological groups was successfully employed to deny compensation to groups of miners. Simultaneously, failure to develop relevant reference classifications for women led to a lack of interest and research into women's lung health. In analysing these historical developments, it is necessary to take an intersectional approach.[57] It is unhelpful to look only at one category (like gender) because by doing so we miss the fact that these categorisation processes are about power more than anything else. And I argue that considering the category of disability makes this clearer. We make use of various reference classes in various situations, but there are challenges in both establishing class membership and establishing class relevance. A further class we might consider is disability and considering the class of disability makes explicit that much of categorisation is about social power, not nature. As we saw previously, there are significant challenges in giving an objective naturalistic definition of disability.

Defining disability

When considering disability, the main proponents of naturalism take a similar position to that developed through the BST's account of normal functioning. The WHO's International Classification of Functioning, Disability and Health (2001) describes disability as entailing 'decrements in functioning': 'disabled people cannot do everything the average human being can do'.[58] A paradigm example of this position in the context of philosophy of disability can be found in Norman Daniels's account, which holds that:

> Disease and disability, both physical and mental, are construed as adverse departures from or impairments of species-typical normal functional organization or 'normal functioning,' for short. The biomedical sciences for humans, like the veterinary sciences for animals, study both the variation in the functional organization typical for our species and the departures from normal functioning that we call disease and disability. The line between disease and disability and normal functioning is thus drawn in the relatively objective and nonevaluative context provided by the biomedical sciences, broadly construed. What counts as disease or disability from the perspective of these sciences is largely free from controversy in the broad range of cases.[59]

This links us back to the second main concept of disease within philosophy of medicine – normativism. The normativist position maintains, against naturalism, that health and disease are essentially value-laden concepts. Historical examples of diseases with a shifting status are therefore reflective of society's changing values. An example of this kind of analysis is hysteria, which, it has been argued, was redefined as a non-disease condition not because of new biological information, but rather due to widespread changes in moral values.[60] Another counterexample often proposed to naturalism is homosexuality, which for most of the twentieth century was classified as a disease in the *Diagnostic and Statistical Manual* (DSM) of the American Psychiatric Association.[61] The naturalist response is that homosexuality and masturbation (a typical defining 'symptom' of hysteria) were never 'real' disorders in the first place, and so this is just a case of erroneous classification.

However, Cooper has convincingly argued that the assumption that disorders must be universal and evident throughout history to be 'real' is unjustified.[62] For philosophers such as Cooper, Boorse's account of disease is fatally flawed. She offers an alternative account which suggests that a disease is a condition that fulfils certain conditions: it is a bad thing to have, it is unlucky that the patient has it and it is potentially medically treatable.[63] By including disability under the category of disease, this account has attracted the ire of many disability scholars who take central issue with the implication that disability is either bad or unlucky.[64]

Disability studies thus poses a challenge to philosophy of medicine, but Kingma has pointed out it also offers a compromise between the two apparently dichotomous positions of naturalism and normativism.[65] Disability studies generally tends towards a social constructivist position, which maintains that classifications originate from social and evaluative considerations, but does not necessarily argue that this means disability is somehow not real or cannot be described in an empirical manner. As philosophers Chin-Yee and Upshur have also pointed out, the disease concept's 'value-ladenness does not preclude the possibility of having a definition informed by empirical science'.[66] Before we attempt to outline such a definition of disability, that is, simultaneously empirically informed and socially constructed, we need to be clear about how disability is conceptualised within disability studies – and there are problems in defining the term disability even within the field. In disability studies, broadly speaking, the consensus on what constitutes disability is not a matter of human bodies but of the society that they are in. This view falls in line with the ideology inherent to social model thinking about disability, a way of thinking which has had a dramatic impact in advancing the political rights of the disabled in Britain.

The UK activism that led to the 1995 Disabilities Act was characterised by its use of the concept of the social model of disability, which presented a dichotomy between the medical and social model of disability. In disability studies, the medical model represents the imperialism of the medical community over the disabled and its attendant treatments and prosthetics. In opposition to this is the social model, a concept which was first coined by Mike Oliver in 1983. It has since become an influential social constructivist ideology that rests on the argument that it is society that oppresses and disables people on top of any impairment. The 'social model' was proposed by the Union of the Physically Impaired against Segregation (UPIAS) network, which was formed by disabled people who rejected the medical model of disability. The network was a small but hardcore disabled activist group with Marxist principles, working to replace segregated institutional facilities with independent living and working.[67] The social model suggests that disability is not so much an abnormality as it is a difference; that there is no fixed 'normal', and instead people exist on a spectrum of ability. Thus, unlike the orthodox philosophical view, which (broadly speaking) tends to view disability as inherently bad, the social model views disability as a primarily socially motivated phenomenon.

This model attributes the difficulties that disabled people experience mainly to societal failures. According to the social model, therefore, the problem of 'disability' derives mainly from society's inability to adapt to a wide range of human capabilities, rather than from an individual's differences from a restricted definition of 'the norm'. Simply, when society treats disabled people as abnormal and consequently excludes them from opportunities in work or education and denies them control over their own living conditions and treatments, then they inevitably experience difficulties. The social model and its neat relocation of the 'problem' of disability in the environment has been an incredibly important tool in advancing the rights of the disabled in the UK and across the world. Its simplicity, however, has been identified by Tom Shakespeare as the 'fatal flaw' of the social model, and he has argued in detail about why he believes the 'strong' social model has become problematic, rigid and exclusionary.[68] It is worth noting here, as Robert Chapman has recently discussed, that the social model as defined by UPIAS still assumes a 'Boorsean' type account in its notion of impairment.[69]

Aligned with Shakespeare, Barnes has argued that the dichotomy between the social and medical model is too strong, and that it does not account for the full variety and divergence within characterisations of disability. In her book, she offers an alternative account, called the value-neutral model, which reframes (physical) disability as 'a way of being a minority body'.[70] Barnes thus argues for a *moderate* social constructivist view. To clarify this point, the social model is a version of social constructivism, but there are other socially constructed explanations of disability. For example, Kuhane and Savulescu's Welfarist account defines disability in a completely revisionary way, as 'a stable personal trait that tends to diminish a person's wellbeing relative to some given context'.[71] It was designed to put greater emphasis on the question of well-being, and to enable clearer thinking in contentious ethical cases involving disability. However, this account results in features of social inequality (such as being a woman in a sexist country) counting as a disability, while other cases of disability considered not to diminish well-being (such as Deafness) do not. For Barnes, this is incompatible with a workable philosophy of disability and should furthermore be dismissed because of its incompatibility with disability studies. That is, 'a philosophical theory of disability shouldn't be in the business of claiming that much of what is said about disability within the disability rights movement is analytically false'.[72]

The definition of disability given by the UN Convention of the Rights of Persons with Disabilities enacted in 2008 was similarly influenced by social constructionism and stated that 'disability results from the interaction between persons with impairments and attitudinal and environmental barriers that hinder their full and effective participation in society on an equal basis with others'.[73] This is similar to scholar Tom Shakespeare's 2006 iteration of disability as predicament, which allows for the idea that we should still try and avoid impairments if possible. He writes:

> We are reminded that disability is extremely diverse and heterogeneous and that generalisations – 'disability is tragic' or 'disability is just another form of difference' – are usually misleading. A second point is that while many limitations experienced by disabled people are externally imposed restriction arising from inaccessible environments and social discrimination, there are also often intrinsic limitations to individual functioning that can only be overcome through the assistance of others, and not always even then. This form of life may not mean suffering, may not be incompatible with a good life, but might entail not being able to do everything that a person might want or hope to do.[74]

However, Barnes points out that if we are really trying to find a metaphysical account of what disability is, then all this view does is shift the burden of understanding from disability to impairment, and attempting to define impairment leaves us in the same position we were in when we critiqued the naturalist account – that is, seeking a metaphysical answer to the question 'what is impairment?'.[75] She also points out that moderate social constructivist positions such as Shakespeare's do not mesh well with the idea of disability pride: 'it's difficult to maintain, simultaneously, that disability is something to be celebrated and that disability is something we ultimately want to get rid of'.[76]

And yet I think one of the reasons that Shakespeare's view is so persuasive is that it appeals to what seems to be an intuitive or common-sense view of what disability is. However, Barnes has countered the temptation to rest our analysis on common-sense suppositions by pointing out that, historically, we have often made assumptions based on common-sense intuitions that we now think of as very wrong, and which were often made by a majority in a way that disempowered a minority.[77] For instance, in the previous chapter we discussed the nineteenth-century science of craniometry and the way in which it was used to demonstrate differences in intelligence between 'races' and between men and women. The apparent 'objectivity' of the scientific data used in this pursuit was deconstructed by Stephen Jay Gould in *The Mismeasure of Man*. As well as arguing that numerical measurements were prioritised as markers of truth, Gould's work also highlighted the pliable ways in which reference classes can be used, particularly when measurement are 'corrected' for the relevant class. To exemplify this, Gould related the story of Paul Broca (1824–80), a renowned French physician and anthropologist, now best known for developing the concept of cortical localisation and the identification of 'Broca's area'. He used lead shot measurements of cranial capacity and weighed brains in order to make the claim that the size of the brain correlated with intelligence. His claims were opposed by the Frenchman Louis Pierre Gratiolet, who argued that the size of the brain bore no relationship to intelligence. Gratiolet's challenge rested on his light-hearted point that 'German brains were on average 100 grams heavier than French brains so therefore brain size could not possibly correlate with intelligence.'[78] However, Broca was able to repudiate Gratiolet by applying corrections to French brains for non-intellectual factors that impact on the brain's size at death, including age, health, manner of death and body size.[79]

This case demonstrates the importance of relevant reference classes and shows how their inclusion or exclusion can allow for easy manipulation of data. Broca never used these corrections in his work on women's brains, for instance, although he realised that their smaller average body size could be impacting on his results. He reasoned that applying corrections to women was unnecessary because of the already established fact of women's inferiority, writing:

> We might ask if the small size of the female brain depends exclusively upon the small size of her body.... But we must not forget than women are, on the average, a little less intelligent than men, a difference which we should not exaggerate but which is, nonetheless, real. We are therefore permitted to suppose that the relatively small size of the female brain depends in part upon her physical inferiority and in part upon her intellectual inferiority.[80]

Broca's rationalisation of women's inferiority would have been considered eminently sensible and fair to many of his contemporary scientists and no doubt to much of the population living at that time. Barnes reasons that remarks like this should show us that we must be wary of relying on our intuitions when defining disability. As Barnes explains, our intuitions are informed by culture, 'And while that might (might!) not matter much when it comes to intuitions about logic or mathematics, it matters a great deal when it comes to intuitions about the well-being of oppressed groups ... And it is particularly suspect when it contravenes the testimony of many members of that disadvantaged group.'[81]

Nonetheless, Barnes's value-neutral model of disability differs from the traditional social model view in that she denies that disability should be considered as on a par with social categories like race and gender. Rather, she argues (again allying herself with Shakespeare on this point) that there is a crucial somatic element to disability. She explains: 'we may not be able to give an account of disability based on objective similarities shared by disabled bodies. And yet what your body is like matters to whether you are disabled. It might not matter for gender or race – I take no stand on that here – but it does matter for disability.'[82] However, Barnes does aver that the categorisation of kinds and the importance we place on them are socially constructed even if the physical features are not. That is, classifying someone as disabled (at least physically) is

> a matter of whether they in fact have particular objective bodily features. But the fact that these bodily features are important to us – the fact that they matter, and are considered relevant to the classification of someone as disabled – is due to the way we think about bodies, rather than some objective similarity between such bodies. And that's what it is, on my view, for disability to be socially constructed.[83]

Thus, she concludes that it is the norms and practices which shape why we take certain bodies to matter that we should be analysing and questioning.[84]

Well-being and disability

Barnes maintains that disability is not something that makes you intrinsically worse off. She points out that there is a great deal of empirical evidence which suggests that

> non-disabled people are extraordinarily bad at predicting the effects of disability on *perceived* well-being. Non-disabled people tend to assume that disability will have a substantial negative effect on perceived well-being, and that the perceived well-being of the disabled will be substantially lower than their own. But a substantial amount of research suggests that this is simply not the case.[85]

The gap between the way that people are defined as disabled and their own identification with this label is a repeated theme in this book. From the miners who believed themselves disabled by dust to the businessmen who argued that their telephones were the real source of their hearing difficulties, we will see multiple cases of individuals contesting the status of their dis/ability. In this section I consider these arguments about well-being and disability more broadly by exploring the concept of the disability paradox. This phrase was coined in 1999 by Albrecht and Devlieger when they introduced empirical evidence supporting the fact that many disabled people rated their quality of life as good or excellent, although external observers imagined them to have an 'undesirable daily existence'.[86] This paper also confirmed that there was a 'decided negative bias in the attitudes and expectations of the public and health-care workers towards people with disabilities' which increased if the disability was visible or associated with stigmatisation and decreased through close contact with the disabled.[87] This phenomenon, the so-called disability paradox, consists, first, in the fact that although the disabled people surveyed reported problems related to discrimination, living activities and society they nevertheless reported excellent or good quality of life.[88] Second, it consists in the fact that the non-disabled, including physicians and healthcare workers, do not believe this to be true and rate the same people as having an unsatisfying quality of life.[89]

Furthermore, non-disabled people, when asked to imagine the well-being of people with certain kinds of disabilities, tend to imagine it to be far worse than it is. More recent studies have shown that even in states of illness that healthy observers rate as being worse than death, the people with the actual conditions reported similar levels of well-being as the healthy counterparts (an exception to this is pain, which does seem to consistently lower levels of happiness).

Findings from the field of hedonic psychology (nicknamed 'the science of happiness') suggest that we are surprisingly bad at predicting what will make us happy and at estimating our levels of happiness in certain situations. I often think that a large (ideally stuffed crust) Domino's pizza is going to make me happy and am inevitably disappointed to feel less than happy after finishing one. One explanation of this phenomenon is that we basically are not good at working out what is going to make us happy. As Wasserman and Asch explain: 'whole disciplines have emerged – hedonic psychology and happiness science – that find that normal functioning and health (as well as wealth and professional success) have far less effect on (self-reported) well-being that commonly assumed'.[90]

A 2010 paper by Ron Amundson explored this in relation to the question of whether we should believe the claims of the disabled about their own levels of happiness. Amundson explored the hedonic psychology studies related to hedonic adaptation: the idea that we adjust our levels of happiness back to their former level after a life event that has raised or lowered them. Related to this is the fact that extreme changes in happiness levels do not tend to last very long. Subjective happiness (he argues) does not result from the accumulation of hedonically positive life factors, but rather from our psychological reactions to those circumstances.[91]

These findings have surprising implications for the way that we think about disability and health, for the way we currently organise funding within the health service and for the priorities we focus on in our own lives. For instance, fluctuations in happiness levels resulting from changing circumstances may not last very long. You may want to win the lottery but any elevated happiness resulting from your win will only last a few years, then you will be back to the same state of mind as before. On the flip side, this also holds for the experience of severe illness or disability.[92] Our health and our wealth may not be as important as our *responses* to the challenges we are presented with. For example, one respondent to the original 1999 survey explained:

> After my wreck with a truck on the Kennedy, I realized I couldn't move my legs. I thought that my life was over. But during rehab and after I came back home I had plenty of time to think. I still had my mind. My body was in a wheelchair but I could still be a father, husband, son, and have friends. I could coach my daughter's softball team and I'm in training to be a counsellor. I can do it. I have a life.[93]

Another respondent elucidated: 'Other people can't understand why I am so happy. They don't have the same appreciation of life. They would have to understand the satisfaction of using all my resources to conquer each day of challenges.'[94] Both these responses highlight the role of challenge as key, which has made some suggest that it is the experience of working towards a goal that truly brings happiness.

More widely, philosopher Havi Carel has discussed more recent studies of objective and subjective well-being that show medical conditions do not generally impact on overall happiness scores.[95] She argues that one of the reasons why there is such a gulf between insider and outsider perspectives of illness is that healthy people weigh the importance of the illness far too heavily based on popular (prejudiced) media representations, a phenomenon known as 'the focusing illusion'. In addition, she points out that the imaginations of healthy people simply do not have the capacity of understanding the lived experience of situations so abstracted from their own lives, or, indeed, the habit of doing so.[96] That is: 'Healthy people spend less time imagining themselves as old and unwell, or diagnosed with a serious illness, than they do imagining themselves playing post-retirement golf in the Florida sunshine.'[97]

However, when presented with the disability paradox, some scholars, particularly in bioethics, have drawn on Jon Elster's 1983 work on rationality, *Sour Grapes*.[98] In this work Elster initially draws on the fable of the fox and the grapes, in which the fox wants to eat some grapes, cannot reach the grapes they desire and so concludes that they were sour and in fact they did not want them after all. Elster's description of adaptive preferences then suggests that while the fox is pretending not to like the grapes he cannot have, a person with adaptive preferences truly does prefer what they can have over that which they cannot. In other words, they do not know what they are missing, having never experienced it.

Barnes counters this kind of criticism, arguing that 'the problem with the adaptive preference model is that it allows us to dismiss certain kinds of testimony as irrational or misleading. And so the adaptive preference model can quickly become a way of defending the moral status quo.'[99] Moreover, Barnes points out that 'it's simply false that all disabled people who express disability-positive views – including the view that they wouldn't want to become non-disabled – don't know what it's like to be non-disabled. And that's because such views are expressed by those with acquired disabilities as well as those with congenital disabilities.'[100] Lastly, Barnes argues that the adaptive preferences notion can hold without necessarily connoting either denial or irrationality, making the point that we all adapt based on the body and environment we are in.[101] Indeed it would be deeply irrational not to do so. For example, I once wanted to be a ballet dancer but considering my aforementioned lack of flexibility, my great dislike of dieting and lack of rhythm, it would seem very strange if I had continued to work towards this goal.[102]

Shakespeare also points out that most of the things that we value most highly for happiness (such as meaningful relationships, being valued, fulfilment of goals) are still accessible to the disabled: 'disability usually does not have to equate to exclusion from most of what makes life good'.[103] Carel relates well-being within illness to adaptation, accommodation and resilience and she explains that there are three main ways in which illness can increase fulfilment. First, there is evidence to show that facing adversity reveals hidden but genuine strengths and creates new confidence. Second, relationships become stronger and more authentic. Third, a new focus on the present moment leads to greater enjoyment of current experiences.[104] She concludes with the beautifully expressed point that:

> If we take seriously the phenomenological approach to illness and the robust evidence that ill people (and others who face adversity) are no less happy than other people, we can conclude that paying close attention to such claims may yield important insights about the experience of illness. If happiness is an achievement that requires thought, planning and work, this view contributes to our understanding of why illness does not affect long-term well-being. Illness provides us with a context and opportunity for the kind of reflection and revaluation that are the condition for and prelude to happiness.[105]

This section therefore reinforces the need for epistemic humility with respect to our pre-theoretical judgements about disability. Furthermore, if part of our theoretical task is to analyse the norms and practices (and in particular the instruments of medical science) which shape why we take certain bodies to matter for being categorised as disabled, then we also need to consider how our judgements about well-being are formed.

Disbelief and epistemic injustice

This reflection on the importance of taking seriously the accounts of others relates to a more insidious response to the disability paradox, which is simply to react with dismissal and disbelief. As Shakespeare brutally but amusingly puts it, 'Perhaps these cheerful people with disabilities are deluding themselves and others.'[106] Such disbelief is a paradigm example of epistemic injustice towards the disabled. Epistemic injustice is a concept developed by Miranda Fricker. She pointed out that in addition to the social or political injustices faced by minority groups, they can also experience epistemic injustice. She splits this into testimonial and hermeneutical injustice. The former is concerned with situations when people are unable to access a shared understanding of their social experience due to prejudiced resources. Similarly, testimonial injustice describes the prejudices that give less credibility to a speaker's assertions because their capacity 'to know' or 'to impart' is doubted. This phenomenon has been explored in relation to healthcare conditions that might specifically reduce credibility, such as chronic fatigue and mental health illnesses.[107] Like invisible disability, the difficulty of securing a trusted instrumental diagnosis exacerbates epistemic injustice. More recently, it has been argued that there are distinctive features of disabled life that promote a specific kind of epistemic injustice.[108] As Barnes points out in relation to disbelief, 'we ought to take disabled people as very good sources of evidence about what it is like to be disabled. Or we at least ought to take them as better sources of evidence than the beliefs of the non-disabled about what is common sense.'[109] And yet, the non-disabled often disagree with disabled people's assessments of their own lives, experiences, needs and knowledges. Jackie Leach Scully has also raised the important point that testimonial injustice can be further inflicted on the disabled through the procedures around claiming social support.[110] And yet, crucially, she elucidates the fact that various kinds of impairments can actually lead to the creation of distinctive knowledge, for example about their condition and the assistive technology that may be associated with it. Not only from their experience and familiarity with their condition, but through their embodied knowledge of exactly what works for them.

This understanding is akin to Margaret Lock's concept of 'local biologies', which denotes the way in which 'the embodied experience of physical sensations, including those of well-being, health, illness, and so on, is in part informed by the material body'.[111] Local biologies are thus linked with both the experience and the interpretation of sensations. This has important ramifications for the way we think about 'lay epistemologies' of health. In this sense, it is not that certain groups do not have symptoms and understandings of their meanings, it is that their interpretations are not heeded by the dominant discourse. In Fricker's conceptualisation of hermeneutical epistemic injustice, marginalised social groups are subjected to epistemic harms due to a silence – a gap in knowledge. Yet these 'local biologies' are most usefully conceptualised within the framework suggested by Kirstie Dotson, which has identified the way that power affects the extent to which the dominant discourse considers 'alternative epistemologies, counter mythologies, and hidden transcripts that exist in hermeneutically marginalised communities *among themselves*'.[112] It is this framework that Braun and Kopinski draw on to explain the normalisation of suffering among communities of mine-workers, arguing that 'publicly-funded science privileges certain accounts of disease and excludes other accounts, such as those of the asbestos workers on the mines'.[113] As Chapter 5 of this book will similarly argue, the miners involved in the researches into pneumoconiosis in south Wales had nuanced and sophisticated awareness of their breathlessness, but the MRC was unable to standardise this type of knowledge into the categorisation systems required for objectivity and compensation calculability. The spirometer was thus embraced as an objective marker of disability that could be utilised in the complex industrial compensation network. Similarly, I argue in Chapter 4 that the audiometer was used over the arguably more clinically useful tuning fork because it provided single-number evidence of hearing levels which could be used to negotiate compensation claims and guard against malingerers and 'hysterical' deafness. Given that social (and indeed oppressive) forces play such a fundamental role in constructing disability, this enhances the possibility of a significant threat of epistemic injustice. If the medical sciences are solely working with a naturalistic conception of disability, this heightens the likelihood of this form of injustice manifesting.

Conclusion

We need to question the extent to which measurements can tell us something 'real or true' about the human body in cases when easily quantifiable measurements of easily recognisable groups are artificially privileged. In this chapter I have argued that the naturalist conception of disability is undermined by the way in which the thresholds of normalcy are statistically constructed. This attack is mounted on two fronts. First, I draw attention to the ways in which the representative subjects used to create the statistical average can distort the threshold of normalcy. This is the situation outlined in Chapter 3, in my exploration of how the measure of normal hearing was defined using the measures of just ten 'normal' male ears. Second, I argue that the varied utilisation of different reference classes creates a problem of misrepresentation, as using arbitrarily defined social groups can promote essentialist thinking about 'natural' differences between these groups and thereby disguise environmental and social impacts on health.

This history should make us cognisant of the danger of essentialising social categories, not only in terms of racial or sexual profiling, but also in terms of disability. My views here are therefore aligned with those of Amundson, who explains that while the concept of normality 'invokes no essentialist casual powers, in that the functional type does not explain biological form. I am concerned, however, that once the concept is introduced and reified, it is itself used in casual explanations of social phenomena. It is used to explain and rationalize the social disadvantages of people labelled abnormal.'[114] Crucially, however, this works two ways. While we ought to be concerned about essentialising social categories, we also need to ensure relevant groups are classified as such *when it matters*. As this book will demonstrate, the pliability and mutability of relevant reference classes meant that these classification systems were integral to the production of biopower in twentieth-century Britain.

Notes

1 Dr Tomas Chamorro-Premuzic has drawn attention to the recent nature of this phenomenon and related it to the impact of individually targeted marketing and especially the specificity of online targeted marketing. He pointed out on BBC Radio 4 that 'this is a fairly recent phenomenon, a hundred years ago if you ask people: "are you destined to be different or destined to be famous or destined to be special?" – about 20 or 30% of people said yes, in the 50s that number went up to 50%, in the 80s it went up to 70% and right now it's about 85%'. BBC Radio 4, 'Average', *The Digital Human*, series 15. Accessed June 2019. www.bbc.co.uk/programmes/m0000qvy.
2 Fricker, M., *Epistemic Injustice: Power and the Ethics of Knowing* (Oxford: Oxford University Press, 2007).
3 Carel, H., and Kidd, I., 'Epistemic Injustice in Healthcare: A Philosophical Analysis', *Medicine, Health Care and Philosophy*, 17:4 (2014), 529–540.
4 Scully, J. L., 'From "She Would Say That, Wouldn't She?" to "Does She Take Sugar?" Epistemic Injustice and Disability', *International Journal of Feminist Approaches to Bioethics*, 11:1 (2018), 106–124.
5 Carel, H., 'Breathless: Philosophical Lessons from Respiratory Illness', *Journal of Medical Humanities*, 6:1 (2014), 1–6.
6 See Barnes, E., *The Minority Body* (Oxford: Oxford University Press, 2016) and Kingma, E., 'Health and Disease: Social Constructivism as a Combination of Naturalism and Normativism', in H. Carel and R. Cooper (eds), *Health, Illness and Disease: Philosophical Essays* (Durham: Acumen Publishing, 2013), pp. 37–56.
7 Kingma, E., 'Paracetamol, Poison, and Polio: Why Boorse's Account of Function Fails to Distinguish Health and Disease', *British Journal for the Philosophy of Science*, 61:2 (2010), 241–264, p. 242.
8 Boorse, C., 'Health as a Theoretical Concept', *Philosophy of Science*, 44:4 (1997), 542–573.
9 Boorse, C., 'Disability and Medical Theory', in D. Ralston and J. Ho (eds), *Philosophical Reflections on Disability* (Dordrecht: Springer, 2010), pp. 55–88, p. 104.
10 Kuhane, G., and Savulescu, J., 'The Welfarist Account of Disability', in K. Brownlee and A. Cureton (eds), *Disability and Disadvantage* (Oxford: Oxford University Press, 2009), pp. 1–37, p. 5.
11 Boorse, C., 'A Second Rebuttal on Health', *Journal of Medicine and Philosophy*, 39:6 (2014), 683–724.
12 Wakefield, J. C., 'The Biostatistical Theory versus the Harmful Dysfunction Analysis, Part 1: Is Part-Dysfunction a Sufficient Condition for Medical Disorder?', *Journal of Medicine and Philosophy*, 39:6 (2014), 648–682, p. 649.

13 Boorse, 'Disability and Medical Theory', p. 69.
14 Ibid.
15 Cooper, R., 'Disease', *Studies in History and Philosophy of Biological and Biomedical Sciences*, 22:2 (2002), 263–282.
16 Boorse does clarify in his 2014 rebuttal that the BST was always meant to be dynamic.
17 My extreme fear that something like this or worse would happen is enough to ensure that I have never indulged in this kind of activity.
18 Kingma, 'Paracetamol, Poison, and Polio', p. 248.
19 Ibid., pp. 248–249.
20 Cooper, 'Disease', p. 263.
21 Cooper, R., 'Shifting Boundaries Between the Normal and the Pathological: The Case of Mild Intellectual Disability', *History of Psychiatry*, 25:2 (2014), 171–186.
22 Amundson, R., 'Against Normal Function', *Studies in History and Philosophy of Biological and Biomedical Sciences*, 31:1 (2000), 33–53, p. 35.
23 Barnes, *The Minority Body*, p. 14.
24 Ibid., p. 15.
25 Ibid.
26 Ibid., p. 16.
27 Ibid., p. 17.
28 Amundson, 'Against Normal Function', p. 45.
29 Boorse, 'A Second Rebuttal'.
30 Kingma, 'Paracetamol, Poison, and Polio', p. 243.
31 Chin-Yee, B., and Upshur, R. E. G., 'Re-Evaluating Concepts of Biological Function in Clinical Medicine: Towards a New Naturalistic Theory of Disease', *Theoretical Medicine and Bioethics*, 38:4 (2017), 245–264, p. 247.
32 Cooper, 'Disease', p. 266.
33 Kingma, E., 'What Is It to Be Healthy?', *Analysis*, 67:294 (2007), 128–133, p. 128.
34 Epstein, *Inclusion*, p. 10.
35 Shim, *Heart-Sick*, p. 18.
36 Ibid., p. 89.
37 Ibid., p. 129.
38 Epstein, *Inclusion*, p. 255.
39 Shim, *Heart-Sick*, p. 194.
40 Epstein, *Inclusion*, p. 11.
41 See Ahrens, K. A., Rossen, L. M., and Simon, A. E., 'Relationship between Mean Leucocyte Telomere Length and Measures of Allostatic Load in US Reproductive-Aged Women, NHNES 1999–2002', *Paediatric and Perinatal Epidemiology*, 30:4 (2016), 325–335, and Szanton, S. L., Gill, J. M., and Allen, J. K., 'Allostatic Load: A Mechanism of Socioeconomic Health Disparities?', *Biological Research for Nursing*, 7:1 (2010), 7–15.
42 Epstein, *Inclusion*, p. 144.
43 Ibid., pp. 210–211.

44 Chow-White, P. A., and Green, J. R., 'Data Mining Differences in the Age of Big Data: Communication and the Social Shaping of Genome Technologies from 1998 to 2007', *International Journal of Communication*, 7 (2013), 556–583, p. 576.
45 Ibid., p. 556.
46 Noble, S. U., *Algorithms of Oppression: How Search Engines Reinforce Racism* (New York: New York University Press, 2018) and Hoffman, A. L., 'Data Violence and How Bad Engineering Choices Can Damage Society', *Medium*, 30 April 2018. https://medium.com/s/story/data-violence-and-how-bad-engineering-choices-can-damage-society-39e44150e1d4. Accessed July 2019.
47 Bowker, G. C., and Star, S. L., *Sorting Things Out: Classification and Its Consequences* (Cambridge, MA: MIT Press, 2000), p. 10.
48 Ibid., p. 110.
49 For comparative arguments about the objectivity and power of numbers in biopolitics see Porter, 'Measurement, Objectivity, and Trust' and Hacking, 'Biopower and the Avalanche of Printed Numbers'.
50 Amundson, 'Against Normal Function', p. 34.
51 Epstein, 'Bodily Differences and Collective Identities', p. 195.
52 Kingma, 'Health and Disease', p. 44.
53 Braun, *Breathing Race into the Machine*.
54 Epstein, *Inclusion*, p. 24.
55 Braun, *Breathing Race into the Machine*.
56 Ibid., p. 205.
57 For the original mapping of intersectionality see Crenshaw, K., 'Mapping the Margins: Intersectionality, Identity, Politics, and Violence against Women of Color', *Stanford Law Review*, 43:6 (1991), 1241–1299, and for more of my analysis using this framework see Chapter 5.
58 Quoted in Shakespeare, T., 'Nasty, Brutish, and Short? On the Predicament of Disability and Embodiment', in J. E. Bickenback, F. Felder and B. Schmitz (eds), *Disability and the Good Human Life* (Cambridge: Cambridge University Press, 2014), pp. 93–112, p. 95.
59 Daniels, N., 'Normal Functioning and the Treatment–Enhancement Distinction', *Cambridge Quarterly of Healthcare Ethics*, 9:3 (2000), 314–315; for a longer explanation of this view see Daniels, N., *Just Health Care* (Cambridge: Cambridge University Press, 1985).
60 Historians and philosophers who have applied this kind of analysis to hysteria include Elaine Showalter in Showalter, E., *The Female Malady: Women, Madness and English Culture, 1830–1980* (London: Penguin Books, 1987); Andrew Scull in Scull, A., *Hysteria: The Disturbing History* (Oxford: Oxford University Press, 2009); and Jan Goldstein in Goldstein, J., *Hysteria Complicated by Ecstasy: The Case of Nanette Leroux* (Princeton, NJ: Princeton University Press, 2010).
61 Cooper, 'Disease'.
62 Cooper, R., 'Are Culture-Bound Syndromes as Real as Universally-Occurring Disorders?', *Studies in History and Philosophy of Science Part C: Studies in History and Philosophy of Biological and Biomedical Sciences*, 41:4 (2010), 325–332.

63 Cooper, 'Disease'.
64 See Barnes, *The Minority Body* and Kingma, 'What Is It to Be Healthy?'.
65 Kingma, 'Health and Disease'.
66 Chin-Yee and Upshur, 'Re-Evaluating Concepts of Biological Function', p. 247.
67 See the introduction to Shakespeare, T., *Disability Rights and Wrongs Revisited* (London: Routledge, 2nd edn, 2013).
68 See Shakespeare, T., 'The Social Model of Disability: An Outdated Ideology?', *Research in Social Science and Disability*, 2 (2002), 9–28.
69 Chapman, R., 'Neurodiversity, Disability, Wellbeing', in N. Chown, A. Stenning and H. Rosqvist (eds), *Neurodiversity Studies: A New Critical Paradigm* (London: Routledge, forthcoming).
70 It is important to note that her book focuses specifically on physical disability, and whether the value-neutral model is valid in cases such as learning disability, chronic illness or mental illness is not clear.
71 Kuhane and Savulescu, 'The Welfarist Account of Disability'.
72 Barnes, *The Minority Body*, p. 12.
73 Shakespeare, 'Nasty, Brutish, and Short?', p. 93 This convention recently condemned Conservative austerity policies *c.* 2008–19 for their overtly negative impacts on the disabled.
74 Ibid., pp. 101–102.
75 Barnes, *The Minority Body*, p. 20–21.
76 Ibid., p. 43.
77 Ibid., p. 72.
78 Gould, *The Mismeasure of Man*, p. 121.
79 This was very troubling for nineteenth-century prison doctors as the brains of the criminals they autopsied tended to be large (because brains expand when a person is hanged).
80 Broca quoted in Gould, *The Mismeasure of Man*, p. 135.
81 Barnes, *The Minority Body*, p. 72 (ellipses added for clarity).
82 Ibid., p. 37.
83 Ibid., p. 38.
84 Ibid., p. 41.
85 Ibid., pp. 71–72.
86 Albrecht, G. L., and Devlieger, P. J., 'The Disability Paradox: High Quality of Life against All Odds', *Social Science and Medicine*, 48:8 (1999), 977–988, p. 977.
87 Ibid., p. 978 and p. 979.
88 Ibid., p. 982.
89 Ibid.
90 Wasserman, D., and Asch, A., 'Understanding the Relationship between Disability and Well-Being', in J. E. Bickenback, F. Felder and B. Schmitz (eds), *Disability and the Good Human Life* (Cambridge: Cambridge University Press, 2014), pp. 139–167, p. 141.
91 Amundson, R., 'Quality of Life, Disability, and Hedonic Psychology', *Journal for the Theory of Social Behaviour*, 40:4 (2010), 374–392, p. 379.

92 Carel, H., 'Ill, but Well: A Phenomenology of Well-Being in Chronic Illness', in J. E. Bickenback, F. Felder and B. Schmitz (eds), *Disability and the Good Human Life* (Cambridge: Cambridge University Press, 2014), pp. 243–270, p. 253.
93 Albrecht and Devlieger, 'The Disability Paradox', p. 983.
94 Ibid., p. 984.
95 Carel, 'Ill, but Well', p. 252.
96 Ibid., pp. 254–255.
97 Ibid., p. 254.
98 Elster, J., *Sour Grapes: Studies in the Subversion of Rationality* (Cambridge: Cambridge University Press, 2016).
99 Barnes, *The Minority Body*, p. 134.
100 Ibid., p. 104.
101 Ibid., p. 125.
102 Barnes draws on Martha Nussbaum's work on capabilities to make this point. See Barnes, *The Minority Body*, p. 128.
103 Shakespeare, 'Nasty, Brutish, and Short?', p. 100.
104 Carel, 'Ill, but Well', pp. 257–258.
105 Ibid., p. 266.
106 Shakespeare, 'Nasty, Brutish, and Short?', p. 97.
107 Carel and Kidd, 'Epistemic Injustice in Healthcare' and Blease, C., Carel, H., and Geraghty, K., 'Epistemic Injustice in Healthcare Encounters: Evidence from Chronic Fatigue Syndrome', *Journal of Medical Ethics* 43:8 (2016), 549–557.
108 Scully, 'From "She Would Say That, Wouldn't She?"'.
109 Barnes, *The Minority Body*, p. 142.
110 Scully, 'From "She Would Say That, Wouldn't She?"'.
111 Lock, M., 'The Tempering of Medical Anthropology: Troubling Natural Categories', *Medical Anthropology Quarterly*, 15:4 (2001), 478–492, p. 483.
112 Dotson, K., 'A Cautionary Tale: On Limiting Epistemic Oppression', *Frontiers: A Journal of Women Studies*, 33:1 (2012), 24–47, p. 31.
113 Braun, L., and Kopinski, H., 'Casual Understandings: Controversy, Social Context, and Mesothelioma Research', *Biosocieties*, 13:3 (2018), 557–579, p. 560.
114 Amundson, 'Against Normal Function', p. 37.

3

THE ARTIFICIAL EAR AND THE DISABILITY DATA GAP

A rabbit vibrating in F

On the evening of Monday, 6 September 1886, Professor William Rutherford travelled from Edinburgh to Birmingham to deliver a lecture to the British Medical Association on a subject that he described as being on 'the borderland between the realm of physics and that of consciousness'.[1] He began by inviting his audience to consider the nature of sound while they listened to a vibrating pendulum and a number of differently pitched tuning forks. After this, he started on his main topic, 'The Telephone Theory of the Sense of Hearing', inspired by the invention of the telephone ten years earlier. He enthused: 'It is, indeed, one of the most wonderful inventions of recent times', and asked his audience, 'can it throw light on the sense of hearing?'.[2] Rutherford had developed a theory of frequency transmission based on the working of the telephone and he postulated that each sound stimulated a corresponding hair cell in the ear, with a correlation between the number of hair cells and the audibility of the transmission. Rutherford had reached this conclusion by taking apart and experimenting with, variously, a telephone, a frog and a rabbit. He boasted: 'I could send as many as 352 impulses per second along the nerve of a rabbit and get a note from the muscle of the pitch of 352 vibrations per second. That is a note of the pitch of F on the lowest space of the treble clef.'[3]

It might not seem that a rabbit vibrating in F has much in common with the British Post Office. Yet not long after Rutherford's experiments, that institution was also trying to discover the extent to which the telephone could throw light on the sense of hearing. Indeed, the Post Office was soon designing telephones specifically for people with hearing loss as part of their government-mandated state monopoly. What happened, in this short space of time, to take British telephone technology from vibrating rabbits to a telephone service for

'Deaf Subscribers'? In some ways very little, as we can see from case studies of users with hearing loss who engaged with the Post Office to improve amplified telephony. The early telephone was very difficult to hear. After failing to access telephony, users with hearing loss responded to its failings by using alternative devices, creating personalised devices or lobbying the Post Office to improve its service. Rutherford's experiments were thus emblematic of the way that the Post Office's amplified telephone service developed, that is, dependent on user experiences and individual experiments, and inextricably tied into the telephone's complicated connection to deafness.

As the Introduction to this book outlined, the telephone was linked to deafness from its 1876 conception: the result of Alexander Graham Bell's desire to teach the deaf to speak. The telephone soon evolved into a hearing testing device in the form of the early induction-coil-style audiometer, which literally commodified the telephone as a device to measure hearing loss.[4] This prioritised quantitative single-number indicators of hearing loss over the qualitative data produced by tuning forks; a development which will be given further consideration in Chapter 4. Here, I argue that the telephone itself was also used as an arbitrator of normal hearing. Moreover, the data used to create a so-called normal level of hearing used in the 'artificial ear' featured what I term a 'disability data gap'. The artificial ear's representation of normal was in fact the ideal (eight normal men with good hearing), to the detriment of those at the outer edges of a more representative average curve. As a result of this, those with less than perfect hearing agitated to demand the Post Office supply telephones that could be used by the majority of the population. The Post Office responded by creating its 'telephone service for the deaf', and the subsequent user appropriation and modification of this service vividly demonstrates the fluid categorisation of deafness that the telephone enabled.

This chapter has three main sections.[5] In the section below on 'The deafened', I explain the ways in which the First World War improved the technology available for use in telephony, while simultaneously creating the conditions of mass deafening that made such technology necessary. Before the First World War, noise-induced hearing loss was mainly a problem for the marginalised working class, but by the eve of the Second World War, hearing loss was regarded as a serious national health concern. This transition was caused by the First World War changing the context of hearing loss. The First World War was the first example of large-scale, industrialised deafening of soldiers. Losing hearing in the service of the country made the condition one that demanded compensation, and this became an issue for the middle and upper classes. During the interwar years the boundaries between deafness and hearing loss were blurred, and definitions depended on the cause and context of the hearing loss.

Vast numbers of newly deafened soldiers prompted an ideological shift concerning attitudes to hearing loss, and the concept of 'the Deafened' emerged during this period as a new term used to categorise adults with hearing loss. Crucially, this kind of categorisation was linked to the way that the Post Office standardised 'normal hearing' using a device called 'the artificial ear' which used data taken from just ten 'normal' male ears. This device was designed as a way of efficiently and objectively measuring and reproducing sound quality without human involvement. This, as I argue in the section on 'The artificial ear', allowed the Post Office to manage the variability of hearing and standardise the norms of human hearing. However, it also featured a 'disability data gap', which meant that the standard of normal hearing was distorted to reflect an idealised average. This impacted on the standards that were used to design 'normal telephones' in Britain. If users did not have the ability to use the normal telephones, then it followed that they had to use the 'telephone service for the deaf'.

Designating the standard of normal hearing in such a narrow mechanistic fashion resulted in increased disconnect between the objective measurement of hearing and the subjective correlate. The resulting problems are discussed in the case studies in the section on 'Individual users versus institutional innovations', which forms the main part of this chapter. Here, I reveal how aspirational users employed a variety of strategies to ensure equitable access to telephony. Users with hearing loss created modified devices so that they could access telephony in a manner sympathetic to their personal experiences of hearing loss. Although the state played a key role in directing Post Office research into hearing assistive devices, the main force motivating the design of the amplified telephone was user activism. Deaf subscribers' personal bodily knowledge was turned into a product that the Post Office could sell on. Yet the interplay between the Post Office and its users was more complex than simple appropriation, especially in the 1920s, when, I argue, amplified telephone technology was in a state of 'interpretive flexibility', with its meaning not yet fixed or defined.[6] That is, during the interwar years the amplified telephone was neither purely medical nor simply technical, and the boundaries between hearing loss and deafness changed with improvements to the technology.

Historian Michael Kay's study of telephone use in the nineteenth century has demonstrated that the telephone's broad inaudibility was one of the main reasons for initial widespread user rejection.[7] For anyone with less than perfect hearing the telephone was inaccessible. This came as a blow to many members of the Deaf community, who had hoped that it could be used like a hearing aid.[8] Subsequently, the first electronic hearing aids were indeed based on basic microphone telephone technology and were often simply called 'phones' or some variant thereof like 'fortiphone', 'magniphone', 'electrophone', 'ossiphone' or 'micro-telephone', or named to indicate their more specialist roles, such as 'operaphones' or 'the "lady shopper's" electric phone'.[9] The 'phone' suffix distinguished these types of hearing aids from the valve-operated hearing aids which developed after the First World War. One man in the US did not wait for these technical developments, and simply walked with an unadorned telephone and his hearing horn attached to him, proffering the receiver to any potential conversationalists.[10] These individualistic solutions were of varying effectiveness, however, and institutional resolutions were soon demanded from the Post Office.

Despite its vast institutional size, the impression historians typically garner of the interwar Post Office is of a monolithic entity with one voice, because any institutional decision had to be agreed by the London headquarters, where the Postmaster General always had the final say. Despite its narrow structure, the Post Office comprised a huge number of individuals who all played a part in different departments that typically had little communication with one another. Its headquarters alone employed 10,000 staff members by 1920, excluding head office personnel.[11] This chapter highlights the division between the research and engineering departments, and between the telecommunications and sales departments, revealing that these two branches had largely divergent views on the necessity of providing amplified telephony. This may have been because the Engineering Department was further removed from the problems that customers were bringing to their local district managers or sales departments. Any problems related to engineering work had to be routed from the local divisions to headquarters in London, which meant any new installations of telephone equipment were mired in interminable complications.[12] Any meaningful decisions regarding amplified telephony were made in the London headquarters, with input from the Research Department. Furthermore, until the 1932 Bridgeman Report prompted reform, the telephone network was severely restrained by the financial constraints imposed by the higher echelons of this massive administrative network, the Postmaster General and the Treasury. Essentially, the Post Office telecommunication services were still being run on the structure of the old National Telephone Company, which the Post Office officially took over in 1911.

This followed on from the 1880 decision that the Post Office (as the government's branch of communications in control of the telegraph system) would take over the trappings and apparatus of the National Telephone Company. The National Telephone Company (NTC) was the Bell and Edison conglomerate which had controlled most of telephony in Britain before the 1880 ruling on the 1869 Telegraph Act mandated a nationalised service – officially instated in 1911.[13] As a result, in the intervening thirty-one years, the National Telephone Company had no reason to invest in its stock, and so let its equipment and researches stagnate. Thus, the company that the Post Office inherited was lagging far behind the telephone companies spreading out across Europe.[14] The Post Office Telecommunications Department barely had three years to consolidate before the First World War broke out, which had a devastating impact on the Post Office's ability to invest in the telephone system.

The First World War generated a new need for telephones for those with hearing loss. The conflict had accustomed a generation of soldiers to the use of telephony, which they then desired to use at home. But their wartime service had also left many of these same soldiers with myriad hearing loss problems, which raised the profile of deafness as a national concern. This development not only made the treatment of deafness a greater priority for the medical profession, but also changed attitudes towards deafness as perceptions of treatment shifted. This shift influenced a move away from treatments derived from eugenics-based ideologies which conceptualised deafness as a purely hereditary condition, to rehabilitation movements based around the theory that noise-induced deafness could affect anyone. War-induced deafness also meant that there was an acknowledgement of social responsibility (manifesting in various charitable movements for disabled veterans) as well as an official policy of state intervention reflected in the establishment of the Ministry of Pensions in 1916.

The Post Office's duty to provide an amplified telephone must be considered in the context of these interwar welfare developments. The Post Office had total control over the telephone network. However, this state backing meant that the Post Office was required to work under the financial constraints of the Treasury and act as an arm of the wider government. The Post Office was a state office of the government, which had increased involvement in the welfare of its citizens from the start of the century, marked through legislation like the National Health Insurance Act (1911) and the creation of the Ministry of Pensions (1916) and the Ministry of Health (1919). The First World War further increased the newly enfranchised public's expectations that the government was responsible for citizen welfare. Disabled veterans returning from the First World War created a need for increased government intervention into public welfare and thus, as an arm of government, the Post Office had to have increased consideration of veterans who had become disabled as a result of their role in the First World War. Amplified telephony was developed according to, and alongside, the emerging priorities of this proto-welfare state. The Post Office's legalised control over the telephone service in Britain meant it was illegal for private companies or individuals to modify or tamper with its apparatus. Crucially, this meant that private hearing aid companies could not attach equipment to Post Office telephones and people with hearing loss could not fit private telephones for use on Post Office lines. Consequently, the Post Office was challenged by aspirational users who desired a telephone that could be used by people with less than perfect hearing.

The Post Office was aware of how hard it was to hear the telephone. In 1923 they proffered advice on how to speak with maximum audibility and effectiveness, counselling subscribers to speak 'clearly' and 'distinctly' and warning that the telephone would blur consonants and elide vowel sounds (see Figure 3.1). As we can see from their advice sheet, accents which blurred vowel sounds were detrimental to clear communication. The telephone consequently worked before and then alongside radio to standardise received pronunciation as ideal for media communication during the early twentieth century.[15] This argument offers parallels with the analysis provided by sound historian Victoria Thaczyk concerning the forced development of a standardised 'normal' media language in Germany in the interwar period, which was, as she shows, facilitated by the gramophone and designed 'to convey an impression of scientific objectivity'.[16] More pertinently for my argument, the Post Office's guidance makes it clear that the process of telephone transmission made speech less comprehensible for those with hearing loss, especially those with noise- or age-induced loss, for whom higher frequencies (the pitch at which the information delivering consonants is delivered) were lost.[17] The Post Office clearly understood the difficulties of using the telephone. Why did they not invest more immediate research into improving sound quality, then? To answer this, we need to understand the historical context influencing the Post Office's structure, and its relationship with the government as a nationalised company.

The deafened

The technology used in amplified telephone equipment developed very much in tandem with the technology used in trench telephony in the First World War. Telephony increased in use and improved in amplification thanks to the valve technology that was used in the trenches and designed by the Post Office. It was this very technology that came to be redeployed in a civilian context to facilitate increased communication for those with hearing loss after the First World War.

Hearing loss was highlighted as a national problem because of the increased attention given and importance attached to hearing during the conflict. For the first time in the First World War the telephone was used as a crucial mode of communication for the British Army, and the Post Office was essential to

POST OFFICE TELEPHONES.

HOW TO PASS AND RECEIVE A TELEPHONE CALL.

PASSING A CALL.

Before passing a call to the Exchange the subscriber should wait until he hears the telephonist's "Number, please?" and then, speaking CLEARLY and DISTINCTLY, with the lips **almost touching the mouthpiece,** he should state the number required.

FIRST the name of the Exchange and THEN the number.

The method of pronouncing numbers in Telephone Exchanges has been devised to guard as far as possible against inaccuracies and a description of the system may be of assistance to subscribers.

It is important to remember that the distinctive sounds of consonants become blurred in the transmission of speech by telephone and words containing the same vowels are apt to sound alike. Greater care is therefore necessary in speaking by telephone than is required in ordinary speech, if mistakes are to be avoided.

0 is pronounced as **"OH,"** with long "O."
1 " " **"WUN,"** emphasizing the consonant "N."
2 " " **"TOO,"** emphasizing the consonant "T" and with long "OO."
3 " " **"THR-R-EE,"** with slightly rolling "R" and long "E."
4 " " **"FOER,"** one syllable with long "O."
5 " " **"FIFE,"** emphasizing the consonants "F."
6 " " **"SIX,"** with long "X."
7 " " **"SEV-EN,"** two syllables.
8 " " **"ATE,"** with long "A" and emphasizing the consonant "T."
9 " " **"NINE,"** one syllable with long "I" and emphasizing the consonants "N."

ANSWERING A CALL.

The call should be answered promptly.

On taking off the receiver, the called subscriber should not say "Hullo!" or "Who's there?" but should immediately announce his name.

A householder would say: "Mr. Thomas Brown speaking."

The maidservant: "Mr. Brown's house."

Mr. Brown, at his office, would say: "Brown & Co., Mr. Thomas Brown speaking."

His clerk: "Brown & Co."

FINISH OF CONVERSATION.

The receiver should be replaced immediately the conversation is finished. Subscribers having Private Branch Exchange switchboards should ensure that adequate arrangements are made for **PROMPT DISCONNECTION AT THE SWITCHBOARD.** Neglect to do this may result in serious inconvenience.

GENERAL POST OFFICE. *October*, 1923.

(43622) Wt. 11863—831 675M 9/23 H.St. G.148
(44376) Wt. 15200—G288 125 10/23 H.St. G.148

Figure 3.1 'How to pass and receive a telephone call', in 'Guidance for Subscribers on How to Articulate and Pronounce Vowels and Consonants, and Phrases to Use When Speaking on the Telephone', October 1923

the development of wartime communications. Most significantly, it supplied telephones specifically designed for the conditions of the trenches.[18] Although the telephone had been taken up by the military soon after its invention, and used in the Second Afghan War in 1879, it was not a popular form of military communication.[19] When the First World War began, the military dismissed the telephone as unimportant and unsafe compared with telegraphy, visual signalling or motorbike couriers.[20] However, the trench warfare conditions that developed as fighting came to a stalemate prompted a rethink over the practicality and utility of telephony. In the dark, underground, isolated trenches, the telephone became a lifeline and an essential tool for communicating and working out what was happening 'over the top'. One corps commander emphasised that the telephone equipment was extremely valuable and ordered that 'the equipment should, therefore, be treated as if it were made of glass, and as if it were as valuable as diamonds'.[21]

Wartime needs put pressure on the Post Office's equipment and researches, but also worked as a catalyst to spur the development of specialised auditory equipment, resulting in concurrent improvements to amplification, audibility and portability. The sudden military demand for telephone equipment could not be met by the small supply originally stored, and the Post Office became the Army's main supplier. In 1920, the total value of the communications equipment the Post Office had supplied was £6,400,000 and included 40,000 protected telephones, designed specially for the trenches.[22] Telephony's usage in warfare thus involved a huge investment from the Post Office, and it was able to use the specific conditions of trench warfare to experiment and test the limits of the equipment.[23] The Post Office's signal services and research departments were integral to the development of specialist telephone equipment for use in a military context. For example, the Post Office designed the hot wire microphones that allowed the British Army to obtain precision sound ranging. Recalling the Post Office's contribution to the war in 1920, Post Office Chief Engineer Sir Andrew Ogilvie explained:

> The assistance of the Post Office was sought by the inventor, and I am proud to say that Mr Pollock, the head of the engineering Research Station, and his assistants not only devised a successful microphone on Capt. Tucker's plan, but also manufactured many thousands in a secret factory in the General Post Office, thus making a practical success of this very important invention.[24]

The Post Office also devised hypersensitive transmitters that were placed on the parapets of opposing trenches and used to spy on enemy conversations and monitor the conversations of prisoners of war.[25] The Post Office's development of these transmitters was directly influenced by hearing aid technology, just as the development of hearing aid technology was influenced by wartime technology.[26]

By 1918 the Post Office had spent an estimated £7,000,000 on the war effort by designing and manufacturing communications equipment for the military as 'Wire, cable, telephones, switchboards and signalling apparatus of new and varied types poured across the channel in ever-increasing quantities.'[27] Yet this innovative technology was not necessarily appropriate for peacetime. In 1919, William Cruikshank, the editor of the Post Office's *Electrical Engineer's Journal*, bemoaned the fact that 'the great proportion of this plant is of special design to meet military requirements, and would be of little use for civilian service if recoverable tomorrow'.[28] The huge amount of equipment supplied to the Army meant that there were domestic shortages as manufacture for home use decreased dramatically. British industrial factories were taken over to produce shells and telephone equipment specifically for the Army. This led to complaints at the end of the war, which the editor of the *Electrical Engineers' Journal* did not receive in good grace, angrily responding: 'He who asks, "Where are the wires to join up my telephone to-morrow, and why are they not available?" will receive the same answer he would have received had he asked, "Where are the men of the old Contemptible Army?" "They lie buried in the soil of France and Flanders".'[29] However, by recycling the technology of the trench telephones into technology for those with hearing loss, the Post Office was able to appropriate the military equipment for civilian use as dedicated equipment for those with hearing loss.[30]

Trench warfare necessitated research focused on improving amplification range and quality while simultaneously creating more portable sets that could be easily carried in soldiers' packs and set up in trenches; civilian telephones did not function well in the damp and mud of a trench.[31] Just as in the case of electric hearing aids, there was constant tension between the ability to improve audibility and retain portability, as an improvement to the latter tended to diminish the former. Amplification of telephony had long been a crucial issue for the Post Office. Its Engineering Department had been working with cathode rays to provide amplification as early as 1908.[32] The *Electrical Engineers' Journal* explained that these experiments were subsequently abandoned due to staff shortages, but were revived in 1913 after the thermionic valve was developed in the USA.[33] John Ambrose Fleming (who also had hearing loss) invented the thermionic valve while working for the Marconi Company in 1904. In 1906 Lee de Forest added a third electrode, meaning that those valves could be used for amplifying electrical currents. This greatly improved long-distance telephony, but it was not until 1915 that they were used in European telephones.[34] A challenge for innovation in the military context arose from the fact that the patent for the thermionic valve was held by Marconi and lasted until 1918.[35] The first valves used in Post Office telephones were 'round' French valves which were incorporated into its earliest telephone instruments. These valves boosted the electrical signal, and thus increased amplification.

The potential power of the thermionic valve as an amplifier was emphasised in the *Electrical Engineers' Journal* in 1919, in which the editor explained how war activities had accelerated development.

> In no branch of the nation's activities – save perhaps in the development of aircraft – has there been such useful progress made during the war as in wireless telegraphy and telephony. The evolution of ... the oscillating thermionic valve, has been one of abnormal progress, and has placed in the hands of the engineer an instrument pregnant with possibilities.[36]

The possibilities of amplification offered by valve technology were realised not only in general improvements to telephone audibility but also ultimately in hearing aid technology and in the telephones designed for users with hearing loss. Moreover, the work that the Post Office did for the government during the First World War signalled the start of an increasingly collaborative relationship between the state and the Post Office. This 'special relationship', as it was often referred to by the Post Office during the interwar years, was integral to motivating the Post Office's development of its amplified telephone service for the deaf. Thus, the technology used in amplified telephone equipment developed very much in tandem with the technology used in trench telephony in the First World War. The same technology was redeployed in a civilian context to facilitate increased communication for the hard of hearing after the First World War.

General attitudes towards the deaf prior to the First World War were formed through segregating the deaf as a separate, problem social group. Care of adults with hearing loss was left entirely to publicly funded charities, so adults suffering from hearing loss in the late nineteenth century were offered little assistance. Treatments for deafness were preventative and often informed by eugenic principles.[37] The state had little involvement in the care of those with hearing loss, although deaf children were cared for in schools established throughout Britain during the nineteenth century. But adults who became deaf later in life had to rely on charitable provision.[38] To meet this need, the National Bureau for the Promotion of the General Welfare of the Deaf (henceforth the Bureau) was established in 1911 by deaf merchant banker Leo Bonn. It was intended to be an umbrella organisation, which would centralise the different charities working independently to help the deafened. It was established partly to ensure that the deaf were not classified as mentally defective under the Mental Health Act of 1913, and partly in reaction to the drop-off in employment of deaf workers that had followed the National Insurance Act of

1911.³⁹ The Bureau was renamed the National Institute for the Deaf in 1924 and was granted the prefix 'Royal' in 1961.⁴⁰ Its work was supplemented during wartime by the National Benevolent Society, which was expressly established in 1918 to meet the needs of deafened ex-service men. The society reported in 1918 that:

> The general public is only just *beginning* to realise as yet that the Deaf are as greatly in need of help as the Blind, and need all our best effort in many directions and our thoughtful care. The 'After Care' work for 10,000 deafened soldiers, sailors and airmen has required incessant and untiring effort and has been widely welcomed by War Pensions, Secretaries, and greatly valued by the men.⁴¹

The government officially endorsed this society in 1919 by licensing it under the War Charities Act to collect funds from the public on behalf of ex-service men.⁴² The National Benevolent Society concentrated initially on administrating the Deafened Ex-Service Men's Fund and providing ex-servicemen with employment advice, loans, re-training and help in claiming pensions and pension arrears, sometimes through specialist re-examination. They were aware that deafness scaled very low in the assessment for pensions, and that large numbers of seriously deafened men received little more than 11s 9d, or 15s 3d, to provide for themselves and their children. Furthermore, like the women working during the war, many deafened men had lost their jobs when men with better hearing returned from the front. Their hearing loss was exacerbated with age and by 1929 the National Benevolent Society reported that there were now 'a good number of cases unfortunately losing their employment owing to increasing deafness, which disability debars a man altogether from employment on the railways, in the mines, and at the docks'.⁴³ This kind of disability was increasingly viewed as a new category of deafening. In 1934 the Bureau reported on the division between the 'deaf-born' and the 'deafened' under the sub-heading 'The Problem before the Institute':

> The deaf fall actually into two general classes, according to the history of their affliction and from the psychic point of view these classes are essentially distinct … The problem before your committee is therefore of a two-fold nature, necessitating separate lines of action to meet the distinctive conditions of the deaf and dumb and the deafened.⁴⁴

This was a key shift in terminology that reflected the growing understanding of hearing loss gained from the war: that deafness could originate from external factors rather than purely hereditary causes or disease. Although there is not scope in this book to fully explore the way that the First World War impacted on changing categorisations of deafness, Graeme Gooday and Karen Sayer's book offers a nuanced and detailed account of these changes, and shows that the spread of telephony and radio after the war to help the war-blinded further alienated the war-deafened.[45]

Increased awareness and understanding of hearing loss was not the only change marked by the First World War, which also demonstrated how important the sense of hearing could be. One of the features that distinguished the First World War from the many conflicts that preceded it was that so much of it could not be seen by the men involved.[46] In dark, troglodytic trenches, hearing was prioritised over sight, and listening became a tactical survival skill with listening posts and sound-ranging techniques (as well as new electro-acoustic technologies) developed to help identify and target the opposition.[47] Therefore, in the First World War trenches, hearing came to occupy a place alongside sight as a crucial sense. The increased importance of sound and hearing in trench warfare was augmented by the impairment to vision. Yet the intense listening required by soldiers was not solely a product of sight deprivation but was also used to map out the surroundings. For example, soldiers could listen to establish the weak spots of enemy defence fortifications and the areas of most intense gunfire.[48]

Ironically, despite the increased importance attached to the aural, it soon became apparent that the tremendous sonic bombardment delivered by shelling and artillery fire was causing widespread hearing loss. Many soldiers who appeared to be suffering from shell shock also presented with symptoms of deafness and deaf mutism. After the conflict it became apparent that this hearing loss was temporary or symptomatic in some cases, permanent or noise-induced in others and only rarely hysterical. But initially all conditions were conflated, and various treatments were devised for their cure. This conceptual shift which saw hearing loss as psychological or functional was marked by the intervention of psychiatry into a domain traditionally dominated by otology.[49] Conceptual concerns about hysterical deafness and the potential for malingerers to feign deafness became embedded in the field of audiometry, which we will discuss further in Chapter 4. But before doing so, we need to understand where the data on normal hearing used in audiometry came from, and for that we need to return to the Post Office telephone service and its instrument for measuring normal hearing – the artificial ear.

The artificial ear

The data used by Post Office engineers in the artificial ear created the standards that were used to design 'normal telephones' in Britain. If users did not have the ability to use the normal telephones, then it followed that they had to use the 'telephone service for the deaf'. Therefore, the data used in the artificial ear and fed into telephone design mediated what we would now think of as a medical condition. Yet deafness was not always conceptualised as such.

In 1908 the National Telephone Company (the NTC) created a 'mechanical ear', which was designed to work in conjunction with an artificial voice. The artificial voice was designed by the NTC by recording and measuring the frequencies of five women who counted the numbers one to five repeatedly – the standard way of making transmission tests. The woman with the most pleasing voice was determined through a vote which the men in the office took part in, and a professional soprano singer was also enlisted to record what was considered to be an *ideal* frequency. Conversely, similar attempts made at Bell Laboratories in the 1940s to make a visual record of the voice used 'a store of examples from hundreds of speakers'.[50] However, in the second half of the twentieth century, the engineers at Bell Laboratories decided that the *patterns* of speech form were more important than frequency for recognising speech and so only used measurements from men and children, the values of which were 'averaged across all the repetitions to serve as the final "typical" value'.[51] Using this kind of statistical approach is why voice recognition machines like Siri and Alexa still have 'significant race and gender biases'.[52] However, it is important to note that Bell Laboratories were pioneering this approach to facilitate speech recognition through a spectrograph, whereas the NTC's mechanical voice was designed as a simple testing device to work in conjunction with the artificial ear. Their final arrangement was measured by an artificial ear that we would think of as more closely resembling a recording device than a replica of a human ear. This allowed for quick and mechanical assessment of the telephone's transmission quality. Its advantage lay in the fact that the telephone circuit was not interfered with, and it gave comparable results to a 'human test' but was 218 minutes faster. The NTC report concluded that: 'There is thus a saving of 67% in time, in addition to the fact that mechanical testing is of course not nearly so exhausting as speech testing.'[53]

The next available report on this subject was produced in 1928, indicating that the Post Office continued using the NTC system during the intervening twenty years.[54] The 1928 report marked a critical change in practice, and in the way that the artificial ear was designed and used. Rather than functioning solely as a testing system, the artificial ear was redesigned by the Post Office to resemble a real ear as closely as possible, replicating the functions of the outer, middle and inner ear, shown in Figure 3.2 from left to right.

The Post Office explained that: 'the present investigation aims at a quantitative determination of the acoustical impedances of a reasonable number of normal (male) ears over a considerable frequency range'.[55] This reasonable

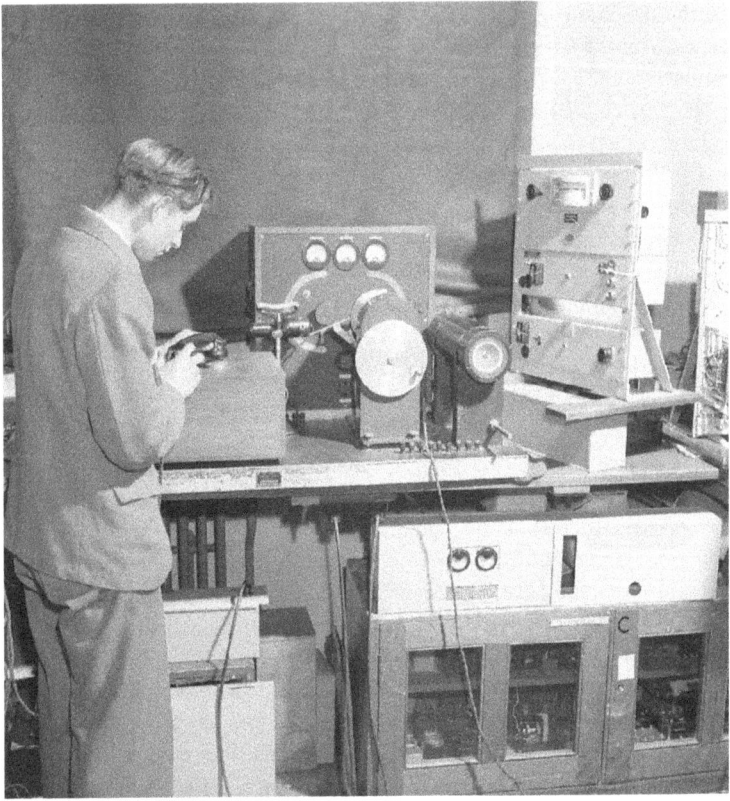

Figure 3.2 The artificial ear, Post Office Research Station, Dollis Hill

number consisted of twelve ears altogether, ten 'normal' male ears and two 'abnormal' ears. The data gathered through tests on the normal ears were used to provide the representative standard of normal hearing. These 'normal' ears were tested for the mean and extreme resistances to different frequencies, with the average value used to design the artificial ear. However, it is clear that there was relevant information garnered from the ears that did not function as expected, as the two abnormal ears were given further tests to establish their 'impedance' values, which meant that the Post Office engineers investigated the extent to which the abnormal ears were able to transmit sound through vibrations:

> During the investigation two ears, which were abnormal in that their hearing was known to be below normal, came under observation. In both cases

the impedances were found to be abnormal, one giving an exceptionally high value and the other an exceptionally low value of absorption at 1100 cycles per second.[56]

Understanding impedance (the conversion of vibrations) was important in improving the artificial ear's design, as the electrical impedance of the artificial ear had previously been adjusted with a real ear.

An artificial ear was considered by the Post Office to be superior to real ears for testing telephone transmission quality for four main reasons. First, it gave quantitative data 'for measurement, in absolute units, of the performance of receivers under their working conditions'.[57] Second, it increased the possibilities of testing volume measurements and comparing different circuits and techniques on that basis.[58] Third, and most importantly, the artificial ear provided a permanent trace, a record that did not depend on consistent reproduction and a large number of tests. Many tests were necessary in any use of real ears for research because of the variability of hearing abilities: 'wide discrepancies between results with different observers necessitates a larger number of tests and observers in order to obtain a representative average'.[59] Such a testing process was felt to be particularly problematic because of its subjective nature, therefore 'the elimination of personal bias by the use of an artificial ear becomes more important'.[60] Thus, fourth, the artificial ear was conceptualised as an objective technology that could be used to manage the variability of hearing. The resulting machine designated standards of normal hearing in narrow mechanical parameters, which led to a situation in which those who did not fit with the Post Office telephonic standards were categorised as deaf, and in need of a 'telephone service for the deaf'. Such telephones were developed during the interwar years through a series of user-forced innovations, as we will see in the following section. Telephone users (such as those with greater hearing loss, different frequency needs or bone-conductive hearing losses) were unhappy with their telephone provision and demanded that the institution fulfil its duty to provide telephone access to all types of citizens. Moreover, the National Institute for the Deaf (the ancestor of the Bureau and henceforth the NID) attempted to improve the provision of electric hearing aids sold during the interwar period by testing them using this machine.[61] It was also used in the design of the first NHS hearing aid, the Medresco.[62] This hearing aid was intended for children and yet data related to children's hearing was not used in the artificial ear.

While it seems strange that this distorted normalcy standard could have remained embedded in the artificial ear between 1928 and 1947, I can find no further investigative reports after the 1928 report, only references to the artificial ear as the standard device against which hearing aids and telephones were calibrated. The Post Office was not a medical institution, and there was no need for it to search for increasingly accurate data. What was wanted was an efficient and successful standard, and, after all, a successful standard is marked out by its invisibility. For instance, Rachel Weber pointed out in 1997 that the only anthropometric data for civilian female populations was from 1940 but was still being used in commercial plane cockpit design.[63] Similarly, Lundy Braun has shown that the spirometric data used for race-specific population standards endured far longer than one would imagine to be appropriate – data gathered by Samuel Cartwright, a Southern physician and slave owner, was used in a germinal study by Benjamin Apthorp Gould that is still cited today by pulmonary researchers.[64] She points out that designing new data sets 'sufficiently large to be scientifically credible' is a drain on time and finances.[65] For the Post Office, the standard of normal hearing was not meant to be medically credible but was simply a useful economic tool: why would they spend time and money on more representative data?

Case studies: individual users versus institutional innovations

Telephony was ultimately used as a tool in the categorisation of disability by the Post Office. The amplified telephone was used by the Post Office to categorise their users' identity as either hearing (could use the standard telephone model), hard of hearing (could use the telephone when amplified) or deaf (could not use the telephone even when amplified). Categorisation largely depended on the efficacy of the technology rather than on the telephone user's level of hearing. The first of these aspirational telephone users were the Smith brothers. The brothers ran an eponymous oil distilling and refining company from 24 Marshgate Lane, Stratford, London, and they opened a dialogue with the Post Office early in 1922. One of the brothers in charge of the company, Mr Worringham Smith, had substantial hearing loss. They wrote to the Post Office in 1922 and advised that their company had lost business because their director was unable to use the telephone, and they pleaded that they were 'willing to pay any sum within reason for facilities which will enable them to interpret their telephone messages'. They added that 'At present they are of the opinion that many orders are lost owing to their defective hearing.'[66] Businessmen were one of the first key groups to embrace telephony in the latter years of the nineteenth century and the Smith brothers demonstrated the negative impact that telephone exclusion had on their business.[67] Their request was initially made in a detailed letter dated 12 January 1922, in which the author (probably Mr Worringham Smith) made two main points to persuade the Post Office to provide this service. First, he pointed out the lack of progress that the Post Office had made since nationalisation in 1912 and compared its service to private companies like the NTC: 'If we were not hidebound by your Authorities regulations – which forbid us – we think we are right in saying a private maker would very soon give us what we want the same as the great National Telephone Company would have done – with an extra sensitive instrument (we do not mind paying).'[68]

This letter pointed out that this was an equity issue, and further argued that the requisite amplification technology was already available and used in telegraphy: 'In wireless telegraphy, as you know, they use amplifiers which greatly magnify the sound. Could not something of the sort be adapted to telephony, so that people with hearing below the normal could be placed on the same footing as those with normal hearing?'[69] The amplified telegraphy referenced in this instance was the repeater system, which used thermionic valves along the line to prevent sound from weakening over distance.[70] The reason that this was in use for telegraphy long before being adapted to telephony is that the repeaters could amplify the static signal used in telegraphy but were unable to work in the same way with the *undulating* signals produced by the voice in conversation.[71]

The original suggestion by the Smith brothers in their 1922 letters regarding amplified telephones for the hard of hearing was entirely feasible, and the Post Office did adapt 'something of the sort' (as the London superintending engineer Mr Purves put it) in response. Purves initially reacted by sending a letter to the engineer-in-chief which asked 'if there are any loud speaking receivers or other suitable devices to meet such cases?'[72] The engineer-in-chief responded to his request by developing specialist amplification apparatus and inviting the subscriber (Mr Worringham Smith) to try it out. Mr Smith wrote that he was 'very favourably impressed' by the instrument and agreed to an annual rental addition of £5 15s to have it fitted to his telephone.[73]

On 10 April 1922 the London superintending engineer wrote to the engineer-in-chief to ask, 'Is it to be understood that this type of apparatus will be available for other subscribers? If so, presumably the Engineer-in-Chief will desire to consider all applications for its provision?'[74] However, the engineer-in-chief replied that: 'it is not desirable that the provision of amplifiers should be suggested to subscribers, but in special cases where a request for such provision is made and it is clear that the subscriber would benefit thereby it will in all probability be possible to supply the required facilities.'[75] This refusal could only plausibly be attributed to the prohibitive costs and exemplifies the way in which the Sales and Telecommunications Department of the Post Office was often at odds with the Engineering Department; the former tended to show more enthusiasm for an amplified service than the latter. The difficulties involved in improving the amplification technology were no doubt a deterrent from an engineering perspective, compounded by the added expense incurred by adding the extra apparatus. Even though this extra cost to the Post Office could be offset by increasing rental, the cost of repairing the delicate valves meant that developing amplified telephony made little fiscal sense.

Reluctance to develop specialist services can also be attributed to the conservative nature of the Post Office institution and the way that the government influenced its attitude towards development. US historian Charles R. Perry has emphasised the extent to which ideology influenced telephony in Great Britain in comparison to the way private telephony companies developed in the USA.[76] The Post Office's reluctance to anticipate demand is the aspect that Perry highlights, and he attributes this to the Treasury, whose ideology was summed up by a clerk who wrote that:

> The sound principle in the opinions of My Lords is that the state, as regards all functions which are not, by their nature, exclusively its own, should, at most, be ready to supplement, not endeavour to supersede, private enterprise, and that a rough but not accurate test is, not to act in anticipation of possible demand.[77]

The Post Office was discouraged from innovation by the government because acquiring new information about as yet non-existent services was expensive.[78] The Post Office's reluctance to innovate and advertise its services in a relatively specialised area such as amplified telephony can therefore also be attributed to the expense of research as well as being in line with broader government policy. The possibility of developing and advertising amplified telephony was consequently only considered after repeated complaints by irate customers who desired access to the service.

The first telephone designed specifically for people with limited hearing was not advertised until 1924, when a brief description of the 'Repeater Telephonic 9A' appeared in a press release that described a telephone 'for the use of "Deaf Subscribers" who experience difficulty in the use of the standard telephone'.[79] This early amplified telephone (the Repeater 9A) featured a controlling key to modify the volume as necessary, which was stored in a separate wooden box, along with the valve amplifier.[80] This aspect of its design was later modified, following customer criticism. The desk-based design reflected the imagined needs of the intended business user, but the box was very unpopular with customers, who found it both cumbersome and stigmatising. The extra rental involved in its hire was also unpopular with customers, some of whom went to great lengths to reduce its price.

We now meet Mr Buckley, a schoolmaster who had lost some hearing in the First World War and worked at Magdalene Court Boarding School in Broadstairs, Kent. He described himself as slightly deaf due to his long war service and in need of telephone access to contact the parents of his boarders (who were usually in London). In the late 1920s, there were still problems with increasing attenuation over long distances which could exacerbate the difficulties of hearing on the telephone, especially for those living in the countryside. Mr Buckley's complaint was not with the efficiency of his amplifier, however, but with the cost of rental. He made a number of points to support his claim that it was overpriced, attacking the Post Office in two main ways: first by highlighting the fact that the institution had a duty to their customers, especially if they had lost their hearing through war service, and second by threatening legal action to remove the Post Office telephone poles on his land.

He started his complaint by writing directly to the Postmaster General on 19 October 1928 with the explanation that he was 'slightly deaf' and struggled to hear country calls clearly.[81] Following on from this he stated that he had enquired into the cost for an amplifier and explained that 'the local engineers who do our wireless tell me that they are not allowed to fix an amplifer; that the actual cost is only a few shillings and that the proposed charge by the local Telephone Manager is exorbitant'.[82] The Postmaster General responded in December, pointing out that 'valve amplifers are relatively costly to maintain', which accounted for the increased rental cost.[83] The Post Office did, however, agree to reduce the original sum demanded and also explained that the Engineering Department were trying to design a cheaper version. This was not enough to placate Mr Buckley, however, and he quickly replied, emphasising the fact that 'the price charged by the Post Office is out of all reason'.[84] His grievance was not just based on the fact that he thought that the Post Office was overcharging for electrical equipment, however, and he explained:

> I considered that it was the duty of the Department to make these charges as little as possible for the convenience of the telephone subscribers, that the necessity for the amplifier arises out of my deafness which is a result of my long war service and for which I am in receipt of a small pension for life.[85]

By referencing his war service and the fact that he received a small pension he pointedly reminded the Postmaster General that the government was taking greater responsibility for the welfare of its citizens. This case came to a close only when the Post Office designed a cheaper version of its amplifier which Mr Buckley agreed to rent at reduced cost with a freehand microtelephone. His resort to legal action and his threats to take the Post Office to court were clear demonstrations of how important the telephone was to him and also indicated his strong belief that on principle, the Post Office should support the men who had lost hearing in the war. Mr Buckley's status as a war veteran gave him more leverage to argue his case thanks to the government's alleged post-war commitment to disabled veterans. The improved amplified telephone (the Repeater 17A) was released in 1934.[86] This was a cheaper amplifier with a freehand microtelephone (see Figure 3.3). As well as being freehand (meaning the volume control was embedded in the telephone itself rather than in a box) this model used a more powerful valve to boost the signal and increase the volume.

The advertisement shown in Figure 3.3 was released in a campaign in 1936 to market the amplified telephone as 'A Telephone for Deaf Subscribers'. The term 'Deaf Subscriber' was itself contrived to group people with limited hearing together, without considering the wide spectrum of hearing abilities.

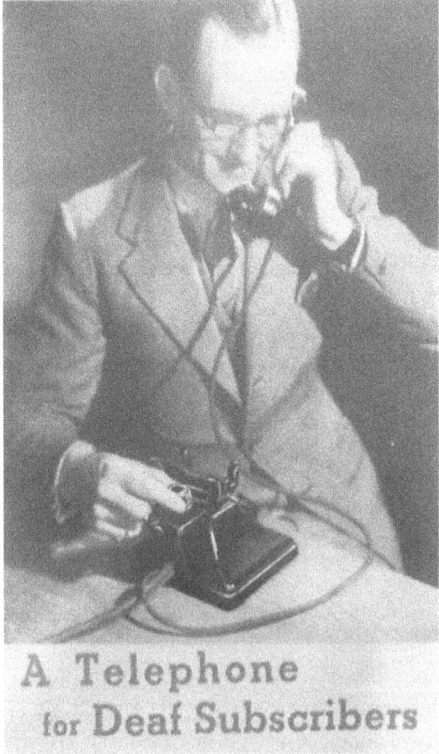

Figure 3.3 Advertising booklet, 'A Telephone for Deaf Subscribers', 1936

During the interwar period, it was understood that hearing limitations varied in intensity, but understanding of the difference between sensorineural and conductive deafness was in its infancy. The need for modification of volume at specific frequency levels was recognised by the Post Office in 1936, when a report on 'Aids to Telephone Reception for Partially Deaf Subscribers' investigated the possibility of designing an aid which would amplify sound alongside an alternative frequency characteristic.[87]

The Post Office's understanding of the variability and individuality of hearing limitations was influenced at this point by its collaboration with the medical scientist Dr Phyllis Kerridge. Her 1935 report on 'Aids for the Deaf' in the *British Medical Journal* was extensively cited in their report.[88] The 'problem of deafness' was thus moving from a problem to be solved by engineers into the realm of medicine. However, the principal group targeted by the Post Office in attempts to popularise amplified telephones would not have automatically identified as deaf and may have passed as hearing in all other aspects of their lives.[89]

Those who desired access to telephony in the interwar years would almost certainly not have recognised the Deaf community and its cultures of the late twentieth century, but less scholarly attention has been paid to those who lost hearing later in life and did not affiliate themselves with the Deaf community. This is in part because there was not an identified community of people with hearing loss, and in part because the stigma surrounding deafness led those with limited hearing to identify as hearing and minimise the significance of their hearing loss.

In modern Deaf culture, hearing loss or limitation is not regarded as disabling. Rather, the Deaf regard themselves as being defined not by their medical status but through their social and political status.[90] The point in emphasising this terminology is to demonstrate the spectrum of deaf experience and note that those who would describe themselves as deaf during this period would likely not have used the telephone, and those who struggled with it would have described themselves as hearing or possibly as hard of hearing. Crucially, the amplified telephone enabled those using it to 'pass' as hearing over the telephone during a period when the stigmatisation of hearing loss was high.[91] The amplified telephone promised to solve issues of both audibility and stigmatisation without being apparent to the caller on the other end of the line. Although the amplifying apparatus used in the design of the modified telephone was bulky and visible to its user, it was invisible to the caller on the other end. The invisibility of the amplified telephone as a prosthetic is particularly salient to hearing loss, itself an invisible disability which is often only revealed by the relevant assistive technology.[92]

However, the integrated receiver of the Repeater 17A, which was a significant change from the older candlestick-style receiver and transmitter, attracted the ire of users with hearing loss who had been using the older models to listen to the telephone using bone conduction – pressing the receivers to their mastoid bone and comfortably listening to the receiver through vibration while speaking into the separate mouthpiece. The Post Office explained that such users 'had been accustomed to holding the bell receiver to the bone at the back of the ear to obtain best reception for his [sic] particular deafness'.[93]

As a result of this problem, Wiltshire-based engineer Mr Raymond Harris designed and built his own personal amplifying apparatus which he used in conjunction with the Post Office telephone and insisted was far superior to even the most recently advertised equipment. As I have discussed in more detail elsewhere, the development of the amplified telephone service involved direct appropriation of the embodied knowledge of telephone subscribers with hearing loss, as we can see in the protracted struggle between Harris and the Post Office.[94] Whilst Harris believed that the Post Office should have been able to provide apparatus at least as good as his own for anyone suffering from hearing loss, the Post Office did not want private apparatus used on its lines, but simultaneously did not want to waste money designing specialised apparatus for a single customer.

After Harris made it clear that he was not satisfied with the new telephone (the Repeater 17A), the Post Office responded by visiting his home to check that its equipment was working. At this point it realised that the newly advertised instrument was not supported in his service area and Harris was still using the Repeater 9A.[95] As well as this realisation, the sectional engineer's visit allowed him to closely examine Harris's personal amplifying device and draw a diagram outlining its design which he then sent to the engineer-in-chief as part of a special report on Harris's design. He explained:

> For his private use the subscriber has an amplifier with associated microphone giving an output much in excess of our instrument. I have called for a special report on this private apparatus and may be able to adapt our amplifier to work in conjunction with it. No mention of this has of course been made to the subscriber.[96]

The Post Office explicitly decided not to inform Harris that they were compiling a special report on his apparatus as this, alongside the absence of patent protection, allowed its engineers to reproduce his design without his knowledge or consent. There was precedent within the Post Office of appropriating designs in this way, as can be seen in the case of the deaf electrical engineer Oliver Heaviside and his interactions with the Post Office in the late nineteenth century.⁹⁷ Like Harris, Heaviside had hearing loss, worked on improvements to telephony (long-distance telephony) and did not protect his inventions because of his altruistic principles. Heaviside also had an acrimonious relationship with the Post Office and his 'open approach' to 'do good to my fellow creatures' was 'in part a reaction against attempts by William Preece, the Chief Electrician at the UK Post Office, to suppress his theories of long-distance telephony'.⁹⁸ Because Heaviside did not patent his innovation and took the same moral stance as Harris regarding the need to share inventions, the Post Office was able to adopt his invention without according Heaviside any recognition.⁹⁹ Like Heaviside, Harris was an innovator but he was also a user. Harris's design was clearly very personal and tailored to his individual body and needs. The disparity between the Post Office's measured approach to the amplified telephone and Harris's personally embodied design was at the heart of the tensions that developed in this case. Harris's correspondence with the Post Office is especially revealing of such inconsistencies between institutional expectations of hearing and user expectations of amplification, as well as incongruities inherent in Post Office policies regarding their 'Deaf Subscribers'. Furthermore, his case highlights how users drew upon personal experience and bodily knowledge to improve the telephones in ways that the Post Office could not.

Although it was created for an individual need, Harris's device was superior to the Post Office's device in providing greater amplification as well as being uniquely suitable for his exact level of frequency loss. The Repeater 9A, the only amplified telephone that could be used in Harris's area, utilised just one single thermionic valve and one dry battery, whereas Harris's circuit greatly increased amplification because it used a triode valve and a pentode valve. The resulting amplification was so great that Post Office engineers reported that it could not be tolerated by a person with normal hearing and that they could not risk putting on the headphones to test it.¹⁰⁰ Although his modified device was perfect for him, it was not accepted by the Post Office because it was not standardised and could not be measured by their equipment or engineers. The level of amplification was perfect for Harris, however, and this aspect of his invention can be usefully considered as a form of embodied knowledge, a type of knowledge intimately linked to a person's specific nature.¹⁰¹

Knowledge of the degree of amplification and tone control needed for Harris to hear on the telephone was something that only he could gauge. His body and his hearing allowed him to mediate the level of amplification in a way that the Post Office engineers physically could not. However, the fact that the Post Office reproduced his amplifier instead of allowing him to use his own indicates that the kind of embodied knowledge gained through disability was not considered legitimate by the institution. Indeed, the decision to move away from equipment designed using personal, embodied knowledge of sound through individual sensory judgement was reflected in larger movements towards standardised measurements of sound in the 1920s and 1930s, which will be explored in the next chapter. Such technocratic approaches represented a developing dichotomy between the divergent needs of users with hearing loss and the decibel-based standards of the Post Office. Although the Post Office admitted that Harris's device provided greater amplification, this dichotomy proscribed Harris's embodied invention as an unmeasurable and unpatented device. His invention could not be tested or trusted by the Post Office engineers. In the context of Harris's innovation, his body was problematised as a reliable source of knowledge because it could only be measured in individualistic terms. Yet it was his personal insight that allowed the Post Office to improve its amplified telephone service. It profited from his bodily knowledge by turning his insight into a commodity that could be exploited for commercial gain. Mills has pointed out that disability can be used in this way to provide a source of technical innovation, but that in the case of telephony and hearing loss, this connection is far deeper and more complicated than simple appropriation.[102] The kind of technical insights that Harris could provide were not welcomed by the Post Office Telecommunication Department, which was trying to provide a standard telephone for the deaf that could be used by a typical 'Deaf Subscriber'.

The Post Office was protected from accusations of plagiarism in cases like this because its work was under Crown copyright, which gave greater protection and secrecy than a patent. Established in 1911, this protected any works created under any government department.[103] Despite the fact that neither the Post Office nor Harris patented their amplified telephones, there were thirteen amplified telephony patents taken out by private entrepreneurs between 1921 and 1935, even though it was illegal to use them.[104] Clearly, the problem of hearing over the phone was widespread and there was felt to be a need for it to be addressed. Private hearing aid companies including Amplivox, Multitone and Ossicaide all invented systems of listening to the telephone via a hearing aid through induced currents.[105] The Post Office viewed private hearing aid firms offering telephonic assistance as a threat to their control and refused to sanction the use of such hearing aid couplers with their telephones. Indeed, it was concerned to such an extent that it advocated completely prohibiting private hearing aids with couplers as illegal infringements, as they had done with Harris's equipment. However, as these devices did not have a physical attachment to the telephones, the Post Office could not completely ban them as they had done with Harris's device, though they were still able to moderate their use.

After the case with Harris was resolved, the Post Office accelerated the development of its telephone for 'Deaf Subscribers' so that a device with greater amplification could be used as standard in *all* areas. This became known as the Repeater 17b and was 13.5 db louder than the 17a and included a tone control button for users like Harris who needed different frequencies amplified (see Figure 3.4).

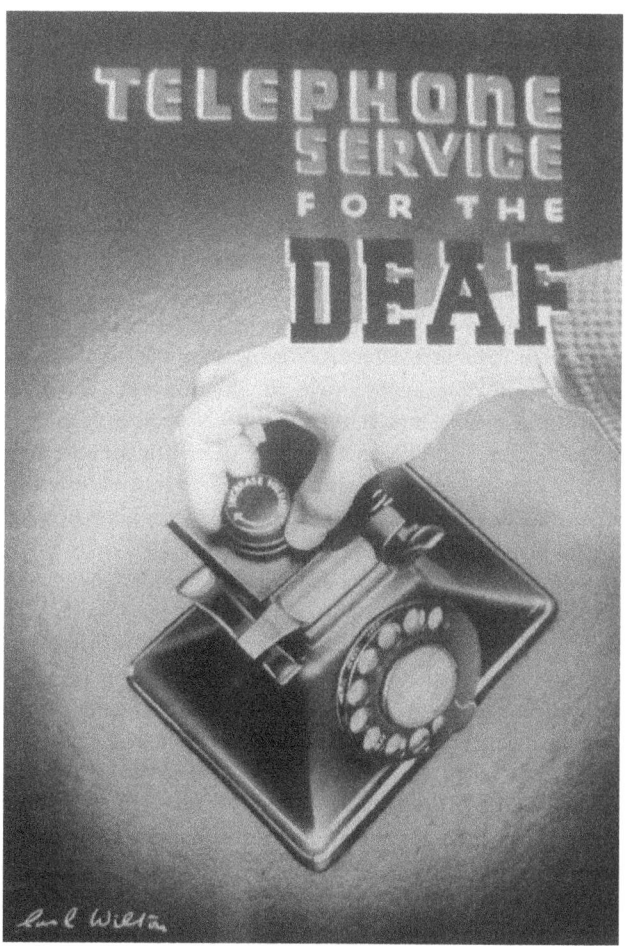

Figure 3.4 'Telephone Service for the Deaf', 1938

Harris was able to use this new telephone even though (according to the Post Office) he was 'extremely deaf'. Categorical terminology like this is a recurring difficulty in such cases, revealing tensions regarding how best to decide who was 'too deaf' to use the telephone, who was 'hard of hearing' and what to call these two groups. The Post Office described those who could use the telephone with extra amplification as 'hard of hearing' and those who could not as 'deaf' or 'extremely deaf'. Categorising deafness in this way meant that the condition of hearing or deafness changed with the improvement of technology rather than through any improvement in hearing. When Harris was able to use the more powerful telephone, he was re-categorised as hard of hearing rather than 'extremely deaf', although his medical level of hearing was unchanged. Categorisation depended on the efficacy of the technology rather than on the telephone user's level of hearing.

The improved amplified telephone (the Repeater 17B) cost £1 more (rental per annum) than the older model. This was not acceptable to users who felt they were being increasingly penalised for their hearing. For example, Mr Mousley, director of the Birmingham company Charles Winn & Co., was outraged at the expense of the more powerful amplified telephone, and refused 'to pay any additional rental in respect of it', and threatened in a letter of July 1938 that if the matter was not given immediate attention he would take the case up with the Postmaster General.[106] He was especially irate at having to pay £3 at his private residence as well as on his business line and in response he withheld his telephone rent, starting on the 9 November 1938.[107] This was an effective strategy. The Telecommunications Department were concerned and asked the Birmingham telephone manager: 'if it is possible to accede to his application. Messrs. Winn & Co. are good customers, the account being in the neighbourhood of £50 per quarter.'[108]

The Sales Department therefore allowed Mr Mousley a three-month trial of the improved amplifier, free of charge. However, their real hope was: 'at the end of that time [to] be able to convince the subscriber that the difficulty that he is experiencing is not due to the service but rather to his affliction.'[109] The sales superintendent in Birmingham also pointed out to Mr Mousley that 'there were a good number of amplifiers existing in the Birmingham telephone area and that he was the only subscriber that complained'.[110] This statement reveals that the amplification service was fairly popular at this time, although it is less clear whether this was due to widespread deafness or particular localised problems with the telephone system in Birmingham. However, at the heart of this case was contestation of the measurement and categorisation of deafness rather than the efficacy of the amplifying technology. For instance, Mr Mousley wrote: 'I resent very much having to pay for an amplifier at all considering the reason is not really my deafness but the inefficiency of some of the Post Office lines and functions.'[111] This was contested by the Post Office, especially when the traffic superintendent discovered that Mousley had started to wear hearing aids for ordinary conversation:

> Mr Mousley now regularly uses special apparatus with which to carry on his normal business conversation. It consists of a headgear receiver connected to a portable valve amplifier, the power being drawn – I am told – from a 2 volt dry battery. The subscriber carries on a conversation apparently without difficulty when wearing the headgear; but in my opinion he is deafer than ever when not utilising this apparatus.[112]

This dialogue provides an example of what I described in Chapter 2 as epistemic injustice of a kind specific to the disabled.[113] The specialist knowledge that the disabled have regarding how their bodies' needs are best met has been consistently undervalued, perpetuating a cycle of injustice which undermines the knowledge claims of the disabled.[114] Not only was the new visibility of Mr Mousley's hearing loss used to discredit his claims about his inadequate telephone provision, his knowledge about the kind of hearing-assistive technology which could have helped him was disregarded.

It is unclear whether this unusual headgear design was provided by a private company or if it was an invention of Mr Mousley's. His company, Charles Winn & Co., did specialise in manufacturing valves (and sewing machines and fire appliances), so he would have had easy access to such materials.[115] Indeed, this kind of innovation was not unusual during this period, and reports of similar designs were outlined in the *British Medical Journal* in 1935. For example, Dr Phyllis Kerridge reported on 'Aids for the Deaf' and explained: 'Amateur wireless constructors have often designed very satisfactory circuits for themselves or their relatives by the method of trial and error.'[116] She gave two examples to illustrate such home-made hearing aids, such as one designed by a laboratory assistant

> so deaf that unaided he could not hear conversation at all. He has a quadruple microtelephone instrument, and wears the microphone hidden under his overall. With this help conversation is possible, and he is able to take instructions and keep his job. He uses one battery a week, and finds that the old ones will light his bicycle lamp after they are no good for the hearing aid.[117]

This example gives us a fascinating insight into the everyday struggles of those trying to use telephone technology to overcome their hearing loss during this period. It is striking how often such apparatus was characterised by user modification. Another example given in the same paper was of an amateur wireless constructor who had

> made himself a valve amplifier set, incorporating a tone control, with which he can hear conversation quite easily. He keeps two sets in working order by him, as he is quite incapacitated without one. He finds the tone control satisfactory for clear understanding, and a further advantage is that he can tune out the unpleasant qualities of voices which he disliked in his hearing days.[118]

This kind of selective hearing and use of hearing aids as a means of power and control has also been noted in the use of acoustic aids such as ear trumpets, which could be effectively manipulated to signal boredom with the conversation and, arguably, to demonstrate control over the conversation.[119]

As the above cases outlined, the development of amplified telephony was marked by tensions between the Post Office's monopoly and the duty it felt to provide a service to citizens with varying hearing needs. The amplified telephone was constructed by the Post Office in a process marked by user input and corresponding design modifications. The selection of cases I have chosen to focus on in this chapter are those which contained more detailed information or forced through specific changes. However, there are many other examples in the archives of such user input, which continued long after the interwar period. For example, on 20 March 1954, William S. Clark wrote to telephone headquarters to point out that 'the present mouthpiece fitted usually to telephone handsets is unsuitable for use for people using deaf-aids'.[120] He explained that

> the usual mouthpiece has a cupped shape. When using a deaf-aid, the earpiece of the handset has to be placed against the deaf-aid microphone. The 'mike' is usually worn on the chest, therefore when using a deaf-aid, the handset is used upside down. This means that the mouthpiece is turned away from the mouth of the speaker.[121]

To illustrate the problem and his suggested solution (changing to standard usage of mouthpiece no. 18) he included a drawing which vividly illustrated the problems he faced in his everyday interactions with telephony (see Figure 3.5). This was another example of user appropriation of technology that had not been anticipated by the Post Office and could not be approved. The engineering department explained that the alternative mouthpiece often led to transmission loss 'during normal use' and argued that 'we should not encourage its use merely for the sake of a slight gain in convenience, and perhaps in relative efficiency, when the handset is used upside down by a deaf person, at the expense of the certain transmission loss to all normal users'.[122]

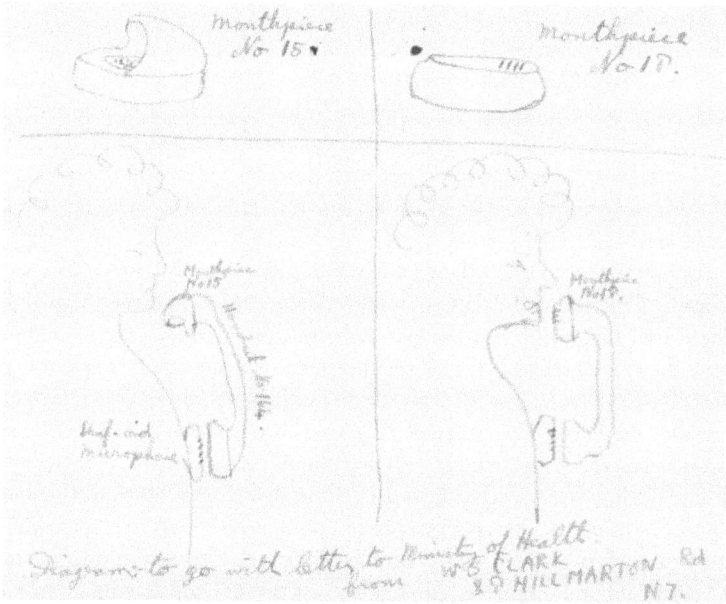

Figure 3.5 'Suggestion that a flat mouthpiece, instead of the normal cupped one, should be provided to facilitate the use of a telephone in conjunction with a deaf aid worn on the chest'. Letter from W. S. Clark to Telephone Headquarters, 20 March 1954

These kinds of suggested improvements to amplified telephony were hampered due to the complexities of matching individual user needs with the Post Office institutional set-up and the way in which individuals' lived experience of hearing conflicted with the Post Office's desire for standardisation. As a government department, standardisation was fundamental to the Post Office's wider ethos regarding its customers, as providing the same service to all was integral to its democratic position.

The aspiration for standardisation was a built-in component of telephone networks more generally and its pursuit was partially driven by technical necessity. Today, telephony is often used by historians of technology to exemplify how a device can create a network effect because the desirability of the telephone directly correlated to the number of subscribers to the same system.[123] However, there were tensions between different exchanges and their networks in the era prior to nationalisation in Britain. For example, local subscribers benefited more from local exchanges, and public exchanges were more expensive for telephone companies to build than private wire systems.[124] But different exchanges that offered different types of connection did not fit with the Post Office's nationalised service ethos. Similarly, though the American Telephone and Telegraph company (henceforth AT&T) did not have a government-mandated monopoly, it still exerted its domination on the lines of communication in a way that has been described as a form of 'American socialism', exemplified by the AT&T slogan: 'One policy, One system, Universal service'.[125]

In opposition to this will towards standardisation, the Post Office's first amplified telephone did not supply everyone with a telephone that they could use: those with hearing loss too great for this Post Office machine were thus redefined as living on the threshold of 'deafness'. This meant that users had to actively engage with the technology on an individual level to pressure the Post Office to create an amplified telephone model that fitted with their level of hearing loss (volume amplification) as well as their type of hearing loss (frequency adjustment). Thus, telephone companies created standards of normal hearing outside of the medical sphere. As Mara Mills has explored, this situation was paralleled through the remit of the private AT&T telephone company. Although no single nationalised company in the United States held a state-sanctioned monopoly over the telephone service as in Britain, AT&T held a practical monopoly over the telephone system in the USA at this time. While AT&T's monopoly was not legislated by the government, in practice it controlled the telephone service and fought off any competition to maintain its position. One seminal example of its monopolistic powers comes from the 1949–68 case of *The Hush-A-Phone Corporation v. The United States*, which centred on the Hush-A-Phone, a device which was attached by the telephone user to the telephone to improve audibility. This was considered by AT&T to be an illegal attachment that infringed on its monopoly and AT&T went to court to successfully ban the Hush-A-Phone device.[126] In contrast the Post Office were advised not to press charges in a similar situation involving private hearing aid companies using couplers to link hearing aids with their telephones on the grounds that these companies were not using *physical* attachments. This was an unusual decision because the Post Office operated a strict blanket ban on any private apparatus on their lines. However, the Post Office did supply amplified telephones for their subscribers with hearing loss throughout the interwar years, and this was a marked divergence from AT&T's policy, perhaps indicating a somewhat more inclusive approach towards those with hearing limitations wrought by UK welfare-state ideologies.

AT&T's specialisation in hearing loss over general telephone lines contrasted with their refusal to provide customers with a telephone system suitable for the deaf, and this became the focus of a widespread campaign in the late 1960s.[127] However, Bell Laboratories did work with the US Public Health Service in 1936 to test the hearing of 9,000 adults using their audiometer.[128] This allowed for testing of the nation's audiological health, as well as providing AT&T with more comprehensive data to set the standard of normalcy. Mills explains that AT&T's study into speech and hearing was wide-ranging and comprehensive, designed for the most efficient telephone service: 'in the hopes of connecting its system to the average ear, and in turn exploiting that ear's limitations to establish the requisites for "intelligible" transmission across imperfect lines (and later still, to transmit compressed speech)'.[129] However, Mills points out that because such surveys sought to identify normal hearing and discounted older people and people with hearing limitations, the resulting average was not the norm but rather the upper quartile of the norm.[130] Like the Post Office, AT&T sought the average of pre-identified *normal hearing* rather than representing the true variability of hearing ability in the population.

The different contexts of nationalisation versus private development meant that the standards in the UK and the USA for normal hearing (the zero line of the audiometer) were different until 1964.[131] This crucial point demonstrates the subtle influence that the classification systems used in technologies like the telephone have on our conception of normal functioning. Comparing AT&T's services for those with hearing loss to the British Post Office's service shows how the drive for standardisation was impacted by both local contexts and commercial imperatives. Mills has demonstrated that there were multiple connections between deafness and the development of telephony at AT&T. First, she illuminates that people with hearing loss were activists, and engaged with AT&T in the pursuit of rehabilitation devices.[132] Second, in turn, the novel concept of *deafening* was appropriated by AT&T as both a useful category and an applied term for telephone engineers. Third, AT&T's audiometric experiments and surveys on levels of normal hearing were utilised in medicine and used to define the 'normal' standard of hearing for the audiograms utilised in hearing tests.[133] That the US norm differed from the UK norm in the interwar period was demonstrated by the much larger (though still not representative) sample used by AT&T to create the standard. Despite these differences, both the USA and the UK telephone companies sought to manage the variability of hearing through mechanisms that promoted a narrow average standard as representative of the norm.

Conclusion: the standardisation of normal hearing

Designating the standard of normal hearing in this narrow mechanistic fashion with idealised averages meant that users were forced to engage with the Post Office to access telephony. User activism was a key force for change in this respect, as aspirational users forced the Post Office to create specialised and affordable technology to allow them to access telephony. As a result, the Post Office became the *de facto* experts in hearing-assistive technology during the interwar period. However, as we will see in the next chapter, data on the expected parameters of 'normal hearing' as the Post Office defined it was gathered by the expanding field of audiometry, which used telephones to measure ears literally through audiometers.[134] Clinicians used the telephone in the form of the audiometer to create standardised levels of normal hearing and defined deviance from that norm as deafness that could be corrected with appropriate hearing aids.

There is a clear feedback loop here, between the engineering of the telephone system and the standardisation of hearing integral to audiometric calibration. This loop was interrelated, working both ways, as deaf ears were used to improve the telephone system just as the telephone system was used to simultaneously define and 'improve' deaf ears. Moreover, the normative standards embodied in such instrumentation became increasingly invisible as they were perpetuated. During the interwar years, the state of being deaf or hearing became defined through the ability, or otherwise, to use certain kinds of telephone – both literally in the form of the audiometer and socially through the ability to engage with the telephone. To retain their hearing identity and not be categorised as deaf, with the corresponding stigma that invoked, people with hearing loss engaged with amplified telephones. Through such interactions, telephony was used as a tool in the categorisation of disability and, in turn, telephone users modified the technology to fit their personal needs, experiences and identities. Yet this promise of improvement was not realised in practice because the Post Office's standard amplified telephone model did not reflect either the significant diversity of users' hearing or the variability of hearing loss. The standardisation of normal hearing and the categorisation of the deafened was therefore both facilitated and created in line with the priorities of the British Post Office's telephone system. This analysis demonstrates the fluctuating and contingent thresholds of normalcy construction and reveals how deafness was socially and technologically constructed in interwar Britain.

As Stuart Blume has elucidated: 'the user "inscribed" in a technology, imagined by its designers, may not correspond with real users in the real world'.[135] Considering user experiences of disability technology often reveals discrepancies between the designed ideal user and the disabled user in real life. Indeed, there is no such thing in real life as the imagined ideal user. However, in the case of the disabled user, the frequent imbalance of power between designer and user can heighten these discrepancies. Analysis of the way these users adapted the telephone to suit their individual needs corresponds to studies concerned with deaf users' relationships to prostheses, especially the way they have been adapted, modified and controlled.[136] Non-use was also a response, and STS scholar Sally Wyatt has clarified the importance of this by dividing this category into four sub-groups: resisters, rejecters, the excluded and the expelled.[137] I add users of the telephone with hearing loss into this analysis as *aspirational* users who wanted to use the telephone and used a variety of techniques to gain access. By following the individual experiences of users, I demonstrate that the telephone was used as a prosthetic to enable users to pass as 'hearing'.

While a growing number of historians of disability examine the multiple ways in which social contexts shape and define disability and ability, this analysis provides a new perspective on the fluid boundaries between hearing and deafness created by the telephone. This neglected episode of early twentieth-century telephony redefines the relationship between technology, communications and disability, and broadens our historical understanding of deafness. Science and technology studies have decisively demonstrated that technologies are not neutral, but rather are shaped by the cultures, contexts and the actors that make them. By focusing on the forces and norms which enact technologies we reveal the socio-cultural and anthropological decisions embedded within them. This is an issue of central concern to disability studies because of the normativising power of technologies like the artificial ear. As this chapter has demonstrated, technology's development is interlinked to the classification and enforcement of normative categories embedded in big data. To explore these topics more thoroughly, in the next chapter I discuss the development of audiometry and its role in shaping the social and technological construction of normalcy.

Notes

1 Lecture by Professor William Rutherford, 'The Sense of Hearing: A Lecture by Professor Rutherford M.D., F.R.S., Professor of Institutes of Medicine in the University of Edinburgh', in Acoustics: Music, Lord Kelvin's Collection, 1886. University of Glasgow Special Collections, Glasgow, Kelvin 119 20 – 1892.
2 Ibid., p. 20.
3 Ibid., p. 21.

4   Enns, A., 'The Human Telephone: Physiology, Neurology, and Sound Technologies', in D. Morat (ed.), *Sounds of Modern History: Auditory Cultures in 19th- and 20th-Century Europe* (New York: Berghahn, 2014), pp. 46–68, p. 62.
5   Parts of this chapter were originally published in McGuire, C., 'The Categorisation of Hearing Loss in Inter-War Telephony', in G. Balbi and C. Berth (eds), Special Issue: 'A New History of the Telephone', *History and Technology* (2019), 35:2, 138–155.
6   Pinch, T., and Bijker, W. E., 'The Social Construction of Facts and Artifacts: Or How the Sociology of Science and the Sociology of Technology Might Benefit Each Other', *Social Studies of Science*, 14:3 (1984), 399–431. See also Bijker, W. E., *Of Bicycles, Bakelite and Bulbs: Towards a Theory of Sociotechnical Change* (Cambridge, MA: MIT Press, 1995) and Pinch, T., and Oudshoorn, N. (eds), *How Users Matter: The Co-Construction of Users and Technology* (Cambridge, MA: MIT Press, 2005).
7   Kay, M., 'Inventing Telephone Usage: Debating Ownership, Entitlement and Purpose in Early British Telephony' (PhD dissertation, University of Leeds, 2015).
8   Esmail, J., *Reading Victorian Deafness: Signs and Sounds in Victorian Literature and Culture* (Athens: Ohio University Press, 2014).
9   These examples are from tenders submitted to the Ministry of Pensions by hearing aid firms between 1924 and 1939. The National Archives, Kew, London (henceforth TNA), 'Supply of Electrophones: 1924–1926'. TNA, PIN 38/450; 'Supply of Electrophones: 1926–1929'. TNA, PIN 38/451; 'Supply of Electrophones: 1938–1939'. TNA, PIN 38/452.
10 Enns, 'The Human Telephone', p. 60.
11 Campbell-Smith, *Masters of the Post*, p. 169.
12 Ibid., p. 271.
13 The 1869 Telegraph Act granted this monopoly over communications and it was confirmed in 1880 that this Act included telephony even though the telephone had not been invented when the Act was first conceived. See Campbell-Smith, *Masters of the Post*, p. 193.
14 Perry, C. R., 'The British Experience', in I. D. Pool (ed.), *The Social Impact of the Telephone* (Cambridge, MA: MIT Press, 1977), pp. 69–96.
15 For an overview of radio and the BBC's impact on accent standardisation see Schwyter, J. R., *Dictating to the Mob: The History of the BBC Advisory Committee on Spoken English* (Oxford: Oxford University Press, 2016).
16 Thaczyk, V., 'Archival Traces of Applied Research: Language Planning and Psychotechnics in Interwar Germany', *Technology and Culture*, 60:2 (2019), 564–595, p. 573.
17 In this book I use the term hearing loss to more accurately reflect the experience of those using amplified telephones during this period as belonging to the new category of those 'deafened' from age or noise-induced hearing loss, who have experienced this change as a loss and tried to recover hearing through technology.
18 Telegraphy, visual signalling and motorbike couriers were considered more important and written proof or an orderly was regarded as more secure. Telephones were only used as Morse receivers or for communicating with surveillance balloons. Bridge, M., and Pegg, J., *Call to Arms: A History of Military Communications from the Crimean War to the Present Day* (Tavistock: Focus Publishing, 2001), p. 39–43.

19 Ibid., pp. 35–40.
20 Hall, B. N., 'The Life-Blood of Command? The British Army, Communications and the Telephone, 1871–1914', *War and Society*, 27:2 (2008), 43–65.
21 Ibid., p. 62.
22 Ogilvie, A., 'Reply: Complimentary Dinner to Sir Andrew Ogilvie', *Post Office Electrical Engineers' Journal*, 12 (1920), 70–81, p. 71.
23 Juniper, D., 'The First World War and Radio Development', *RUSI Journal*, 148:1 (2003), 84–89.
24 Ogilvie, 'Reply', p. 72.
25 Haigh, A., 'Post Office War Research. "To Strive, To Seek, To Find": Post Office Engineering Research from the Experimenting Room to "Dollis Hill", 1908–1938' (PhD dissertation, University of Leeds, forthcoming).
26 The 'Acousticon' transmitter was originally designed as a hearing aid but was developed into the hypersensitive transmitters used by the Post Office. See ibid.
27 Ogilvie, 'Reply', pp. 70–81.
28 Bridge and Pegg, *Call to Arms*, p. 176.
29 Cruikshank, W., 'Editorial Notes and Comments', *Post Office Electrical Engineers' Journal*, 12 (1919), 173–178, p. 175.
30 Such appropriation of military equipment for civilian use has been explored by Mara Mills in relation to the miniaturisation of hearing aids in the context of the Second World War. See Mills, M., 'When Mobile Communication Technologies Were New', *Endeavour*, 33:4 (2009), 140–146.
31 Bridge and Pegg, *Call to Arms*, p. 42.
32 'Editorial: The Telephone Repeater', *Post Office Electrical Engineers' Journal*, 12 (1919), 7–8, p. 7.
33 Ibid., pp. 7–8.
34 Hall, 'The Life-Blood of Command?', p. 46.
35 Arapostathis, S., and Gooday, G., *Patently Contestable: Electrical Technologies and Inventor Identities on Trial in Britain* (Cambridge, MA: MIT Press, 2013).
36 Cruikshank, 'Editorial Notes and Comments', p. 79.
37 See Gooday and Sayer, *Managing the Experience of Hearing Loss*; Virdi [Virdi-Dhesi], J., 'Curtis's Cephaloscope: Deafness and the Making of Surgical Authority in London, 1816–1845', *Bulletin of the History of Medicine*, 87:3 (2013), 347–377.
38 Branson and Miller, *Damned for their Difference*.
39 See ch. 6 of Gooday and Sayer, *Managing the Experience of Hearing Loss*.
40 In 2011, the charity became Action on Hearing Loss to better reflect its target users.
41 The National Benevolent Society for the Deaf, 'Hon. Central Secretary's Report, 1918–1919'. UCL Ear Institute and Action on Hearing Loss Library, London (hereafter AOHL). Emphasis in original.
42 The National Benevolent Society for the Deaf, 'Annual Report 1919'. AOHL.
43 The National Benevolent Society for the Deaf, '11th Annual Report 1929'. AOHL.

44 National Bureau for the Promotion of the General Welfare of the Deaf, 'Report of the Third Annual Meeting, Wednesday November 11th 1914'. AOHL. See also National Bureau for the Promotion of the General Welfare of the Deaf, reports of annual meetings between 1911 and 1922.
45 Gooday and Sayer, *Managing the Experience of Hearing Loss*, p. 27.
46 Hendy, D., *Noise: A Human History of Sound and Listening* (London: Profile Books, 2013), p. 36.
47 Van der Kloot, W., 'Lawrence Bragg's Role in the Development of Sound-Ranging in World War I', *Notes and Records of the Royal Society*, 59:3 (2005), 273–284, p. 278.
48 Enke, J., 'War Noises on the Battlefield: On Fighting Underground and Learning to Listen in the Great War', *German Historical Institute London Bulletin*, 37:1 (2015), 7–21.
49 Also see Hurst, A. F., Letter to the Editor, 'War Deafness', *The Lancet*, 192:4955 (1918), 218–219, and Turner, W. A., 'Remarks on Cases of Nervous and Mental Shock: Observed in the Base Hospital in France', *British Medical Journal*, 1:2837 (1915), 833–835.
50 Li and Mills, 'Vocal Features', p. 136.
51 Ibid., p. 152.
52 This is also a problem for anyone with a non-standard accent. Being both Scottish and a woman I find voice recognition nigh impossible and once memorably accosted a gentleman passing me on Woodhouse Lane in Leeds and exhorted him to speak my registration number into my mobile so I could use the voice recognition system to park my car as I was running late for a job interview. Comedians Iain Connell and Robert Florence vividly demonstrated this issue in 'Voice Recognition Elevator in Scotland' from the BBC Scotland sketch show *Burnistoun*, which ends with two frustrated men stuck in a voice-activated elevator screaming 'Eleven' at an unyielding microphone. https://web.archive.org/watch?v=sAz_UvnUeuU. Accessed July 2019. See also, Bajorek, J. P., 'Voice Recognition Still Has Significant Race and Gender Biases', *Harvard Business Review: Technology* (10 May 2019). https://hbr.org/2019/05/voice-recognition-still-has-significant-race-and-gender-biases. Accessed July 2019.
53 The National Telephone Company, Engineer in Chief's Department, 'The Selection of Suitable Substitutes for the Human Voice and Ear in Transmission Testing,' 26 February 1908, p. 29. BTA, TCB 22 T0339.
54 The Post Office kept the structure of the NTC and inherited all its outdated equipment because the company stopped investing in its stock when they realised that they would have to hand it over to the government. The Post Office also had to invest enormous amounts of material and research in the war, which would account for this gap in research and development.
55 Alridge, A. J., and West, W., 'Measurements of the Acoustical Impedance of Human Ears', Research Report No. 4697, Research Station at Dollis Hill, May–September 1928, p. 2. BTA, TCB 422 04697. Acoustical impedance was defined in the report

as 'the ratio of alternating pressure to alternating rate of volume displacement, i.e. if a piston of area is vibrating with velocity v and a pressure p per unit area is developed at its surface due to its contact with the medium (air)'.
56 Ibid., p. 15.
57 Alridge, A. J., and West, W., 'An Artificial Ear', Research Report No. 4946, Research Station at Dollis Hill, 21 October 1929, p. 7. BTA, TCB 422 04946.
58 Ibid., p. 8.
59 Ibid.
60 Ibid.
61 The Post Office tested hearing aids at the Dollis Hill Research Station on behalf of the National Physical Laboratory and in conjunction with the NID. See Wharry, H. M., and Crowden, G. P., 'Correction of Hearing Defects', *British Medical Journal*, 1:3727 (1932).
62 Plans for an NHS hearing aid began in 1947. The Medresco was a contraction of 'Medical Research Council', and this name has led to overemphasis on the MRC's role in its creation, with attendant erasure of the work of the Post Office. Instead of designing a new amplified telephone alongside the NHS hearing aid, the Post Office engineers designed an adaptor to link the new hearing aids with telephone receivers. This would allow users to link into any telephone and not just their home sets. See McGuire and Carel, 'The Visible and Invisible'.
63 Weber, 'Manufacturing Gender', p. 240.
64 Braun, *Breathing Race into the Machine*, Introduction, p. xxvi.
65 Ibid., p. xvii.
66 Smith Brothers & Co., Letter to The Engineer, London Telephone Service East Exchange, 12 January 1922. BTA, POST 33/1491C.
67 Kay, 'Inventing Telephone Usage'.
68 Smith Brothers & Co., Letter to The Engineer. His reference to the NTC is interesting as the government takeover of the telephone system was generally popular with the British public, who wanted a regulated, cheaper telephone service. However, a regulated government service may not have been the best outcome for those who had specific needs that a private company might have provided for. The reference to using a private maker related to the threat of private hearing aid companies.
69 Ibid.
70 Hong, S., *Wireless: From Marconi's Black-Box to the Audion* (Cambridge, MA: MIT Press, 2001), pp. 163–167.
71 Ibid., p. 9.
72 Letter from Superintending Engineer (London Engineering District) to the Engineer in Chief, 30 January 1922. BTA, POST 33/1491C.
73 Secretary for the Engineer in Chief, Memorandum dated 10 March 1922. BTA, POST 33/1491C.
74 Note to the Engineer in Chief, 1922, from Superintending Engineer. BTA, POST 33/1491C.

75 Memorandum attached to the above note. BTA, POST 33/1491C.
76 Perry, 'The British Experience', p 85.
77 Ibid.
78 Rosenberg, N., *Exploring the Black Box: Technology, Economics, and History* (Cambridge: Cambridge University Press, 1994), p. 5.
79 Memorandum from Accounts to the Superintending Engineer, 23 October 1924. BTA, POST 33/1491C.
80 Memorandum from the Engineer in Chief (Accounts) to the Superintending Engineer Concerning Insuring the Repeater 9A, 23 October 1924. BTA, POST 33/1491C.
81 Correspondence between H. C. Buckley and Postmaster General, 19 October 1928. BTA, POST 33/1491C.
82 Ibid.
83 Correspondence between Secretary and the Postmaster General and H. C. Buckley, December 1928. BTA, POST 33/1491C.
84 Correspondence between H. C. Buckley and Postmaster General, 12 December 1928. BTA, POST 33/1491C.
85 Ibid.
86 McGuire, C., 'Inventing Amplified Telephony: The Co-Creation of Aural Technology and Disability', in C. Jones (ed.), *Rethinking Modern Prostheses in Anglo-American Commodity Cultures, 1820–1939* (Manchester: Manchester University Press, 2017), pp. 70–90, p. 74.
87 'Aids to Telephone Reception for Partially Deaf Subscribers', Research Report No. 9150, Post Office Research Station, 21 April 1936, precis. BTA, TCB 422 09150.
88 Kerridge, P. M. T., 'Aids for the Deaf', *British Medical Journal*, 3886:1 (1935), 1314–1317.
89 Esmail, *Reading Victorian Deafness*. On passing, see Cureton, A., 'Hiding a Disability and Passing as Non-Disabled', in A. Cureton and T. E. Hill, Jnr (eds), *Disability in Practice: Attitudes, Policies and Relationships* (Oxford: Oxford University Press, 2018), pp. 15–32.
90 For an overview of d/Deaf history and the history of hearing loss see Gooday and Sayer, *Managing the Experience of Hearing Loss* and Davis, *Enforcing Normalcy*.
91 Brune, A., and Wilson, D. J., *Disability and Passing: Blurring the Lines of Identity* (Philadelphia: Temple University Press, 2013).
92 For consideration of how this affects user rejection of assistive technology, see McGuire and Carel, 'The Visible and Invisible'.
93 'Aids to Telephone Reception'.
94 For the full article, which contains more details of the Harris case, see McGuire, 'Inventing Amplified Telephony'.
95 It could be used in CB and automatic areas but not in the Magneto and CBS areas. At this time, the telephone service was divided into service areas which were

abbreviated according to the system they used. They were either CB (central battery working), CBS (central battery signalling), Magneto (using crank generators) or the Automatic exchanges, which were becoming more common after 1920. CBS and Magneto were old and outdated systems by the 1930s, which explains why the newer amplified telephones did not work in areas using these systems. They also had batteries at their end rather than at the exchange, which would have further complicated adding extra apparatus.

96 W. G. Luxton, Bristol Sectional Engineer, to the District Manager, 5 August 1936. BTA, POST 33/1491C.
97 Arapostathis and Gooday, *Patently Contestable*, pp. 106–110.
98 Ibid., p. 107.
99 Ibid., p. 110.
100 Letter from W. G. Luxton, Sectional Engineer, to the Superintending Engineer, 28 September 1936. BTA, POST 33/1491C.
101 Fourcade, M., 'The Problem of Embodiment in the Sociology of Knowledge: Afterword to the Special Issue on Knowledge in Practice', *Qualitative Sociology*, 33:4 (2010), 569–574, p. 571.
102 Mills, M., 'Deafening: Noise and the Engineering of Communication in the Telephone System', *Grey Room*, 43 (2011), 118–143.
103 Green Paper, 'Crown Copyright in the Information Age', Section 2.5 (1998). www.opsi.gov.uk/advice/crown-copyright/crown-copyright-in-the-information-age.pdf. Accessed April 2019.
104 Accessed using Directory of European Patents, European Patent Office. http://worldwide.espacenet.com/mydocumentslist?submitted=true&locale=en_EP. Accessed April 2019.
105 Letter from Edwin Stevens/Amplivox to the Chief Engineer, 7 July 1938. BTA, TCB 2/171–2/172.
106 Letter from Mr Mousley to Telecommunications Department, 28 July 1938. BTA, TCB 2/171–2/172.
107 Letter from Charles Winn & Co., 9 November 1938. BTA, TCB 2/171–2/172.
108 Letter from Telecommunications Department, 2 November 1938. BTA, TCB 2/171–2/172.
109 Letter from Sales Department, 30 July 1938. BTA, TCB 2/171–2/172.
110 Memorandum from Acting Sales Superintendent in Birmingham, 17 November 1938. BTA, TCB 2/171–2/172.
111 Letter from Mr Mousley to the District Manager, 20 April 1938. BTA, TCB 2/171–2/172.
112 Letter from the Traffic Superintendent, April 1938. BTA, TCB 2/171–2/172.
113 Scully, 'From "She Would Say That, Wouldn't She?"'.
114 McGuire and Carel, 'Stigma, Technology and Masking'.
115 The letterhead on the Charles Winn & Co. stationery also indicates that Mr Arthur Mousley held an MBE.
116 Kerridge, 'Aids for the Deaf'.

117 Ibid.
118 Ibid.
119 Gooday and Sayer, *Managing the Experience of Hearing Loss*.
120 'Suggestion that a flat mouthpiece, instead of the normal cupped one, should be provided to facilitate the use of a telephone in conjunction with a deaf aid worn on the chest'. Letter from W. S. Clark to Telephone Headquarters, 20 March 1954. BTA, TCB 2/172, folder 'Telephones for Deaf People'.
121 Ibid.
122 Ibid.
123 Agar, *Constant Touch*, p. 64.
124 Kay, 'Inventing Telephone Usage', pp. 150–180.
125 Sterling, B., 'The Hacker Crackdown: Evolution of the US Telephone Network', in N. W. Heap (ed.), *Information Technology and Society* (London: Sage, 1995), pp. 33–40, p. 37.
126 George, G. F., 'The Federal Communications Commission and the Bell System: Abdication of Regulatory Responsibility', *Indiana Law Journal*, 44:3 (1969), 459–477, pp. 460–462. I am grateful to Mara Mills for drawing this case to my attention.
127 This struggle has been documented in Lang, H. G., *A Phone of Our Own: The Deaf Insurrection against Ma Bell* (Washington, DC: Gallaudet University Press, 2000). This book also repeatedly emphasises the difficulty of working with the British Post Office.
128 Mills, 'Deafening', p. 132.
129 Ibid., p. 120.
130 Ibid.
131 Noble, W. G., *Assessment of Impaired Hearing: A Critique and New Method* (New York: Academic Press, 1978).
132 Mills, 'Deafening', p. 121.
133 Ibid., pp. 118–143.
134 Virdi and McGuire, 'Phyllis M. Tookey Kerridge'.
135 Blume, S., *The Artificial Ear: Cochlear Implants and the Culture of Deafness* (London: Rutgers University Press, 2010).
136 For example, see Blume, *The Artificial Ear* and Virdi, J., 'Between Cure and Prosthetic: "Good Fit" in Artificial Eardrums', in C. Jones (ed.), *Rethinking Modern Prostheses in Anglo-American Commodity Cultures, 1820–1939* (Manchester: Manchester University Press, 2017), pp. 48–69.
137 Wyatt, S., 'Non-Users Also Matter: The Construction of Users and Non-Users of the Internet', in T. Pinch and N. Oudshoorn (eds), *How Users Matter: The Co-Construction of Users and Technology* (Cambridge, MA: MIT Press, 2005), pp. 67–79, p. 76.

4

THE AUDIOMETER AND THE MEDICALISATION OF HEARING LOSS

Units of sensation

When I was around seven years old, we went on a family trip to Aberdeen Science Centre. My memory of that day has largely faded, but I now know that something significant happened on that trip. One of the exhibitions featured an umbrella-style speaker used to demonstrate the normal ranges of human hearing. Human hearing is, as this book should have already made clear, a complicated topic. What we can hear depends both on loudness (decibel levels) and pitch (frequency levels), as well as a variety of other factors. This speaker was set up to gradually increase in frequency, so that it progressed from tones such as those you would hear on a standard piano, through to higher sounds like that of a microwave beeping, to end with barely audible tones of around 20,000 Hz. While Dad, my brother and I were laughing and joking about how long we could hear birdsong and so on, Mum was realising her hearing range had cut out long before ours. It was a strange way, no doubt, to find confirmation of one's deafness.

The kind of technology that was used in this display relies on the standardisation of electronic sound, which was perfected and pursued in the interwar years as the audiometer was embraced as an objective tool to define noise limits and thresholds. Its utilisation of fixed thresholds for the normal ranges of hearing were also, as I explain in the section that follows, fixed through 'the telephone as audiometer'. The audiometer was elevated as a tool for testing both noise levels and hearing loss, I argue, because it provided an objective numerical inscription, which could be used to guard against malingering and to negotiate compensation claims for hearing loss. It was also as utilised in the prescription of hearing aids and, as I show in the section on 'The telephone as hearing aid', the interwar period featured an explosion of hearing aids based on telephone technologies, which led to the increased medicalisation of deafness as the medical community sought to temper the 'quack' hearing aids flooding the market. However, the medicalisation of hearing aids was no simple matter. Such medicalised prescription was complicated by conflicts over categorisation, the status of hearing aids as medical devices and the question of which institutional bodies were responsible for the 'problem of hearing loss'. The Post Office, telephone engineers, hearing aid manufacturers, the Ministry of Health, the MRC and the NID were all embroiled in this debate, as each body sought to temper the explosion of hearing aid devices available for those with hearing loss in the interwar period. Even the Ministry of Pensions was involved in their distribution, as it started supplying hearing aids to deafened ex-servicemen as a supplement to or replacement for a full pension. Moreover, because hearing aids were variously categorised as either medicines, prosthetics or technological apparatus, their categorisation was mutable and subject to politicisation. In the section on 'Advertising hearing aids', I explain that this meant that the Post Office was able to legally advertise so-called 'quack' hearing aids with impunity. Simultaneously, the Post Office engineers' growing expertise in auditory technologies meant that they were concurrently involved in the design of the first NHS hearing aid – the Medresco. In the section on 'Putting the user in the picture', I analyse the ending of the Post Office's amplified telephone service, and argue that their failure to consider user input or the reality of hearing aid usage from the perspective of the 'deaf subscriber' led to their failure to provide an NHS adjunct for telephony. In the conclusion to the chapter, I argue that this has had profound consequences on our elevation of access to face-to-face speech above access to sound technologies such as telephony or music.

In the previous chapter, we explored the extent to which the British Post Office's artificial ear technology defined normal hearing in the telephone system. In this chapter, we move beyond the Post Office to reflect on the way that this mechanistic understanding of hearing impacted wider society, by analysing how the audiometer developed from the telephone, worked to medicalise hearing loss and was used to calibrate and prescribe hearing aids.

Inventions including the microphone, the vacuum tube and the condenser transmitter ushered in a new wave of electro-acoustic tools over the course of the 1920s; these were tools which 'not only provided acoustical researchers new means by which to study sound' but also 'new models for thinking about it'.[1] In the early 1920s, sound was measured in ambiguous noise or sensation units. These were obtained through the use of a rudimentary audiometer, which the recorder would turn up until the tone was loud enough to mask the ambient noise around them.[2] This gave a proxy measure for the environmental noise levels. But this was inadequate, as Post Office research engineer W. West explained in a 1933 lecture to the Post Office Telephone and Telegraph Society of London.[3] West argued that although instruments could be constructed to record objective measurements of noise, this kind of measurement would not capture frequency levels, nor the quality of noise disturbance as perceived by an individual, therefore, 'this reading will not necessarily bear any close relation to the loudness as heard by the ear'.[4] A better method, he proposed, made use of an 'observer' provided with: 'a standard tone – say a pure tone at 1000 cycles per second in a telephone receiver – and if he has also an attenuator to vary the magnitude of this tone by known amounts, he can adjust the attenuator until he judges the standard tone to be as loud as the noise to be measured'.[5] He argued that this could be done by a number of observers, with the average results giving the 'frequency characteristics of normal hearing'.[6] Thus, this method, originally used by telephone engineers to measure electrical noise on transmission lines, was used to measure noise levels in the city.[7] West further pointed out that by the 1930s, an objective measurement of sound was becoming more important, as 'the standardization of noise units and loudness units is at present under discussion in this country'.[8] Indeed, this kind of individual subjective measurement was gradually superseded during these decades with the rise of decibel measurement, a term coined in 1923 by Bell Laboratories in the US and then gradually adopted by the UK.[9]

These broad shifts towards increased objectivity and accuracy in sound measurement were also apparent in hearing testing, as the interwar years featured a broader drive for a standard criterion of sound.[10] The Post Office Engineering Department was particularly motivated to replace data based on the kinds of individual patterns of use we discussed in Chapter 3 with more quantifiable data concerning sound, hearing and hearing aids. Simultaneously, standardisation of the measurement and definition of sound was necessary to provide proof of the levels of noise pollution, which was of intensifying concern during the interwar period. Emily Thompson has shown that instruments designed to measure noise actually worked to redefine the meaning of sound, as the 'problem of noise was further amplified in the 1920s by the actions of acoustical experts'.[11] For an example of this, we can look back at West's Post Office paper, which included a 'noise chart' showing the progression of noise levels in different types of spaces, ranging from the 100 decibel 'noisy aeroplane cabin', the 60 decibel 'steam train (window open) to the 40 decibel 'quiet saloon car (30MPH)'.[12] However, his measurements included decibel units as well as indicators of the 'threshold of feeling', which was measured in dynes per sq. cm.[13] Thus, units of sound measurements were unstable in 1933, yet by the latter years of the 1930s the decibel was fixed in use to describe sound and hearing loss both in the telephone system and in the human body. As this chapter will explore in more detail, the decibel standard for measuring hearing loss was fixed in large part as a result of the influence of the telephone companies. These shifts in quantifying and assessing sound levels echoed deeper changes in the way that hearing was conceptualised by both engineers and otologists. Post Office engineers wielded great influence in building such new mechanistic models of sound, which were then incorporated into their interpretation of what constituted hearing loss in the medical sphere.

The telephone as audiometer

A way of using objective technology to define and diagnose deafness was sought out long before the field of audiology professionalised after the Second World War. In this section, I outline the longer history of using technology to diagnose deafness through discussion of the beginnings of otology, before elucidating how the audiometer was eventually embraced as a trusted instrument to secure levels of hearing loss for compensation in numerical terms in the industrial/military context.

Treatment and diagnosis of deafness in the early nineteenth century was difficult, and this difficulty fostered instability in the fledgling field of otology and in aural surgery.[14] Historian Jaipreet Virdi has explained that one of the ways that nineteenth-century aurists attempted to legitimise their work as scientific was by appealing to their use of technology.[15] Later in the century otology established itself as a specialism, and its practitioners began using tuning forks to establish both frequency loss and type of hearing loss.[16] Tuning fork tests thus gave qualitative as well as quantitative results. However, it was the 1879 invention of the audiometer by Welsh scientist David Edward Hughes (1831–1900) that ushered in the means to make large-scale quantitative surveys on hearing loss.[17] Hughes's instrument attached the telephone to a horizontal bar adorned with two coils, which set up an induction current linked to a battery and microphone, meaning that the current could be heard through the telephone as a tone.[18] When the induction coil was nearer one end of the bar (and the larger coil) the sound was louder, and the sound decreased when it moved in the opposing direction.[19] Hughes introduced his instrument to the medical profession and emphasised to the Royal Society 'the value of the instrument as an *absolute measure* of our hearing powers'.[20] This early version of the audiometer measured hearing on a scale based on the division of the bar into 200 parts, so hearing could be tested from the maximum of 200 units to absolute zero.[21] However, as historian Michael Kay has pointed out, the nineteenth-century audiometer was largely rejected by practitioners, who disliked its expense, complexity and inconvenience.[22] Tests using tuning forks, the watch tick test or the spoken voice (Snellen) test were considered by most clinicians to be far simpler. Debates over the utility of these tests intensified in Britain after the First World War, when doctors were faced with treating soldiers suffering from both noise-induced hearing loss and temporary hearing loss caused by shell shock.

Rather than in its initial iteration, it was therefore during the interwar period that the audiometer was repeatedly lauded as a significant advance in the diagnosis and classification of deafness.[23] In 1928, the aural surgeon (and founder member of the Socialist Medical Association) Mr Somerville Hasting advocated in the *British Medical Journal* for the need for standardisation, emphasising that 'from the point of view of scientific advance, arbitrary units of hearing must be given up'.[24] The audiometer's ability to provide quantitative units of hearing ability and to allow for their comparison was especially valuable in achieving this, as one American otologist explained: 'The invention of the telephone and its universal use offered a means for producing a sound which could be standardized and measured.'[25] This was a clear advantage compared to the more commonly used voice test, which could not be standardised and necessitated the involvement of the clinician's own (variable) body. In 1931, the NID's medical sub-committee highlighted the importance of standardisation to argue that hearing should no longer be tested through the unreliable and subjective medium of the voice:

> In view of the improvement in the making of gramophone records, in gramophone and in methods of transmission of speech sounds to the ear by telephone, the committee feel that it should be possible so as to standardise gramophone records and the speech intensity delivered to the ear so as to produce a standard of hearing for speech ... Inasmuch as the decibel index of speech sounds by telephone has been adopted by international agreement between the various telephone services, the committee recommend that this index should be the basis of measurement and description of standard speech intensities used for testing hearing for speech.[26]

The above quotation highlights the extent to which hearing testing was actively influenced by developments in sound recording technologies and especially by telephony and telephone companies.

Moreover, the audiometer produced an audiogram, through which otologists could establish at last the 'facts' of 'normal hearing'.[27] The audiogram rendered the 'quantitative measurement of hearing' in graphical form, allowing for the recording, reproduction and graphical comparison of hearing.[28] For some of its proponents, the value of this inscription for research purposes lay precisely in the fact that it circumvented the need to rely on the testimony of those with hearing loss, for example in instances where, as a report in *The Lancet* explained, 'the effect of drugs may be recorded graphically instead of having to rely on the statements made by patients'.[29]

As a result, I argue that the audiometer can be considered as a model instrument to wield in promotion of the kind of 'mechanical epistemic injustice' explored in Chapter 2. Related to this was the audiogram's status as an 'objective test' that could be used to prevent malingering, which deafness had long been associated with. The suspicion attached to deafness in the interwar years was compounded by its invisibility, alongside

> the fact that there is no known objective test by which hearing power or its absence can be measured. With the blind the statement of the person under examination can be subjected to corroboration by instrumental tests in which he has no say; but the deaf subject must be left to give his answers unchecked, even when the watch or whisper tests, or the use of graded tuning-forks are employed. In fact the only way to detect the malingerer is by the familiar test of making a loud noise behind the subject in order to elicit a surprise.[30]

Hearing loss thus posed a problem related both to the subjectivity of the individual body and its invisibility *outside* of the individual body. The lack of tests to catch supposed malingerers became particularly problematic in the First World War because of the difficulty of diagnosing 'hysterical' deafness in soldiers. In 1915, Dr William Alden Turner wrote to the *British Medical Journal* to describe 'Cases of Nervous and Mental Shock' and included a section on 'Deafness and Deaf-Mutism'.[31] Turner was influential, acting as consultant neurologist for the War Office from January 1915 and later becoming the adviser for the Ministry of Pensions on matters concerning neurology after the war.[32] Turner noted that this kind of deafness comprised 'one of the clinical surprises of the war' and that 'examination of the sense of hearing reveals deafness of the nervous type'.[33] Wartime hearing loss was thus considered to be psychosomatic or 'functional', which meant that the underlying pathological cause could not be seen, but, crucially, was supposed to exist. Such an ideology was in line with psychiatry's long-standing insistence that there was a fundamental bodily cause for all mental illness.[34] In 1917, the editor of *The Lancet* similarly expressed the opinion that 'the present war has made us acquainted with new varieties of deafness'.[35]

Treating hearing loss alongside shell shock in the First World War led to conflict between psychiatry and otology.[36] Hearing loss gained new visibility within the public consciousness and became a high-profile issue precisely because it was intimately bound up with the visible and disturbing new condition of shell shock. As it became increasingly apparent that shell shock had psychological origins, the idea that hearing loss was also psychological gained increased credence within psychiatry. This led to a wave of new theories about the causation of hearing loss, and correspondent new treatments to test and treat the malingerers so that, as historian Julia Enke has put it, 'after the noise, the soldiers' ears were beleaguered by medicine'.[37] Treatments and diagnoses of these new varieties of deafness were split between more traditional treatment favoured by aural surgeons and the treatments favoured by psychiatric practitioners. On the side of traditional otology, aural surgeons Dr A. Logan Turner and Dr P. McBride (ear and throat surgeon and consulting surgeon respectively, at Edinburgh Royal Infirmary) classified hearing loss purely as injuries of the internal ear, middle ear or tympanic membrane and considered middle-ear deafness to be nerve deafness.[38] Turner and McBride wrote to *The Lancet* in 1918 to criticise the new ideas about deafness circulating within the wider medical profession. They made the case that wartime hearing loss was organic, and argued that: 'very grave injustice might be done if the dictum were accepted that given a man deaf from explosion, if he reacts to the vestibular tests in what his examiner considers a normal manner he is therefore either a malingerer or the victim of hysteria'.[39]

However, differentiating between malingering and hysteria was itself difficult, as we can gather from neurologist Arthur Hurst and aural surgeon E. A. Peters's attempts to test one of their sleeping patients by 'by shouting "fire", and by banging a poker against a coal-scuttle within a few inches of his head'![40] The category of 'hysterical' deafness was particularly fraught in the military context, as medical officers were generally highly suspicious of 'malingering' and hysteria was often considered to simply be a form of unconscious malingering. The audiometer offered a more reliable way to test malingering, and instructions to this effect were given as part of the kit for the 1940s commercial Amplivox audiometer shown in Figure 4.1. Amplivox was a successful hearing aid company and would have used an audiometer like this primarily to prescribe hearing aids. However, the instructions accompanying it emphasised its utility to those involved in moderating contested hearing loss and they explained that 'malingerers feign deafness in various degrees and for various reasons'.[41] Several strategies could be adopted to detect and confound the malingerer, including hiding the front panel from the patient's view, using the tone interrupter (Figure 4.1, bottom right) so that the patient would be unable to remember previous tone intensities, and by switching tones from ear to ear and from air to bone conduction, which 'easily confuses the subject and makes it practically impossible to deceive the operator'.[42]

Similarly, the audiometer enabled detection of those who could 'pass' as hearing by lip-reading.[43] This was especially valuable in the testing of

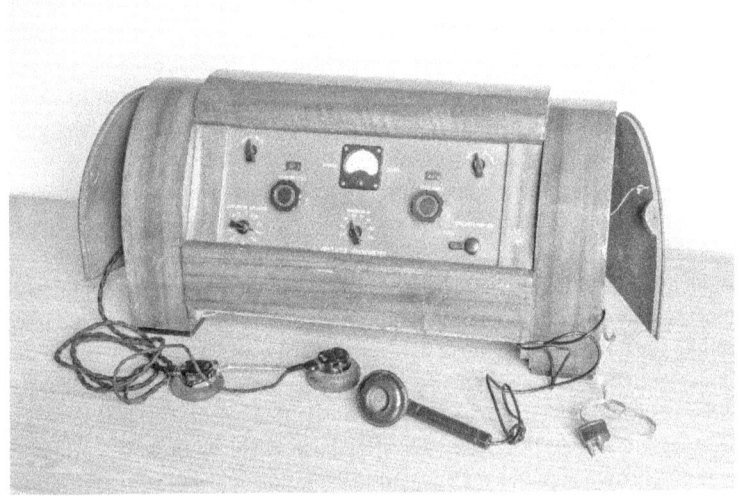

Figure 4.1 Audiometer

school-children, who could be tested rapidly and in larger groups with the audiometer.[44] This resulted in an increase in the more 'precise' sorting of children, 'who were found to be defective' and so reclassified.[45] In this way, the audiometer worked as an inscription device, an apparatus whose end-product was the audiogram and the creation of 'Normal Hearing' and, crucially, its counterpart.[46] We can see in this way how the power of the audiometer as a classifying device influenced the social construction of disability, which was reinforced as the audiometer created more data on normal hearing, a process I now discuss in more detail.

As historian Mara Mills has shown, the necessary data came first from American telephone companies, who produced the Western Electric 1A audiometer in 1922, considered to be the first commercial electronic audiometer.[47] This was lauded by many British otologists as a great step forward. For example, leading British otologist Dr Wharry Crowden acknowledged that the Bell Telephone Company had 'helped the medical profession greatly by producing a reliable audiometer which is now being effectively used'.[48] One of Bell Laboratories' foremost researchers, Harvey Fletcher, clarified that a unit for measuring sound in a standardised fashion was necessary for the telephone business, in which 'the commodity being delivered to the customers is reproduced speech'.[49] The standard unit eventually adopted was, of course, the decibel, ten of which make up a bel – named for Alexander Graham Bell.[50] As I have previously argued with Virdi, through this standardisation the audiometer came to represent 'a new mechanistic understanding of auditory perception, one that merged a physical instrument with a more precise and measurable way of tracking perceptions of sound.'[51]

As *The Lancet* recognised in 1933, advances in audiometry interrelated with developments in sound reproduction techniques more broadly, which were used not only in telephony but also in radio.[52] For example, the vacuum tube (in American English) or valve (in English) was essential in advancing the construction of radios, audiometers and telephony during this period. Yet, as the NID's medical committee noted in 1926, such technical advances were utilised in sound technologies which further isolated those with hearing loss:

> The frequent press references to wireless telephony as a curative agent in deafness induces your Committee to make the following observations on the matter. Wireless is of no use to the deaf-mute. In cases of hardness of hearing, those who hear through the ordinary telephone will hear wireless through its earphones; and those who have difficulty with speech, heard through the air, will have the same difficulty with the loudspeaker. There is, no doubt, a percentage of hard of hearing persons who experience pleasure from listening to wireless speech and music but the sensational promises of relief, often disseminated through the Press, lead only to disappointment and add to the burden of the affliction.[53]

Nevertheless, such technical developments were incorporated into otology alongside techniques for testing transmission quality pioneered by the British Broadcasting Company (the BBC).[54] For the MRC, the audiometer offered a way to 'merge clinical research with scientific efficiency', and it became central to their interwar hearing committee's projects on normal hearing and its potential restoration.[55]

The audiometer was also critical to the interwar commitments of deaf educators and especially fuelled the legitimacy of the commitment to oralism, an educational method that prioritised speech and lip-reading to 'normalise' deaf children and force their integration into the hearing world.[56] It was further embraced by the industrial/military nexus as a way of arbitrating compensation for hearing loss, as it was determined to be useful as a means of identifying 'impaired hearing' and hence 'the unfitness of applicants for insurance policies, automobile licenses, and for enlistment in the Army and Navy, also in the life protection tests of railroad and steamship companies, and in the health corrective examination of schools, colleges, and gymnasiums'.[57] Indeed, the field of audiometry frequently identifies its origins as truly lying in the Second World War, when it was embraced by the US military for compensation purposes to provide a numerical assessment of hearing loss before and after service, which was critical to the management of compensation claims. In the military it was necessary to test many people quickly and have a numerical result that could be compared before and after service in order to award or refuse compensation for noise-induced hearing loss. Audiology then solidified as a field through the work done with deafened ex-service men during the war.[58] That compensation required the creation of numbers to indicate critical thresholds of disability is a key component of this book's main thesis, as this process worked to categorise disability, and did so in a way which discounted the need for individual testimony.

Despite the fact that the Second World War is frequently cited as the starting point for audiology, there are clear precursors to its development in the interwar years; in audiologist Berger's terms, the field 'existed some years previously, but without a special name'.[59] One contemporary clinician wrote in *The Lancet* in 1934 that 'the great advances in the precision of electrical instruments for amplifying and transmitting sounds have all been made since the War'.[60] As Emily Thompson has shown, the First World War worked as a catalyst to stimulate acoustical researches in America, which in turn stimulated the design of new instruments to detect and measure sound.[61] In Britain, however, the nascent field of audiometry primarily developed in the interwar years through the encouragement of the scientist Dr Phyllis Kerridge, who perhaps more than anyone else advocated for more scientific methods for testing hearing.[62] Kerridge was the first person in Britain to own a Western Electric (pure tone) audiometer, and she used this to conduct statistical studies on hearing thresholds, moving hearing loss into the realm of medicine by considering hearing loss as a 'legitimate scientific problem worthy of technocratic intervention'.[63] Kerridge's plans to define 'normal hearing' were based on her faith in precise and 'exact measurement' and she introduced her MRC investigation on *Hearing and Speech in Deaf Children* by invoking the infamous 'curse of Kelvin' (discussed in Chapter 1).[64] She used this investigation to compare different methods of testing hearing, and questioned the validity of the 'normal' level of hearing set by the audiometer, noting that:

> There is no indication in the literature of the degree of variation among the 'normals'. The same remark applies to the 'normal' bone conduction line. Further, it is an assumption that lines are the same for children as for adults.[65]

As Kerridge was using a Western Electric audiometer this meant that the average threshold level was set according to the Bell Laboratories.[66] Normal hearing was calibrated to 'the average child in the average classroom'.[67] As her remarks make evident, Kerridge not only recognised the danger of equating the average with the normal, but also highlighted the need to use different normalcy levels for different groups, such as children or the elderly (see Chapter 2). She questioned the assumption that the zero line representing normal hearing was universal for all peoples of all ages and sexes, and 'demonstrated the arbitrariness of its construction'.[68]

Kerridge's pioneering techniques were used in the prescribing and moderation of hearing aids, which she argued needed to be standardised within medicine.[69] In the spring of 1937, she opened the first hearing aid clinic in Britain, where she fitted patients for hearing aids based on their audiograms, taking the responsibility of hearing aid prescription away from commercial firms.[70] Kerridge thus addressed the lacuna that Dr D. F. Fraser-Harris (professor of physiology) had highlighted in 1934, when he noted that

> strange as it may appear, there is no body of persons qualified to interpret an aurist's prescription for a deaf patient, and to supply the appropriate deaf aid instrument, as there are opticians able to read an oculist's prescription and to provide the spectacles specified. Just as it requires a specialist – the oculist – to ascertain the precise nature and amount of departure from normality in vision, so it requires a skilled person to ascertain the precise kind and degree of deafness from which a deaf patient may be suffering. The reason for this difference is that the science of optics has been developing for about the last two hundred and fifty years.[71]

In contrast, as the next section will outline, regulation of hearings aids was in a state of flux during the interwar years, as the viability of electrical hearing aids rapidly improved during this period.

The telephone as hearing aid

From their initial instantiation as 'micro-telephones', electric hearing aid devices became increasingly viable in the interwar period.[72] This increase in viability is evident in analysis of the hearing aids distributed to deafened ex-service men by the National Benevolent Society (discussed in the previous chapter), which administered the Deafened Ex-Service Men's Fund. Use of electrical hearing aids by their members increased rapidly year upon year according to the society's reports: from no reports of use between 1921 and 1923, to 73 earphones issued in 1932 and 162 in 1939.[73] This increase could be explained by the technical developments that led to increased manufacture of electrical hearing aids during the 1930s. However, the National Benevolent Society itself attributed the increase to 'so many of the slightly deafened men of twenty years ago becoming so deaf that they are in danger of losing their employment'.[74]

The first mention of their use came in 1924, in a testimonial from a soldier who wrote, 'I have great pleasure in informing you that I have been fitted with a Stools [sic] electrophone by the Ministry of Pensions'.[75] The government had advocated lip-reading for deafened ex-servicemen since 1917 because of growing concern about national productivity, as the 'industrial effectiveness [of soldiers] has been seriously impaired by deafness due to military service'.[76] Centres of instruction for lip-reading were set up in response, but very few ex-servicemen applied for classes or accepted them when offered. This prompted the Ministry of Pensions to set up a special aural board, which became instrumental in allocating the distribution of hearing aids and pensions.[77] The first official ministry ruling on hearing aid supply came in 1922 in response to an enquiry from the commissioner of medical services for the ministry, who asked whether hearing aids could be charged to their account.[78] Sir Dundas-Grant (1854–1944), director general of medical services, wrote in response that

> [if the hearing aid has] been recommended by a specialist member of the board which examined him [then] supply is admissible at the public expense and the article may best be obtained from the Stols Electrophone Company ... with whom the Ministry have a special arrangement and who are prepared to supply these appliances to our order at a discount of 20% on the list price.[79]

Supply of batteries was also subsidised by the ministry but was closely controlled, with a restricted number of batteries (soldiers were allowed two a month), which presumably also restricted the level and type of usage. Many hearing aid firms wrote to the ministry to try and solicit its endorsement and stressed that they offered one price to the ministry and the medical profession and another price to the public. As the Mears earphone manufacturers put it, 'we only hand these to Medical Men, not to the public'.[80] This meant that, as in the case of charitable provision, deafened servicemen were given consideration and support that did not extend to deafened civilians.

In 1922 the Ministry of Pensions spent £100 on hearing aids, but three years later this figure had risen to just over £136 2s 9d.[81] The sum spent on hearing aids was to increase exponentially throughout the interwar years as electrical aids were increasingly used by the ministry as supplements or alternatives to a full pension, and as a means of reintegrating vast numbers of ex-servicemen with hearing loss into the workforce. The ministry's relationship with hearing aid suppliers offers a fascinating snapshot of how state hearing aids were provided *before* there was a state hearing aid. Moreover, it demonstrates that state intervention into hearing loss increased alongside developments in hearing aid technology that were thought to provide a quick and cheap 'fix' for deafness. Yet before the instigation of the NHS, there were still great discrepancies between the care given and the care needed. As Gooday and Sayer point out, most of the government pensions granted to ex-servicemen were dedicated to 'those who had lost limbs, eyes, or been facially disfigured'.[82] Charitable provision was left to address the needs of the others. The records of the National Benevolent Society in 1928 reported that 'the latest official figures show that 33,768 men were discharged from the Army and Navy on account of deafness'.[83] The increased visibility of deafness in returned soldiers helped to normalise hearing loss and make the deafened more of a priority for social welfare. Indeed, the classification of those with hearing loss solidified after the First World War into a new category – the 'deafened'. As Gooday and Sayer have argued: 'Deafened combatants were not treated as being genetically predisposed to loss of hearing, but the honourable victims of the damaging percussive effects of artillery.'[84] Yet the stigma associated with deafness was still high, especially for women and the congenitally deaf, who were targeted in this period as a problem for eugenicists.

That the stigma surrounding deafness during the interwar years was still great is evident from the lengths that those with limited hearing would go to in order to identify as hearing and minimise the significance of their hearing loss. It is further manifest in the rhetoric attached to advertisements for hearing aids during the interwar period. Hearing aid companies made exaggerated claims, using vivid language and images to persuade customers of their devices' effectiveness. These advertisements relied for their effectiveness on the socially constructed imperative that such disability should be concealed.[85] This imperative was exacerbated at the start of the twentieth century as stigmatisation of deafness increased alongside industrialisation's demands for standardised practices. As Gooday and Sayer explain, this demand meant that deaf people had to 'adapt to the hearing world's oral norms or face marginalisation in unemployment'.[86]

A common trope in such advertisements was to draw on the stigma of deafness to sell the product by emphasising the inconspicuousness and invisibility of the hearing aid.[87] The 'micro-telephone' by the Stols Electrophone company, for instance, was advertised as such:

> [F]or those who require a hearing aid that can be worn inconspicuously we recommend the micro-telephone illustrated above. In use, it can be concealed under the coat or blouse, and a midget ear-piece no large than a sixpence can be applied to fit closely in the ear and which, in the case of a lady can be completely concealed by the hair.[88]

Similarly, the makers of the fortiphone urged its users to be, 'free from the embarrassment associated with clumsier devices'.[89] One American otologist hyperbolically underscored the fact that 'the public is not wont to employ people with a telephone stuck on one side of their heads'.[90] For women, there were additional imperatives driving concealment. For example, the 'Mears Ear-Phone' was depicted in one advertisement held like a delicate fan against the ear of a beautiful woman with an ornate hairstyle, while the gentleman next to her leaned close to her and whispered (into her other ear!). Below this image was the caption 'A complete success: enjoy the pleasures of sound again.'[91] This exemplifies the additional gendered imperative that such advertisements frequently invoked, which compelled women to wear hearing aids that would conceal their hearing loss and allow them to compete and 'succeed' on the marriage market.

The stigma attached to conditions like hearing loss was complicated by the fact that it was ostensibly invisible, and offered the potential to remain so for the sufferer who chose not to accept assistive equipment.[92] Hearing loss was only apparent if the person with hearing loss chose to expose it, which was not always the best course of action.[93] Moreover, in the case of hearing loss there was an added pressure to use hearing aids so as to avoid inconveniencing others in conversation.[94] As Mills has argued, the hearing aids construction as a 'stigma symbol' drove the increased miniaturisation of electrical aids, while their increased usage augmented the number of those who identified as 'hearing' or 'hard of hearing' rather than Deaf.[95] It is worth noting, however, as Gooday and Sayer have discussed, that there are always 'two stories' that can be told about hearing aids. And while a story about increased miniaturisation and stigma is certainly evident (particularly during the interwar period), it runs alongside the stories of those who wielded their hearing aids as powerful prosthetics that allowed them to dictate the terms of the conversations they were involved in and the people that they allowed to engage with them.[96] Indeed, Mills stresses that there are many examples of hearing aid users controlling and directing conversations, and that, 'Deaf and hard of hearing people played shaping roles as early adopters, inventors, retailers, and manufacturers of miniaturized components.'[97]

Yet the growing popularity of electric hearing aids led to a subsequent proliferation of unscrupulous electrical hearing aid manufacturers; the controversial practices of some of these firms resulted in the medical profession taking a more active interest in the regulation of their distribution. Such divisive practices included the work of those who were widely derided as 'quacks', that is, hearing aid vendors who exaggerated their ability to cure deafness in a way that sparked the ire of the medical community.[98] As Kerridge baldly put it in 1935: 'The commercial hearing aids may be roughly divided into those that are frauds and those which are not.'[99] The electrical hearing aids designed 'on the telephone principle' were criticised by Kerridge on a number of points. They magnified sounds only by about 20–60 decibels and this magnification took place 'mostly in the middle frequencies', despite the fact that most adults with hearing loss were unable to access the *higher* frequencies.[100] As a result, she noted that 'they have been the cause of such a lot of hope and disappointment to deaf people'.[101] They also gave the voice a less natural, more mechanical quality, and Kerridge quoted one of the children she had lent such an instrument to, who responded that it 'made her teacher sounds like a "movie star" '.[102]

By the 1930s, valve technology had advanced sufficiently to allow for hearing aids that could be worn directly on the body (rather than necessitating batteries carried in separate bags) and this led to a rise in their usage and popularity.[103] These, Kerridge conceded, gave a better quality sound and she noted that she had 'recently met two deaf physicists who have made very good sets for themselves and who are anxious to help other deaf people'.[104] However, the medical profession recognised growing concerns about the administration of these devices, and in 1937 *The Lancet* pointed out that 'the conditions under which hearing-aids are supplied to the public should include tests of the patient's response to pure tones by the audiometer, and a standardised articulation test with the instrument which it is proposed to supply for a period of trial'.[105]

The practices of such hearing aid manufacturers were of great concern to the NID because of their business practices, which the NID regarded as unethical. But they did not condemn the hearing aids because they did not work. Rather, firms were criticised for concerns surrounding unethical business practices – not allowing free trials or refunds, and for using intrusive advertising strategies. In 1935 the NID complained about the lack of government legislation to regulate these issues, which meant that:

> It is therefore open to any person, if sufficiently base, to pretend to cure deafness and to set up clinics for this purpose … They appear in various places under different names and are sufficiently versatile in the healing art to undertake to treat other defects, such as rheumatism or asthma, when the supply of deaf persons willing to be duped in any particular locality runs short. Scarcely less despicable than the practices of quacks are the proceedings of those who take advantage of the deaf under the guise of helping them through aids to hearing. In the exaggeration of their advertising and other literature, there is little to choose between them. Hearing aids are now advertised by sandwich boards and hawked from door to door. Nothing like this is associated with any other affliction.[106]

Edwin Stevens of Amplivox attempted to defend his profession by forming the Hearing Aid Manufacturers' Association, which only included firms on the NID's approved list who would cooperate with the medical profession in their selling of hearing aids.[107] He described his decision to do this in *The Lancet* in 1938, when he argued that advertising was linked to fraudulent practices and emphasised the increasing importance of the decibel measurement as the ideal standard for the purposes of testing hearing as well as measuring noise levels.

There are, on the other hand, certain commercial firms who advertise continuously and flamboyantly in the daily press and whose sole object is to exploit the deaf public for all it is worth. Their prices are exorbitant and they charge fees for trial which are not allowed for when a purchase is made. These firms do not worry about decibels, possibly because they have not yet heard of them.[108]

Advertising hearing aids

For an example of one of the most sustained campaigns against hearing aid manufacturers' predatory behaviour, we return once more to the Post Office, and its use of advertising in stamp books. Stamp books were initially conceived of as a way of holding sheets of stamps together but were soon discovered to be a lucrative form of advertising. These small booklets contained stamps alongside pages of advertising features, and in the interwar period these advertisements were pervasive. In 1920, nearly 6 billion items were posted in Britain.[109] These booklets were therefore highly visible publications that constituted a uniquely ubiquitous form of advertising which could target a spectrum of postal users, crossing boundaries of age, sex and class. They were utilised by various companies for advertising purposes. Indeed, certain hearing aid firms, including Ardente and Ossicaide, had long-term lucrative subscriptions to the Post Office to advertise their products within them. These were not like the advertisements discussed in the previous section, because their appearance in a Post Office publication legitimised them to the public as reputable products. Thus, these small objects had a powerful impact on driving regulation of the hearing aid industry.

Many of the people who bought the kind of cheap hearing aids advertised in the stamp books were unhappy with the devices they had purchased and complained variously to their MPs, their ministers, doctors and to the NID. Many were especially incensed because the advertisement's appearance in the Post Office stamp books had indicated to them a crucial governmental stamp of approval. For instance, one minister in Canterbury, whose wife had hearing loss, wrote to the Post Office Public Relations Department asking:

> I should like to know what guarantee can be given either by the PMG or the firms advertised on enclosed extracts from books of stamps that THE DEAF WILL HEAR. These firms are well known in London to exploit the deaf and their friends for their own profit and it is degrading to a Government department

to lend any encouragement to such people. Papers like 'The Times' will never admit advertisements of quack remedies such as appear in your stamp books.[110]

The Post Office's repeated inclusion of such advertisements led to a protracted campaign by the NID, the medical community, the press and several political figures, who aimed to persuade the Post Office to remove them. The NID initiated this campaign in 1936 with the emotive indictment, 'No government publication should be used to attract afflicted persons to seek relief from firms whose practices are incompatible with those usually observed in treating human suffering.'[111] It then went on in 1937 to request that the Post Office insert a disclaimer absolving itself from endorsement or responsibility for the devices. The Post Office refused to do so.[112] In the NID's correspondence with the Post Office, it emphasised the special position that the Post Office had in terms of public influence and stressed that:

> These advertisements appearing in the Stamp Books acquire an added importance in the minds of the public who seem to think that such appearance in an official publication implies a government guarantee of the articles advertised. Indeed we are often told by deafened people who have been attracted by these advertisements, 'I saw it in the Stamp Books so I thought it was all right.'[113]

The NID's concern about the Post Office's ability to influence the public was echoed in Parliament where the stamp book problem was brought up on numerous occasions. The first of these took place on 2 June 1933, when Sir Harold Sutcliffe, the Conservative MP and ex-serviceman, asked the Postmaster General how much revenue the Post Office derived from advertisements for hearing aids in books of stamps.[114] The Postmaster General responded that 'the financial loss from the exclusion of advertisements to hearing would be upwards of £3000 a year.'[115] In an internal report, however, we find more specific figures: 'The revenue derived by the Post Office from advertisements in the books of stamps for the year ending 30th of September, 1936 (an average year) was £16,492 of which a very significant proportion – £3073 or 18.63% – related to advertisements of appliances for the deaf.'[116]

On 30 March 1936, Labour MP Mr William Thorne questioned the Postmaster General again about the unfair and exaggerated stamp book advertisements.[117] Again the Postmaster General denied institutional responsibility, arguing that, 'Unless and until Parliament enacts further legislation making all advertisements of this kind illegal, I do not feel that there is any adequate ground on which the Post Office can refuse advertisements.'[118] On 7 December 1936, Conservative MP Sir Robert Cary also questioned the Postmaster General on this point, making reference to the 1914 Report of the Select

Committee on Patent Medicines and arguing that hearing aid advertisements should be prohibited under its terms.[119]

These objections made repeated appeal to the ruling of the Select Committee on Patent Medicines, paragraph 58(2), and the Postmaster General explained that this included fraudulent remedies such as

> a large class, having an extensive sale, often at high prices, consisting of abortifacients, of alleged cures for cancer, consumption, diabetes, paralysis, locomotor ataxy, Bright's disease, lupus, fits, epilepsy, rupture (without operation or appliance), deafness, diseases of the eye, syphilis, etc. ... There should be little difficulty in identifying remedies of this class, and their treatment in the public interest need involve no doubt or hesitation. They are, and are known by their makers to be, cruel cruel frauds; and the sale and advertisement of them should be prohibited under drastic penalties.[120]

The Post Office's response hinged on a technicality of categorisation: that hearing aids were apparatus, not medicine. As the Postmaster General explained, 'Though deafness is mentioned, the reference is to medicines. Advertisements of medicines purporting to relieve or cure deafness are not accepted for insertion in the books of stamps; but advertisements of appliances to assist the deaf are not rejected for they do not claim to cure the disease.'[121] This reveals the tension over the categorisation of hearing devices as either medicines, prosthetics or technological apparatus. In this context, the label given depended very much on the agenda of the advertiser. The hybrid status of hearing aids themselves was crucial to the way they were advertised. If hearing aids were categorised as medical devices, then they would have fallen under the jurisdiction of the medical profession and the NID. By referring to them specifically as apparatus, the Post Office was able to advertise them without contradicting the Patent Medicines Act. The provision of vitamins was similarly interpretative during this period, as they were classified variously as foods or as medicines depending on fluctuating chemical categorisations.[122]

False advertising of medical equipment was deliberated by Parliament in 1936 in the context of a new Medical and Surgical Appliances Bill designed to restrict the sale and advertisement of medicines and surgical appliances. This bill was designed to extend and support the findings of the select committee on patent medicines by considering medical advertising in the widest possible sense. It caused controversy, however, because it was perceived as a means of protecting and ensuring the monopoly of professional doctors over all aspects of the medical profession. This private member's bill did not get a second reading and it was suspected at the time that those opposing the bill resented the stronghold of the medical profession and their vested financial interests in its success.[123]

However, the campaign for the removal of hearing aid advertisements was supported by the British Medical Association, which made its position on the matter very clear, stating that 'the committee deplores the continued appearance in books of stamps of advertisements of hearing aids'.[124] This definitive statement was reported widely as part of the press campaign against the stamp book publications. The campaign was reported across a spectrum of publications and locations, receiving coverage in *The Times* and *John Bull*, as well as in the *British Medical Journal*, all of which condemned the hearing aid advertisements as 'misleading' and their producers as 'quacks'. Many of the articles highlighted the fact that it was especially those on lower incomes who were conned into buying useless hearing aid products. For instance, an article in *John Bull* explained that: 'Ex-servicemen and domestic servants are constantly induced to throw away pounds they cannot possibly afford on some of these worthless "inconspicuous aids to the deaf"'.[125] This article was particularly detailed and condemnatory in its style, using emotive language in its depiction of the 'innumerable instances – pathetic in their detail and hardship – where poor people have been despoiled of their savings in a vain search among the quacks for promised relief to their deafness'. It outlined those most afflicted: 'poor people, old age pensioners, ex-servicemen and domestic servants' as well as the heroes whose 'deafness [was] brought on by war service'.[126]

The conservative MP Sir Francis Fremantle (1872–1943) was a crucial campaigner in these debates. He was an active figure in a variety of British medical services and an influential campaigner on issues concerning public health both within Parliament and during war service. He was a Medical Officer of Health and held presidential roles at the British Medical Association and the Incorporated Society of Medical Officers of Health, and was an active member of the NID and the Deafened Ex-Service Men's Society.[127] Fremantle portrayed himself as representative of the medical profession and was prolific in writing on and campaigning for improved public health. On 24 November 1937 he wrote to ex-Postmaster General Sir Kingsley Wood to argue that:

> To claim 'amazing results' from any apparatus even in the most acute cases of Middle-ear Disease and 'Stone Deafness' is a wicked lie, a danger to life and a deliberate fraud. And yet the government broadcasts this wickedness in order to obtain a few shillings more than they would from an honest advertisement.[128]

The Post Office's continued refusal to remove these advertisements even in the face of this popular campaign was in part due to the flexible definition of hearing aids in this period. However, it was also linked to the way in which the Post Office's profits were used. In 1919 the British government had invoked a ten-year rule to reduce funding on defence, following domestic and political pressure to lower defence estimates and reduce taxation.[129] By 1935, however, Germany had commenced rearmament and defied the Treaty of Versailles, which prompted a rethink on the part of the British government on the subject of defence spending, with such spending duly increased throughout the 1930s.[130] This, combined with the massive public debt following on from the First World War, meant that the Treasury struggled with the armed forces' demands for increased funding and the financial implications of potentially impending war. In 1938, the Post Office public relations officer, Colonel Crutchley, reflected on the fact that 'Wars are notoriously expensive and when it becomes necessary to pay for them one of the first services to be tapped for revenue is the Post Office.'[131] Thus, although there was pressure on the Post Office to remove these contentious advertisements, the Treasury control of the Post Office and reliance on its revenue made their removal impossible in the impoverished interwar financial context. The outbreak of war temporarily prompted the end of stamp book advertising, as civilians were encouraged by the government not to use the Post Office services during wartime. Perversely, use of the postal system increased during these years and stamp books were summarily reintroduced because of their potential for vast income generation.[132]

Putting the user in the picture

With the advent of the British National Health Service (NHS), the Post Office decided to modify its amplified telephones (discussed in detail in Chapter 3) so that 'deaf subscribers' could use the telephone with their new NHS hearing aids. This eventually led to the ending of the amplified telephone service and this case provides a microcosm of the issues at stake when designers produce prosthetics without consulting the users. As this chapter has argued, the increased mechanisation of hearing loss, hearing aids and hearing tests took place alongside a gradual silencing of the voices of those with hearing loss. As well as perpetuating the mechanical epistemic injustice discussed in Chapter 2, loss of user input impacted on the feasibility of the Post Office's electroacoustic services.

Plans for an NHS hearing aid were raised in 1947 after the Second World War and this device became known as the Medresco, a contraction of 'Medical Research Council'.[133] In 1946 the Post Office Engineering Department reported to the Telecommunications Department that the Ministry of Health was developing a government-sponsored hearing aid, which had not been announced to the public at that point. The quotation below outlines the Post Office's commitment to telephony for all and highlights its acknowledged expertise in hearing-assistive technologies at this period.

> The present position in this respect is very different from that which existed before the war when the original enquiry was proposed, as at that time the Post Office was working practically single-handed. It now seems likely that almost all deaf people will become users of the Government sponsored hearing aid and that the best solution of the problem of affording them telephone facilities will be to design an adaptor for associating the microphone of the hearing aid acoustically with the receiver of a telephone.[134]

Therefore, instead of designing a new amplified telephone, the Post Office engineers decided to design an adaptor to *link* the new hearing aids with telephone receivers. This, they believed, would have the advantage of allowing users to link into any Post Office telephone rather than restricting their telephone usage to the home. Once the Engineering Department decided an adaptor was the most suitable solution, two means of adaption were considered: an acoustic adaptor or electrical induction.[135] Electrical induction had several disadvantages and it was deemed liable to be inefficient and variable in performance as a result of electrical interference or 'howling'. Moreover, the Engineering Department was constrained because the MRC had mandated that the frequency response characteristic of the Medresco had to be maintained across all conditions of use.[136] This part of the Engineering Department's report notes that this would also affect the ability to use induction 'pick up' between the Medresco and the radio. The report concluded that the hearing aid was 'primarily designed for speech'.[137] Building in speech as a priority over and above the need to access music or telephony was to have a long-lasting negative effect on people with hearing loss, as the aural landscape of the hearing aid users was constrained by the Medresco's focus on speech and its standardised design, which also did not allow for bone-conductive usage.

Several design constraints were imposed on the project because of the Ministry of Health's restrictions, and this was exacerbated because the Medresco was never designed to function in conjunction with the telephone; the crystal microphone precluded the use of electrical induction technology and it was impossible to make changes to the moulded case of the hearing aid to facilitate an adapter, as this would delay production, meaning they would miss the deadline for release on the NHS.[138] However, the Ministry of Health emphasised that no delays or changes to the initial design of the Medresco would be tolerated. The crystal microphone would need to be redesigned to operate with an electrical 'pick-up' coil. This stipulation further restricted the Engineering Department's ability to experiment with electrical induction. On the other hand, the only disadvantage of the acoustic adaptor was that it would have to be physically coupled to the hearing aid and telephone every time it was used. This was therefore deemed to be the most advantageous design and so the Engineering Department began to create an acoustic coupler to link the amplified telephone with the Medresco.

Subscribers already using the amplified telephones were not consulted before the telephone was designed, because 'as far as likely users are concerned the subjective conditions likely to be met with will be extremely varied and cannot be satisfied equally'.[139] This was perhaps one of the legacies of users modifying their own telephones in the 1920s. Although there was recognition of the diverse needs of people with hearing loss, the design of the telephones was conducted entirely to the specifications of the engineers, with no input from relevant users. Although interviews had initially been considered, in 1946 the Public Relations Department declared that: 'no useful purpose would be served by undertaking interviews with deaf persons as was originally proposed'.[140]

In addition to technical difficulties, the funding of the device was a major source of contention. There were questions from the start of this proposal over how the service would be funded and distributed. Colonel McMillan of the Research Branch in the Engineering Department raised the issue of how the telephone would be distributed in relation to the new hearing aid, asking:

> Is it the intention to give a hearing aid to any person who needs it, as part of the National Health Service? It is a question whether free distribution of the adapter ought to follow as a complementary feature of the deaf aid service, and if so on what basis the distribution should be made, and by whom. As it is understood that the adapter will be capable of use with a coil office telephone as well as a subscriber's telephone, it seems clear that the distribution could not be limited to subscribers. The question of need might be determined simply by application i.e., a person having a deaf aid might be supplied with an adapter on demand.[141]

The Post Office obviously considered that the amplified telephone should be offered to people in receipt of a hearing aid as part of the NHS. Clearly, at this point, the Post Office conceptualised the amplified telephone as a *medical* device that should be free as part of a national *health* service. Yet still the Post Office was unwilling to cede control of the device to the Ministry of Health

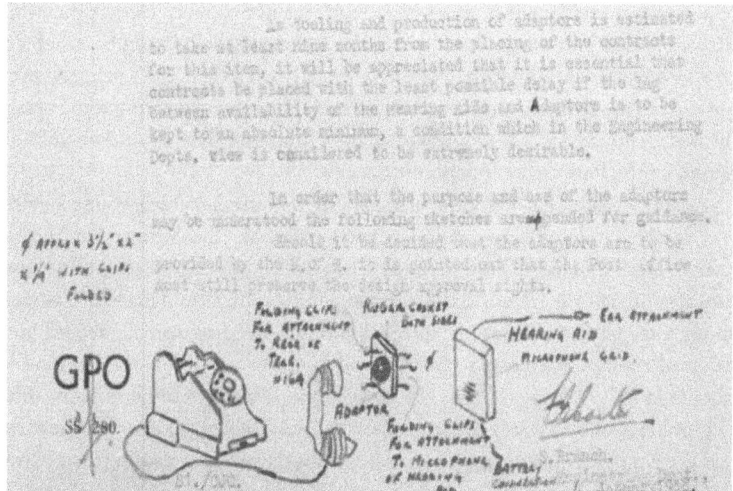

Figure 4.2 Engineer's drawing of the hearing aid adaptor, 1947

and so attempted to categorise the device as an adjunct to the telephone rather than a hearing aid, and reminded the ministry that: 'It would perhaps not be reasonable to contemplate selling the adapter when the hearing aid itself is issued free.'[142]

Once the conditions of supply of the state hearing aid had been determined the Engineering Department resumed investigations and sent the sketch shown in Figure 4.2, illustrating how the device would work for the Ministry of Health with the proviso that 'the Post Office must still preserve the design approval rights'.[143] While this design does illustrate clearly how the circuit would work from a detailed technical perspective, it does not actually show anyone talking on the telephone or wearing the hearing aid. The user is utterly absent. By failing to put the user in the picture, the engineers neglected to consider the social context in which the device would be used. This is in contrast to the earlier period of amplified telephone explored in Chapter 3, during which changes in design were instigated by the user and moulded to their expectations.

While the Engineering Department attempted to perfect the design, the Telecommunications Department was receiving letters from subscribers paying the excess rental for their amplified telephones declaring that they would now refuse to pay this surplus. For these 'Deaf Subscribers', the amplified telephone naturally fell under the remit of the NHS. However, the Post Office's request for grants for those who needed the repeaters was rejected by the Ministry of Health out of hand, as 'this is not a charge which could be accepted by this department under the National Health Service ... Their primary purpose is not medical but simply to enable a telephone conversation to be heard through a hearing aid. It would seem, therefore, that they should be sold or rented by the Post Office Telephone Service.'[144]

Again, we see that the categorisation of the amplified telephone device was flexible, and subject to different party interests. The Ministry of Health reacted in a bemused fashion to the idea of a hearing aid for the telephone, and explained that: 'We have had difficulty in getting clear Otological [sic] advice about a telephone attachment to the Medresco Hearing Aid ... Would you be good enough, therefore to have a model sent to us, so that we can have it examined by Otologists?'[145] As the body responsible for government healthcare policies, the Ministry of Health felt that the adaptor designed for hearing loss should rightly have been handled by medical experts in hearing loss. However, the amplified telephone had been designed in response to user demand, by engineers. What is abundantly clear is that users were not included in any part of this process.

It was at this point in 1949 that the Ministry of Health asserted its position regarding the need to provide telephones to the deaf. As well as deeming amplified telephony to be outside its remit, it also decreed the adaptor to be unnecessary, and one minister complained to the Post Office that: 'Under the National Health Service Act we have no power to sell "gadgets".'[146] A vitriolic dispute between the two government bodies ensued. A similar struggle over prosthetic provision was ongoing at this time between the Ministry of Health and the Ministry of Pensions, as both bodies argued that wheelchairs were not part of their remit.[147] The Post Office was adamant that access to telephony was an essential aspect of the health and well-being of the deaf, in accordance with its long experience in providing such apparatus. It was also quick to recognise that the issue at stake was whether the adaptor was categorised as medical or not, as this would determine which body took responsibility for enabling the deaf to access the telephone. The Post Office emphasised that it anticipated a large demand for the adaptor, and that the Ministry of Health should sponsor it:

> If it decides to the contrary we could hardly sell or rent an article for attachment to an aid provided free by another Government department. If you decide that an aid to hearing ordinary conversation is medical, whilst an aid to hearing telephone conversation is not, you will have some difficulty in providing suitable answers.[148]

The Ministry of Health disagreed and argued that access to *speech* was essential to health and social well-being, but access to *telephony* was not. Nevertheless, it recognised that this distinction was tenuous:

> There is some distinction between providing a hearing aid for restoring the sense of hearing, thus enabling a person to take his part in social life – important from the health point of view – and proving apparatus to enable that person to use the telephone; we feel the latter is not for us. This distinction is one which would be difficult to make in a manner convincing to the public who would be slow to understand why we provide aids free but make a charge for the adaptor. We are hoping that we may be able to persuade you to regard this adaptor as a fitment enabling a telephone to be used with a hearing aid rather than as a fitment enabling a hearing aid to be used with the telephone.[149]

The Ministry of Health interpreted the 1946 National Health Act to include 'provision of surgical, medical, and other appliances'.[150] Despite the decree that amplified telephony did not quite fit any of these headings, the adaptors were produced.[151] In fact it was a letter from the NID offering to arrange user trials of the device that rang the death knell for this project.[152] When people actually used the adaptor, it became clear that the engineers had not considered the reality of hearing aid use, particularly from a feminine perspective. Most women concealed their devices under clothing. While men would easily conceal the aid in jacket or shirt pockets, women disguised the aid under skirts, making use of stockings and suspender belts to attach the aid to their body. The failure of the engineers to envision such usage meant that the clip-on attachment was very difficult for women concealing the aid to use without partially undressing to use the phone.

Reviews on performance were therefore overwhelmingly negative. Background noise was also considered to be a major problem. In terms of increased audibility, the adaptor was considered by its users to be inferior in comparison with the Repeater Telephone 17a, the standard model still available. The Post Office had capitulated to the Ministry of Health with respect to payment, and so asked testers if they would pay 4d to 5d for the adaptor. Most testers deemed this cost excessive. However, the most problematic issue was the fact that the adapter had to be attached to the microphone of the hearing aid, which was usually embedded within garments. The first tester to respond was a woman who explained, 'I consider the aid unsuitable for a girl who wears the aid concealed under clothing as I do.'[153] The second respondent also emphasised the fact that 'if, like myself, the user wears the aid concealed, it means that one has to detach the microphone case from the inside of ones [sic] apparel each time it is used'.[154] Similar objections were made by all the female correspondents, but perhaps the most succinct expression of the problem came from the head postmaster in Malton, Yorkshire, who had been using an amplified telephone for his work at the Post Office for years. He asked if he could test out the adaptor and responded to its trial with a detailed letter. While he felt the adaptor was useful for his purposes, he candidly pointed out that:

> Now, how a woman would manipulate the phone and where she would fit her aid is up to her, but she could hardly be expected to partly undress, and women are a bit keen to undisclose the aid outside, but to me – a man – I don't mind in the least as it is results I am concerned about. I must hear at all costs – regardless of sight of plastic bands etc.[155]

The adaptor perfectly suited the needs of its designers but not the needs of their so-called 'Deaf Subscribers'. By choosing not to consult people with hearing loss who wore hearing aids and desired to use the telephone, the Post Office had engineered a device that was completely unsuitable for the everyday lived reality of hearing loss. In fact, they had designed an aid that was inconvenient for everyone. Everyone, that is, *except* for a stereotypical man working in an office for the Post Office. Figure 4.3 shows such idealised use of the telephone

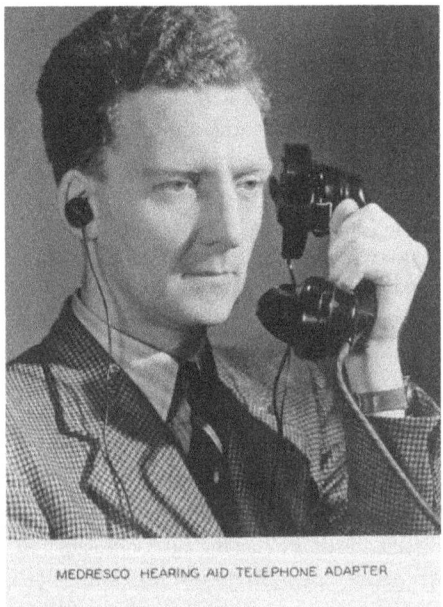

Figure 4.3 The Medresco hearing aid telephone adapter

adaptor, with a man wearing work clothes hiding the microphone easily in his pockets.

I have previously argued, with philosopher Havi Carel, that this is a 'paradigmatic case of intersectionality, in which hearing loss and female identity intersected to produce an inability to access assistive technology which was particularly harmful to women with hearing loss'.[156] As demonstrated in the postmaster's quote, the extra obligation on women to hide their hearing aid amplified their difficulties in accessing amplified telephony. Women were both subjected to a more powerful social requirement to conceal hearing loss and were further impacted by the fact that the device could not be used by women wearing dresses in the way it could by men wearing suits.[157]

The engineers' purely technical approach did not allow for consideration of the social aspects of deafness. There was no awareness of the stigma that surrounded hearing loss or the difference that gender made to the way people wanted to use such devices. In the case of the head postmaster in Yorkshire, he had to simply *hear* at all costs, whereas for the female correspondents, concealment was prioritised over efficiency. Thanks to the overwhelmingly negative feedback from users, the Post Office cancelled the project. The decision not to consult end users at the start of the design process meant that the product was not acceptable to people with hearing loss who desired access to telephony.

Conclusion

I began this chapter by writing about my Mum, and my thoughts turn to her again as I conclude it. Recently she explained to me that she prefers to talk to me on the phone only while in the car – even while sitting stationary on the driveway – because by routing her mobile through the car's speaker system via Bluetooth she can ensure that she can hear me. Out of the car, she makes sure she hears the phone ringing by linking it with her smartwatch, so she can both feel and see incoming calls, alarms or texts. These are innovative individual solutions to an issue that is not widely considered to be problematic. Although there are now some mobile phones designed for the elderly which feature higher volume levels, these are notably expensive and certainly not something one could get state assistance to access. Yet during the interwar years, access to telephony for those with hearing loss was considered by the Post Office to be a crucial part of the health service. Solutions for hearing loss are now often focused on individual fixes designed to enhance access to conversation and one wonders if this would be the case if we had prioritised equitable access to a wider world of sound in the interwar period, including access to telephony, recorded music and cinema.

In many ways, the failure to do so rested on the categorisation of speech as crucial to health, while access to sound more broadly was not so categorised. This chapter has emphasised contested categorisation issues throughout, by highlighting the different technical, medical and social influences which impacted on the categorisation of hearing aids and hearing loss during the interwar period. The drive to consider hearing as quantifiable was impacted by the need to compensate for hearing loss occasioned by warfare. Audiometry was therefore embraced as an objective test of hearing loss, which could confound malingerers and allow for quick testing of large groups of people. Furthermore, this more precise testing method expanded the numbers (particularly children) who could be categorised as deaf. This more scientific method of testing was also applied to the prescription of hearing aids, as administration was taken over by the field of medicine, despite the protestations of hearing aid manufacturers and advertisers, who emphasised the status of hearing aids as unregulated 'apparatus'. A similar interpretation of the amplified telephone as an 'adjunct' was invoked by the Ministry of Health as a way to ignore their responsibility for providing access to telephony under the NHS. While this marked the end of the Post Office's amplified telephone service, it also signalled a more technocratic approach to hearing loss, which could now be measured objectively and numerically. As the next chapter will demonstrate, strict instrumental measurement of normal sensorial functioning simultaneously defined firm thresholds of disability, which did not necessarily connect with the lives and experiences of those categorised as such.

Notes

1 Thompson, E., *The Soundscape of Modernity* (Cambridge, MA: MIT Press, 2002), p. 96.
2 Ibid., p. 148.
3 West, W., *Room Noise and Reverberation* (Post Office Green Paper No. 2) (London: His Majesty's Stationery Office, 1934).
4 Ibid., p. 4.
5 Ibid., pp. 6–7.
6 Ibid., p. 7.
7 Thompson, *The Soundscape of Modernity*, p. 148.
8 West, *Room Noise and Reverberation*, p. 7.
9 Kerridge, P. M. T., *Hearing and Speech in Deaf Children* (Medical Research Council: Reports of the Hearing Committee, Special Report Series No. 221) (London: His Majesty's Stationery Office, 1937), p. 20.
10 Concert pitch was also standardised as A = 440 in the 1930s. See Gribenski, F., 'Negotiating the Pitch: For a Diplomatic History of A, at the Crossroads of Politics,

Music, Science and Industry', in F. Ramel and C. Prévost-Thomas (eds), *International Relations, Music and Diplomacy: Sounds and Voices on the International Stage* (Cham: Palgrave Macmillan, 2018), pp. 173–192.
11 Thompson, *The Soundscape of Modernity*, p. 119.
12 West, *Room Noise and Reverberation*, p. 6.
13 Ibid., p. 5.
14 Virdi [Virdi-Dhesi], 'Curtis's Cephaloscope', p. 349.
15 Ibid. For more on the professionalisation of aurists see Virdi [Virdi-Dhesi], J., 'From the Hands of Quacks: Aural Surgery, Deafness, and the Making of a Surgical Speciality in 19th Century London' (PhD dissertation, University of Toronto, 2014).
16 What we would now determine as either sensorineural or bone conductive. Mills, 'Deafening', p. 125.
17 Sterne, *The Audible Past*.
18 Hughes, D. E., 'On an Induction-Currents Balance, and Experimental Researches Made Therewith', *Proceedings of the Royal Society of London*, 29:196–199 (1879), 56–65, p. 58.
19 Kay, 'Inventing Telephone Usage', p. 52.
20 Hughes, 'On an Induction-Currents Balance', p. 58. Emphasis added.
21 Richardson, B. W., 'Some Researches with Professor Hughes' New Instrument for the Measurement of Hearing: The Audiometer', *Proceedings of the Royal Society of London*, 29:196–199 (1879), 65–66, p. 65.
22 Kay, 'Inventing Telephone Usage', p. 55.
23 Fraser-Harris, D. F., 'The Treatment of Deafness', *The Lancet*, 224:5792 (1934), 481–483, p. 481.
24 Report of Societies, 'Tests and Classifications of Hearing', *British Medical Journal*, 10:2/3540 (1928), 845–848, p. 847.
25 Bunch, C. C., 'Methods of Testing the Hearing in Infants and Young Children', *Journal of Paediatrics*, 5:4 (1934), 535–544, p. 537.
26 'Minutes of the Meeting of the Medical Committee of the National Institute for the Deaf, 6th of March 1931'. AOHL.
27 Fraser-Harris, 'The Treatment of Deafness', p. 482.
28 Balbi, C. M. R., 'The Audiometer and Its Application to Medical Research', *The Lancet*, 205:5305 (1925), 954–956, p. 954.
29 Ibid.
30 Anon., 'The Problem of the Deaf', *The Lancet*, 220:5703 (1932), 1347–1349, p. 1347 [summary of report by Dr A. Eichholz CBE to the Ministry of Health and the Board of Education].
31 Turner, 'Remarks on Cases'.
32 Clark, B. M. J., 'The Rejection of Psychological Approaches to Mental Disorder in Late Nineteenth-Century Psychiatry', in A. Scull (ed.), *Madhouses, Mad-Doctors, and Madmen: The Social History of Psychiatry in the Victorian Era* (London: Athlone, 1981), pp. 271–312.
33 Turner, 'Remarks on Cases', p. 834.

34 Linden, S. C., and Jones, E., '"Shell Shock" Revisited: An Examination of the Case Records of the National Hospital', *Medical History*, 58:4 (2014), 519–545, p. 531.
35 Anon., 'War Injuries and Neuroses of the Ear', *The Lancet*, 189:4878 (1917), 304.
36 The complex condition of shell shock has been described very well by a number of scholars so will not be repeated here. See, for example, Barham, P., *Forgotten Lunatics of the Great War* (New Haven, CT: Yale University Press, 2004); Reid, F., *Broken Men: Shell Shock, Treatment and Recovery in Britain 1914–30* (London: Continuum, 2010); Meyer, J., 'Not Septimus Now: Wives of Disabled Veterans and Cultural Memory of the First World War in Britain', *Women's History Review*, 13:1 (2004), 117–138; and Scull, *Hysteria*.
37 Enke, 'War Noises on the Battlefield', p. 13.
38 McBride, P., and Turner, A. L., 'War Deafness, with Special Reference to the Value of Vestibular Tests', *The Lancet*, 192:4951 (1918), 73–74. Logan Turner's 1924 book on *Diseases of the Ear, Throat and Nose* is still in print today and its 11th edition is considered essential reading.
39 McBride and Turner, 'War Deafness'.
40 Arthur Hurst (1879–1944) is now best known for his MRC-sponsored filming of shell-shocked patients at Seale Hayne Hospital in Devon. See Hurst, A. F., and Peters, E. A., 'A Report on the Pathology, Diagnosis and Treatment of Absolute Hysterical Deafness in Soldiers', *The Lancet*, 190:4910 (1917), 517–519, p. 517.
41 'Malingering Tests' section of instruction booklet attached to audiometer, accessed at the Thackray Medical Museum, Leeds.
42 Ibid.
43 Crowden, G. P., 'Measurement of Deafness in School-Children', *The Lancet*, 218:5650 (1931), 1324–1325, p. 1324.
44 Anon., 'The Problem of the Deaf', p. 1347.
45 Bunch, C. C., 'Methods of Testing the Hearing in Infants and Young Children', *Journal of Paediatrics*, 5:4 (1934), 535–544, p. 539. For the point about precision see Anon., 'The Hearing Power of School-Children', *The Lancet*, 222:5754 (1933), 1328.
46 Latour and Woolgar refer to the end product as 'literary inscription' in Latour, B., and Woolgar, S., *Laboratory Life* (Princeton, NJ: Princeton University Press, 1979), p. 63.
47 Mills, 'Deafening', p. 129.
48 Anon., 'The Hearing Power of School-Children', p. 1328.
49 Fletcher, H., 'Physical Measurements of Audition and Their Bearing on the Theory of Hearing', *Journal of the Franklin Institute*, 196:3 (1923), 289–326, p. 297. This article was written while Fletcher was working at the research laboratories of AT&T in New York.
50 Kerridge, *Hearing and Speech in Deaf Children*, p. 20.
51 Virdi and McGuire, 'Phyllis M. Tookey Kerridge', p. 128.
52 Anon., 'Hearing-Aids: A Report to the Medical Research Council', *The Lancet*, 229:5919 (1937), 340–341, p. 340.

53 Minutes of the NID Medical Committee, 31 March 1926. AOHL.
54 Fry, D. B., and Kerridge, P. M. T., 'Tests for the Hearing of Speech by Deaf People', *The Lancet*, 233:6020 (1939), 106–109, p. 106.
55 Virdi and McGuire, 'Phyllis M. Tookey Kerridge', p. 130.
56 Esmail, *Reading Victorian Deafness*.
57 'Ears Good?', p. 370, quoted in Thompson, *Soundscape of Modernity*, n. 137.
58 Berger, K. W., 'Genealogy of the Words "Audiology" and "Audiologist"', *Journal of the American Audiology Society*, 2:2 (1976), 38–44, p. 38.
59 Ibid., p. 40.
60 Fraser-Harris, 'The Treatment of Deafness', p. 481.
61 Thompson, *The Soundscape of Modernity*, p. 89.
62 For a full review of Kerridge's contributions to the standardisation of audiometry see Virdi and McGuire, 'Phyllis M. Tookey Kerridge' and the forthcoming book on Kerridge by the same authors.
63 Ibid., p. 126.
64 Kerridge, *Hearing and Speech in Deaf Children*, p. 8.
65 Ibid., p. 29.
66 Noble, *Assessment of Impaired Hearing*, p. 176.
67 Kerridge, *Hearing and Speech in Deaf Children*, p. 24.
68 Virdi and McGuire, 'Phyllis M. Tookey Kerridge', p. 134.
69 Ibid., p. 139.
70 Berger, 'Genealogy of the Words "Audiology" and "Audiologist"', p. 40.
71 Fraser-Harris, 'The Treatment of Deafness', p. 481.
72 The first electric hearing aid was created by Miller Reese Hutchinson in 1891 through combining the telephone with the carbon transmitter. For more on the evolution of electric hearing aids see Mills, M., 'Hearing Aids and the History of Electronics Miniaturization', *IEEE Annals of the History of Computing*, 33:2 (2011), 24–45, p. 27.
73 The National Benevolent Society for the Deaf, Annual Reports, 1918–1952. AOHL.
74 The National Benevolent Society for the Deaf, Annual Report 1938. AOHL.
75 The National Benevolent Society for the Deaf, Annual Report 1924. AOHL.
76 Discharged Soldiers (Deafness), HC Deb 2 July 1917, vol. 95, cc. 741–742. http://hansard.millbanksystems.com/commons/1917/jul/02/discharged-soldiers-deafness#S5CV0095P0_19170702_HOC_98. Accessed via Hansard, March 2015.
77 Ibid.
78 'Supply of Electrophones: 1938–1939'. TNA, PIN 38/452. The Disablement Branch was a dedicated branch that had been concerned with advances in prostheses before this point and had been involved in or aware of the testing of soldiers for deaf pensions, but it was only in 1922 that it became involved with hearing aids. For example, see Inter Allied Committee for the Study of Questions Concerning the Disabled, 'Review of the Technical and Scientific Institute of Prosthesis and Surgical Apparatus', January 1922. Wellcome Library, London, MS 9200, Box 440.

79 Letter from Director General of Medical Services to the Commissioner of Medical Services, MOP, Northern Region, 1922. TNA, PIN 38/449/9. Dundas Grant was also the Honorary Consultant Aurist to the Ministry and became a KBE in 1920 for his work in this respect. He tried to instantiate the use of the unit of 'percentage hearing' but his efforts were criticised in Kerridge, *Hearing and Speech in Deaf Children*, p. 27.
80 Letter from Mears Ear Phone Co., London to the MOP, 1922. TNA, PIN 38/450/23.
81 See reports: 'Aural Appliances Electrophones – supply of: 1920–1923'. TNA, PIN 38/449; 'Aural Appliances Electrophones – supply of: 1924–1926'. TNA, PIN 38/450; 'Aural Appliances Electrophones – supply of: 1926–1929'. TNA, PIN 38/451; and 'Aural Appliances Supply of Electrophones 1938–1939'. TNA, PIN 38/452.
82 Gooday and Sayer, *Managing the Experience of Hearing Loss*, p. 110.
83 Ibid.
84 Ibid., p. 108.
85 Mills, 'When Mobile Communication Technologies Were New', p. 144.
86 Gooday and Sayer, *Managing the Experience of Hearing Loss*, p. 84.
87 Mills, 'Hearing Aids and the History of Electronics Miniaturization'. See also stamp book advertisements for hearing aids sent to the Post Office from complaining customers. British Postal Museum Archive, London (BPMA), POST 33/3481B.
88 Stols electrophone advertisement booklet sent to the MOP. 'Aural Appliances Electrophones – supply of: 1924–1926'.
89 Fortiphone advertisement sent to the MOP. 'Aural Appliances Supply of Electrophones 1938–1939'.
90 Hays, 'The Social and Economic Importance of Deafness', p. 303, quoted in Virdi, J., 'Prevention and Conservation: Historicizing the Stigma of Hearing Loss, 1910–1940', *Journal of Law, Medicine and Ethics*, 45:4 (2017), 531–344, p. 535.
91 This situation could only have been deemed a success if the woman was in fact trying to deliberately waste her admirer's time and avoid having to listen to him. Mears earphones advertisement sent to the MOP. 'Aural Appliances Electrophones – supply of: 1924–1926'.
92 McGuire and Carel, 'The Visible and the Invisible'.
93 Cureton, 'Hiding a Disability and Passing as Non-Disabled'.
94 Virdi, 'Prevention and Conservation', p. 533.
95 Mills, 'Hearing Aids and the History of Electronics Miniaturization', p. 30.
96 Gooday and Sayer, *Managing the Experience of Hearing Loss*. I thank Karen Sayer for taking the time to explain this point to me in more detail.
97 Mills, 'Hearing Aids and the History of Electronics Miniaturization', p. 30.
98 For a fully detailed history of this phenomenon see Virdi, J., *Hearing Happiness: Fakes, Frauds, and Fads in Deafness Cures* (Chicago: University of Chicago Press, forthcoming).
99 Kerridge, P. M. T., 'Can Physics Help the Deaf Child?', *The Lancet*, 225:5811 (1935), 104–108, p. 106.

100 Ibid., p. 107.
101 Ibid.
102 Ibid. This observation also gives an interesting insight (or inear?) into the sound quality of 1930s cinema.
103 Mills, 'Hearing Aids and the History of Electronics Miniaturization', p. 30.
104 Kerridge, 'Can Physics Help the Deaf Child?', p. 108.
105 Anon., 'The Limitations of Hearing-Aids', *The Lancet*, 229:5920 (1937), 395–396, p. 395.
106 'The Eleventh Annual Meeting of the National Institute for the Deaf, July 30, 1935'. AOHL (edited for length).
107 Stevens, A. E., Letter to the Editor, 'Hearing Aids for Deafness', *The Lancet*, 231:5988 (1938), p. 1307.
108 Yearsley, M., Letter to the Editor, 'Hearing Aids for Deafness', *The Lancet*, 231:5981 (1938), p. 914.
109 In 1920, 5,716,000,000 postal packets were delivered according to F. H. Williamson, 'Post and Postal Services', BPMA, POST 72/211. 'Post Office Statistics', The Postal Museum. www.postalmuseum.org/discover/collections/statistics/. Accessed May 2019.
110 'Mr Smailes, minister of the Methodist church, at The Knoll, Elham, near Canterbury, Kent, to the Public Relation Office, May 23, 1938'. BPMA, POST 33/3481B.
111 Letter from the NID to the Postmaster General, 8 April 1936. BPMA, POST 33/3481B.
112 Letter from the NID to Major Tyron, Postmaster General, 16 December. BPMA, POST 33/3481B.
113 Letter from the NID to the Post Office, Major Tyron, Postmaster General, 13 May 1938. BPMA, POST 33/3481B.
114 House of Commons Sittings, 2 June 1933, vol. 278, c. 2237. http://hansard.millbanksystems.com/commons/1933/jun/02/post-office-advertisements#S5CV0278P0_19330602_HOC_4. Accessed via Hansard, November 2014.
115 Response to Mr Sutcliffe, Thursday, 29 July 1937. BPMA, POST 33/3481B.
116 Internal report, Postmaster General, Slip G. Undated but judging by context 1937. BPMA, POST 33/3481B.
117 House of Commons Debate, 30 March 1936, vol. 310, c. 1609. http://hansard.millbanksystems.com/commons/1936/mar/30/advertisements#S5CV0310P0_19360330_HOC_68. Accessed via Hansard, November 2014.
118 Internal memorandum. BPMA, POST 33/3481B.
119 House of Commons Sitting, 7 December 1936, vol. 318, c. 1624. https://api.parliament.uk/historic-hansard/commons/1936/dec/07/advertisements#S5CV0318P0_19361207_HOC_82%3E. Accessed via Hansard, May 2019.
120 Postmaster General Major Tyron, 6 December 1937. BPMA, POST 33/3481B.
121 Postmaster General Major Tyron, 11 December 1936. BPMA, POST 33/3481B. It should be noted that the Post Office did refuse to endorse various products and

the list of prohibited advertisements included: alcoholic liquor, temperance (antiliquor), lotteries, imitations of Post Office marks, bookmakers, football pools, betting and gambling, birth control and rubber goods, clairvoyants, astrology and palmistry, foreign agricultural produce, offers of employment, private telephone installations, money lenders, illustrations of Royal Family, questionable or controversial books and periodicals, political advertisements, offers of employment, annuity business and patent medicines. They further restricted advertisements for building societies, anti-vivisection, electro-radiant treatment, parcel deliveries and corsets and lingerie. See 'Restriction to Post Office Advertising'. BPMA, POST 33/3481B.

122 Bramwell, E., 'Rethinking Patent Medicine Culture in Britain, 1909–1949' (PhD dissertation, University of Lancaster, forthcoming).

123 'The Bill has the support of the medical profession and the pharmaceutical and advertisement trades, but opponents of the Bill seemed to suspect them of a financial interest in its success, and to resent the rigid conservatism of the medical profession'. See report 'Patent Medicines', *The Spectator*, 3 April 1936. www.archive.spectator.co.uk. Accessed March 2016.

124 Letter from the Council of the British Medical Association to the Postmaster General, 23 February 1938. BPMA, POST 33/3481B.

125 Sir Wyndham Childs, 'Warning to 2,000,000 Deaf', *John Bull*, 7 March 1936, p. 19. BPMA, POST 33/3481B.

126 Medical and Surgical Appliances (Advertisement) Bill, House of Commons Sitting Deb, 27 March 1936, vol. 310, cc. 1563–1600. http://hansard.millbanksystems.com/commons/1936/mar/27/medicines-and-surgical-appliances#S5CV0310P0_19360327_HOC_7. Accessed via Hansard, November 2014.

127 'Fremantle, Sir Francis Edward', in Royal College of Surgeons, *Plarr's Lives of the Fellows*. http://livesonline.rcseng.ac.uk/biogs/E004111b.htm. Accessed December 2014.

128 Sir Francis Fremantle to Sir Kingsley Wood (passed to Major Tyron). BPMA, POST 33/3481B.

129 Peden, G. C., *British Rearmament and the Treasury: 1932–1939* (Edinburgh: Scottish Academic Press, 1979), p. 3.

130 Ibid., p. 9.

131 Crutchley, E. T., *GPO* (Cambridge: Cambridge University Press, 1938), p. 78.

132 'The Divergence of Postal/Telecom Profits'. BPMA, Post Office Statistics. www.postalheritage.org.uk/page/statistics. Accessed February 2020.

133 The naming of this device has led to overemphasis on the MRC's role in its creation, with attendant erasure of the work of the Post Office. Medresco was also the name used for the MRC in telegram correspondence.

134 Letter from the Engineering Department to the Telecommunications Department, 30 September 1946. BTA, TCB 2/172.

135 Memorandum, Ministry of Health Hearing Aid. 'Hearing Aid Adaptor to Permit Use of the Aid with the Telephone in Special Apparatus Fitted on Telephone Exchange Lines Rented by Deaf Subscribers'. BTA, TCB 2/172.

136 Engineering Department, Branch S Memorandum, Ministry of Health Hearing Aid. 'Hearing Aid Adaptor to Permit Use of the Aid and the Telephone'. BTA, TCB 2/172. See also MRC, *Hearing Aids and Audiometers* (Special Report Series No. 261) (London: His Majesty's Stationery Office, 1949).
137 Memorandum, Ministry of Health Hearing Aid. 'Hearing Aid Adaptor'.
138 Ibid.
139 Public Relations Department memorandum to Engineering Department, 27 July 1946, in 'Special Apparatus Fitted on Telephone Exchange Lines Rented by Deaf Subscribers'. Henceforth SA, BTA, TCB 2/172.
140 Ibid.
141 Memorandum, September 1947. SA, BTA, TCB 2/172.
142 Telecommunications Department to the Engineering Department, 29 July 1947. SA, BTA, TCB 2/172.
143 Letter from the S. Branch Engineering Department to the Telecommunications Department, 'Ministry of Health Hearing Aid', 27 July 1946. BTA, TCB 2/172.
144 Ministry of Health to the Post Office 30 April 1949. SA, BTA, TCB 2/172.
145 Ministry of Health to G. P. Wooley, Telecommunications Department, 26 May 1948. SA, BTA, TCB 2/172.
146 Letter from Ministry of Health to Post Office, June 1949. SA, BTA, TCB 2/172.
147 Woods, B., and Watson, N., 'In Pursuit of Standardization: The British Ministry of Health's Model 8F Wheelchair, 1948–1962', *Technology and Culture*, 45:3 (2003), 540–568, p. 554.
148 Post Office to the Ministry of Health, 14 May 1949 (emphasis added). SA, BTA, TCB 2/172.
149 Ministry of Health reply to the Post Office, June 1949 (emphasis added). SA, BTA, TCB 2/172.
150 Woods and Watson, 'In Pursuit of Standardization', p. 555.
151 Although they were designed by the Post Office research and engineering departments, the Plessey Company provided the equipment to make the prototypes.
152 This trial was with members of the London League for the Hard of Hearing (which was also testing out the Medresco).
153 Letter from NID to Post Office Headquarters, St Martin's Le Grand, London, 16 October 1950. SA, BTA, TCB 2/172.
154 Letter from NID to Post Office Headquarters, St Martin's Le Grand, London, 13 December 1950. SA, BTA, TCB 2/172.
155 Letter from Head Post Office, Malton to R. W. Clarke (Sales Division), 26 April 1951. SA, BTA, TCB 2/172.
156 McGuire and Carel, 'The Visible and the Invisible'.
157 Ibid.

5

THE SPIROMETER AND THE NORMAL SUBJECTS

Normal breathing for whom?

During one of the Life of Breath project research meetings in 2018, consultant Dr Sara Booth recounted the story of a school teacher who felt such pressure to consistently hold her stomach in when standing in front of the class that her subsequent propensity to breathe costally (from her chest) impacted on her ability to breathe in fully – with the result that her respiratory problems were exacerbated. As I sat listening to Dr Booth talk, I wondered: how much does such lived experience of being a woman in the world impact on the ability to fill our lungs? Are we not taking our fair share of air? I argue here that we must also consider how life experiences might impact on respiration.

The way that we experience breathlessness is moderated by both the mind and the body. Furthermore, levels of breathlessness cannot be consistently linked to discrete phases of illness.[1] Yet attempts to capture this experience with objective measures such as those offered by spirometry have obscured this multi-dimensional quality.[2] As a result, the measurement of breathlessness in a strictly medical paradigm has privileged the physiological symptoms of breathlessness in a way that fails to account for the lived experience of the patient.[3] Increasingly, researchers have demonstrated disconnect between the subjective individuality of breathlessness and its numerical correlation.[4] In this chapter I argue that considering the *history* of the measurement of breathlessness sheds light on this recurring disjunct between objective and subjective measures. This chapter explores how the drive to translate breathlessness into quantifiable, scalable measures has been influenced by complex historical interactions between medical expertise, industrial interests and compensation schemes. Considering these historical interactions highlights the related processes by which we have variously decided which groups counted as medically distinguishable populations. In other words, whose bodies mattered for these measurements. Who were the normal subjects? And was normal breathing universal or varied between groups?

As I show in the first section, spirometry was developed in the nineteenth century as a physiological test designed first to measure the volume of air that an individual could exhale and second to express this as a number indicating individual 'vital capacity'. Although these tests later developed to account for residual air in the lungs and now include a timed component, in its initial iteration the spirometer simply measured lung volume through measuring individuals' exhalatory ability to displace a volume of water measured in litres.[5] This became known as a person's 'vital capacity'. As medical historian Lundy Braun explains, this meant that for the first time: 'with the help of this new, refined instrument, "lung capacity" became a discrete entity that could be measured, quantified, and ranked'.[6] The spirometer thus presented vital capacity as lung capacity. Yet using vital capacity to determine health, or even levels of breathlessness, was immediately problematic for clinicians – especially when measuring women, for reasons explained in the section on 'Breathing like a girl'.

In the following sections, I track the changing normal values used in spirometry. These values will be refracted through the prism of two groups considered to be significant categories at different points in the twentieth century – women and miners. Taking this thematic approach highlights the interactions between race, class and gender in spirometry. In each case I move from the end of the nineteenth century to the present day, allowing for a fruitful comparison between the groups. By considering the first group, women, I demonstrate how difference in lung function between men and women was established, and the varying extent to which such differences were attributed to biological or societal causes. Similarly, analysing the efforts to define normal lung function for miners, my second group, highlights the extent to which abnormal lung function was attributed to the essential nature of the miner's body, and underlines the impact of politics on the classification of respiratory disability.

As the definitive essay 'Throwing Like a Girl' by I. M. Young, which has inspired one of the section headings for this chapter, argued, there are 'certain observable and rather ordinary ways in which women in our society typically comport themselves and move differently from the ways that men do'.[7] That such ways of being in the world might impact on health is the implication in Janet Shim's work on how the categories of race, gender and class are used in epidemiological studies of heart disease. For example, she concludes that for most of the researchers she interviewed, differences between men and women were regarded as simple and clearly *binary* biological differences.[8] However, one epidemiologist did postulate that 'processes related to gender discrimination and perhaps the stress of both attempting to conform to as well as resist normative gender roles could be reasonably hypothesized to affect cardiovascular health'.[9] It is this position that the people living with heart disease overwhelmingly expressed in Shim's interviews. That is, they 'understood gender relations as relations of power and experienced their manifestations as embodied sources of distress, grief, regret, and anger that they explicitly constructed as significant risks to their cardiovascular health'.[10] Such power relations intersected with race and class to produce chronic, structural oppressions and stresses that extracted a corporeal cost to health.[11] Braun's work on the racialisation of spirometry has similar implications, as she outlines the growing evidence pointing to the importance of considering social and environmental explanations as causal explanations for difference in lung function over genetic difference. Indeed, Braun's book memorably concludes with the exhortation that we must consider lung health as reflective of individual lived experience and intersectional oppressions.[12] As the pioneering work of researchers such as Anna Louise Kirkengen has established, the cumulative impact of successive strains can be considered using an 'allostatic load' model, which suggests that overload to the body's stress responses overtaxes the immune system, the hormonal system and the central nervous system, leading to subsequent body pathologies.[13]

If this is the case, we might see that certain disease causations linked to the biological traits of a group may in fact be the result of specific ways of living as a member of that group, as I argue was the case with the measurement of miners. How, then, should we classify this group – if indeed they should be so classified? And if we decide on a suitable reference class, how would we then define and assess normalcy in that group? In this chapter I use historical case studies to argue that the selection of healthy subjects to create a standard of normalcy worked as a powerful way to manipulate the categorisation of disability as well as obscuring its true causes.

The development of spirometry

John Hutchinson (1811–61) coined the term spirometer and defined vital capacity as 'the *volume* of air that a man can force out of his chest'.[14] For most of the twentieth century spirometry was used as part of large clinical or anthropometric studies rather than becoming incorporated into routine patient diagnostics in the way that the stethoscope was. Only a very few spirometers from the early twentieth century remain, which indicates that these were not ubiquitous diagnostic tools. The spirometers from this period that we do have

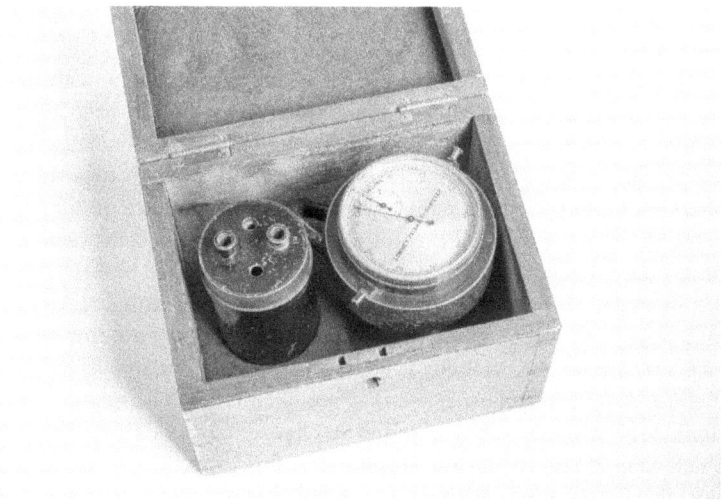

Figure 5.1 Lowne spirometer, 1904

are large, to the extent that it is impossible to fit them in most museum display cases used at the Royal College of Surgeons and the Thackray Museum. They are also heavy and cumbersome, difficult for an individual to carry. The Lowne spirometer from 1906 shown in Figure 5.1 retailed at four pounds and fifteen shillings (around £371) and was kept in a heavy, mahogany, felt-lined box that further indicated its expense and rarity.

The word 'spirometer' translates literally as breath measurer. However, this translation greatly simplifies the working of this instrument, which only estimates lung capacity as 'vital capacity'. Yet actuaries were able to wield spirometers to accurately predict premature mortality, and indeed Hutchinson had originally suggested that they should be used in military assessment and in actuarial prediction for life insurance policies.[15] Similar devices, known as pulmometers, had been used previously in clinical investigations, for example by Charles Turner Thackrah (1795–1833) in his 1832 study of the industrial workers of Leeds.[16]

However, Hutchinson is regarded as the inventor of vital capacity because he found that with every inch of height vital capacity increased by 8 cubic inches.[17] He arrived at this conclusion after using the spirometer to collect data from over 4,000 test subjects, categorised by variables including occupation and class. He divided his subjects into types, including paupers, sailors, firemen, grenadier guards, mixed classes, diseased cases, gentlemen and pugilists.[18] Hutchinson then created corresponding tables showing what the ideal vital capacity ought to be for height. Hutchinson argued that the measure of vital capacity was impacted by attributes including height, attitude, weight, age and disease.[19]

Nineteenth-century attempts to accurately measure and scale lung capacity through the spirometer were complicated by the need to first define the measure for normal breathing – there can be no abnormal without an initial definition of the normal. Classification and categorisation of relevant group varieties perpetuated scientific acceptance of difference between these groups, and the notion that these groups constituted distinct natural kinds.[20] This phenomenon was first identified by Braun, who demonstrated that correcting for race in spirometry cemented acceptance of difference between racial groups.[21] The classification of entities such as race, sex, disease and disability is highly controversial and important, as in the process of being constructed they are often fashioned as natural divisions. As scholars such as Bowker and Star have attested, this is not so much a reflection of reality as it is a shaping of reality.[22] Yet the objectivity and trust that we associate with numerical scales means that their related classification schema become invisible as categories are replicated as though they are inevitable and natural.[23] The attempt to standardise the parameters of normal breathing has thus long been complicated by the drive to categorise the social groups that should represent the standard of normal breathing *for* that particular group.

Hutchinson's ideal vital capacity tables represented the standard data sets for assessing normal lung function until after the First World War, when Georges Dreyer (1873–1934) asserted in 1919 that lung capacity standards for pilots needed to be more strictly measured.[24] Vital capacity offered a quick and easy way to assess physical fitness and so was used as a routine test in the examination of candidates for the Royal Flying Corps, with the results leading to either rejection or acceptance based on an arbitrary minimum standard. Men with superior respiratory capabilities were sought out for their capacity to withstand the atmosphere of the open cockpits.[25] Incidentally, these open cockpits had noise levels of up to 125 decibels, which meant many First World War pilots ended their careers with substantial hearing loss.[26] As a result, 'the Americans considered letting deaf men fly, reasoning that pilots could not hear anything anyway'.[27] While hearing was not considered relevant for successful piloting, lung capacity was. Dreyer argued that Hutchinson's results did not give enough credence to the impact of weight on lung capacity and so he created new data tables.[28] In collaboration with the MRC, he published *The Assessment of Physical Fitness by Correlation of Vital Capacity and Certain Measurements of the Body* in 1920 and dedicated the book to John Hutchinson. This was a large volume, as it chiefly comprised hundreds of tables indicating the normal ranges for weight and height, and their correlation with vital capacity. Dreyer's epigraph for the book demonstrated that it was clearly created as part of an effort to improve the nation's physical fitness, with the military particularly in mind.

Dreyer started the book with the assertion that the First World War had made physical fitness an issue of national importance. He prophesied that: 'it is only when the meaning of "the normal" with respect to these measurements is understood, and when the limits of the normal have been properly defined, that it will be possible to study with any prospect of accuracy or success the deviations from the normal'.[29] Dreyer categorised his results by grouping people into three classes – A, B and C – which represented the conditions of perfect, medium and poor physical fitness. These groupings corresponded closely with social class, with boys in public school placed in class A against children in upper-class schools who were categorised as class B. However, the impact of social class, Dreyer believed, could be transcended or depreciated by occupational training, and so Army and Navy personnel and blacksmiths were placed in class A while upper-class clerks remained in class B. Indeed, in an article published the year before in *The Lancet* Dreyer had warned against biological essentialism by emphasising that it was clear that 'difference in vital capacity exhibited by different classes has nothing to do with fundamental bodily deficiencies, but is simply a result of conditions depending upon occupation and mode of life'.[30]

Using his system, the person being measured would first be placed into their appropriate division, and then their vital capacity percentage ascertained for that group.[31] This allowed for the comparison of the reference class groupings relevant to Dreyer: age, sex, class and occupation.[32] Dreyer argued that if someone was found to have 'as much as 10 per cent less vital capacity than is normal for his class, it is probable that he is suffering from some health-depressing condition, and if he is as much as 15 per cent below the normal limit it is practically certain that he is abnormal in this respect'.[33] As Horrocks and Smith have argued, Dreyer's standardised method for classifying individuals' health was particularly appealing to the MRC because of its emphasis on standardised laboratory medicine, and its lack of reliance on a clinician's subjective opinion.[34]

Despite indicating 15 per cent as the limit of normality, Dreyer was concerned more with identifying fitness levels than with defining illness. His measurements were interpreted thus by C. B. Heald, the medical adviser to the Department of Civil Aviation, who viewed spirometry as a valuable method of measuring physical fitness, providing, as he put it, 'a scale upon which individuals can be placed in order of physical fitness'.[35] His understanding echoed earlier military observations about the utility of spirometry for assessing the general fitness of recruits. As early as 1860 an MD reported to the *British Medical Journal* that 'a vital capacity below the average may be considered rather as indicating a generally feeble organisation, less capable of resisting the deteriorating influences to which a soldier is exposed'.[36] While some accordingly saw the spirometer as providing a numerical estimation of a person's overall fitness, it was recognised by others that the spirometer could be used to identify and monitor illness progression, and that there was a subsequent need to collect comparable data on hospital patients. In 1922, Dr Charles Cameron, the medical officer working at the Ochil Hills Sanatorium in Glasgow, made such an attempt by using the Dreyer method to determine the normal vital capacity for 223 male patients. Cameron questioned Dreyer's vital capacity as being fixed arbitrarily to represent what he termed, 'the probable normal'. His observations were designed to fill this disability data gap by giving standards for patients with pulmonary tuberculosis.[37]

In 1920, Wing Commander Martin Flack argued that the vital capacity value could not adequately describe what was normal for any one individual and proposed the addition of a breath-holding test, which he believed could assess psychological fortitude as well as giving evidence of the healthy lungs needed for flying.[38] It is likely that this psychological addition was designed to identify applicants at risk of developing shell shock, which was of increasing public concern at that time, as well as working to mitigate against the fear of malingering. The potential for malingerers to abuse the spirometry test by failing to cooperate was noted as a key concern in many studies using spirometry during this period.[39] For example, miners who complained of breathlessness were often dismissed as malingerers, or their respiratory trouble was diagnosed as being of psychological origin, as we will see in the section below on 'Normal breathing for miners'.[40]

By the 1930s, Dreyer's standards had been largely discredited by statisticians.[41] In 1932, Dr Alan Moncrieff asserted that a more straightforward means of assessment was needed and pointed out (quite correctly) that the literature was strewn with disregarded methods and standards. Although he described breathlessness as 'essentially a subjective phenomenon', his view was that quantitative measures were necessary for evaluating the success of cardiovascular surgery and silicosis disability: 'The advantage of such methods is that they provide a numerical statement of the degree of respiratory efficiency or failure, but the grave disadvantage is present for all of them that normal figures may provide a too rigid standard, and wide deviation may be possible in health.'[42] Like Cameron, Moncrieff argued that 'the standards set out by Flack for the Air Force appear to be far too high for the ordinary population attending hospitals.'[43] Furthermore, he demonstrated that 94 per cent of the women he tested failed to reach the average standard for a 'normal' person.[44] As a result of such discrepancies, those wielding the spirometer began to seriously question the extent to which deviation occurred between the sexes, as discussed in the next section.

Breathing like a girl

Hutchinson had not addressed vital capacity in women in his 1846 publication, and in his second work of 1852 he admitted that he was frequently asked whether his table could also be applied to women. He responded that it was unnecessary to differentiate vital capacity measures from men to women and explained that 'we see no reason why their vital capacity should not correspond with that of men, for their chest mobility seems to exceed that of men.'[45] As we saw in Chapter 2, measuring women was simply perceived as more difficult than measuring men, and Hutchinson elaborated that 'we do not know the vital capacity of women, nor is it easy to determine it', and mused upon the extent to which the use of corsetry impacted on women's breathing: 'when clothed, as women in this country are wont to attire, they all seem to breathe the same volume as if they lived under one uniform tightness in dress.'[46] He elaborated on the potential impact of tight stays further when he noted: 'Observations upon females are more difficult. We never heard a woman acknowledge that she wore her clothes tight, and we have put this question to thousands, and yet we believe a certain number do wear tight dresses.'[47]

As the dressing habits of Victorian women remained mysterious to him, Hutchinson chose to use the vital capacity of men as standard for women rather than making separate studies. However, this was an unusual move to make in a medical milieu fascinated by the science of difference. Others soon called for representative studies to clarify the normal range of vital capacity in women. The influential statistician and eugenicist Francis Galton (discussed in Chapter 1), for instance, separated his anthropometric studies by sex, as in the 1883 Final Report of the Anthropometric Committee of the British Association for the Advancement of Science, which included breathing capacity standards for boys and girls.[48] But difficulties in measuring women abounded. Galton decided against measuring women's heads when they visited his anthropometric laboratory at the international health exhibition because 'it would be troublesome to perform on most women on account of their bonnets, and the bulk of their hair, and that it would lead to objections and difficulties.'[49] Again, women proved too 'troublesome' to measure easily.

Yet unconventional sexologist Havelock Ellis made use of the spirometer in his 1904 study of 'man and woman'. He started his chapter on respiration with the claim that 'it is well recognised that the "vital capacity", as the breathing power indicated by the spirometer is commonly called, is decidedly less in women than in men'.[50] He elaborated that vital capacity was 3 litres in women compared to 3½ litres in a man of equal height, and that height increased vital capacity in men to a greater extent than in women.[51] Ruminating on the causes for this discrepancy, Ellis attributed it to the fact that women had 'a less keen need of air' and noted that they fared better both at high altitudes and in occupations working in front of hot stoves.[52] Various theories were espoused to explain the lower lung capacity of women. One of the most enduring theories was that men's respirations naturally stemmed from the diaphragm while women breathed from the chest (costal breathing). This point was raised by Hutchinson in 1846 in his reported remarks to the Royal Medical and Chirurgical Society: 'The breathing in women differed from men only in one respect, their ordinary breathing being chiefly costal and not abdominal. Whether this was due to gestation or not he could not say; he thought there was some doubt of its being caused by the peculiarities of their costume.'[53] Ellis also believed that women breathed costally (from the chest) rather than from the diaphragm, noting that 'The characteristic costal breathing of women begins, according to Sibson, about the tenth year of life.'[54] However, such breathing was, for Ellis, largely attributable to the constraint of corseted dresses.

The association between corsets and costal breathing meant that this type of breath was linked, at least for Ellis and his correspondents, with civility and racial purity. Costal breathing was connected only with women of the more civilised races.[55] For example, Ellis published his correspondence with Dr J. H. Kellogg (of cornflakes fame), who wrote:

> I observed the breathing of 20 Chinese women and the same number of Indian women, and I found the abdominal type very marked in every case ... I examined several of the Cherokee and Chickasaw women in the Indian Territory. These women had all worn civilised dress, and some of them had worn corsets. Those who had worn corsets and tight dresses gave tracings like civilised women; those who has only worn loose dress gave normal tracings.[56]

While costal breathing was thus largely regarded as an artificially created difference caused by 'the evils of tight-lacing', one of Ellis's correspondents explicitly elucidated the links between thoracic breathing and sexuality. In what was acknowledged by Ellis as intended as a private letter to him, Dr Louis Robinson expressed his feelings that one of the reasons (and there must be strong ones) for the persistent habit of tightening up the belly-girth among Christian damsels is that such constriction renders the breathing thoracic and so advertising the alluring bosom by keeping it in constant and manifest movement. The heaving of a sub-clavicular sigh is likely to cause more sensation than the heaving of an epigastric or umbilical sigh.[57]

Ellis also included remarks from Dr Sargent of Harvard University, who had used the spirometer to demonstrate the negative impact of corset wearing to his students by showing that 'The average lung capacity when corsets were worn was 134 cubic inches; when the corsets were removed the test showed an average lung capacity of 167 inches – a gain of 33 cubic inches.'[58] The spirometer thus became a tool used to demonstrate the negative impact of corsetry and tight stays. In a similar vein, a British textbook giving practical guidance for singers and speakers cautioned in 1891 against wearing corsets, based on evidence showing increased vital capacity measures of women free from corsets.[59] Its authors – vocal surgeon and voice trainer Lennox Browne and physiologist Emil Behnke – explained that they extrapolated a normal female measure by subtracting a percentage from the male standard.

> Until quite recently no experiments have been made in any large numbers of females, and a deduction of 33 per cent has been made for the 'weaker sex.' We have for many years been in the habit of making an allowance of only 25 per cent. for females; and more recent experience leads us to believe that even this difference is greater than would be justified by fact in normal subjects undeformed by fashion.[60]

As the inclusion of 'undeformed' indicates, the writers were extremely critical of corsets and their tendency to produce costal breathing or what they sometimes termed 'collar-bone breathing.'[61] Spirometry was invoked by the authors in order to demonstrate the injurious effects of corsets. Using a breathing capacity table from the Anthropometric Committee of the British Association for the Advancement of Science, Browne and Behnke took spirometry readings from women with and then without corsets in order to show the numerical gain from breathing without restriction. The authors explicitly appealed to the sensibilities of their female readers by explaining that corsets could cause the 'horror' of 'fat' accumulating due to suppression of natural breathing:

> If, as Mr. Lennox Browne has shown, a lady with normal lung capacity of 125 cubic inches, reduces this to 78 inches by means of her stays, and attains 118 inches all at once on leaving them off, it is certain that her prospects of becoming fat and flabby ... are greatly increased.[62]

Uncertainty about whether corsets were restricting breathing to the extent that they were altering vital capacity remained.[63] Indeed, the Lamarckian theory of inheritance (which argued that the changes made to an organism in its lifetime could be passed on) was invoked to show that corsetry had led to costal breathing becoming 'fixed by heredity into a secondary sexual character'.[64] This observation encapsulates the element of *blurriness* between biological and environmental causes of difference between men and women crucial to the creation of spirometric standards.

The MRC intervenes

The trouble with girls was recognised by the MRC Pneumoconiosis Research Unit (PRU) in south Wales in 1975 when they proposed conducting studies that for the first time would stipulate the respiratory values of normal women in Britain and thus allow for the monitoring of respiratory health of women working in industry. The initial commission draft was prepared for the newly formed Health and Safety Executive's Employment Medical Advisory Service (henceforth HSE) and explained that 'it is important that in any industry where there is a respiratory hazard it should be possible to compare lung function to women with a normal value'.[65] Yet, as this draft emphasised, 'There are at present no reference values in the UK for healthy women with which abnormalities can be compared.'[66] Of course, this may be partially due to the fact that women (since 1842) were prohibited from working in mining, which was the industry that (as we explore in the next section) was subject to most of the UK's clinical investigations of lung function in attempts to establish the cause of miner's lung.[67] However, even considering their exclusion from mining, and disregarding the work of women in potentially toxic industries like munitions factories during the First World War, it is still remarkable that there were no accepted normal values for women's lung function in Britain until 1979.[68] Consider that by 1844 not only did we have normal lung function values for men but we had normal lung function values for subdivisions of men: male policemen, firemen, wrestlers, grenadier guards, miners, aristocrats, small men, tall men and every man in between.

The 1975 attempt to redress the (by then) 131-year imbalance was initially part of a broader remit of research on lung function conducted at the MRC Pneumoconiosis Research Unit, where researchers hoped to obtain further funding for their work from the HSE. Unfortunately, the HSE was not prepared to accept work on the initially proposed *general* topic of lung function and asked the PRU to split the original proposal into two separately defined commissions. Pioneering lung function expert Dr John E. Cotes (1924–2018) was the main researcher working on lung function and he found it very difficult to deal with the bureaucracy that the HSE demanded, as Dr Joan Faulkner's note on their visit with Dr Alan MacAuslan to the PRU made explicit:

> It became clear from the start of our discussion that Dr Cotes was going to be very difficult. I had already explained to him in a previous interview that the exercise in which we were engaged was largely a paper one but if we collaborated, it was likely to make things much easier in the long run. I knew that he was incensed about the fate of the proposed work on small airways obstruction in the slateworkers' survey but I had shown him Dr Norton's letter to Dr Owen and also emphasised that Dr MacAuslan had been in no way involved in the decision. Nevertheless, he mentioned it on several occasions during the day and although Dr MacAuslan behaved in a civilised, sympathetic and placatory manner, I found the discussion exceedingly difficult to manage The main trouble was that Dr Cotes repeated over and over again that what he did formed a continuum and that it was virtually impossible for him to split off any part of his work to form one or more specific commissions. His irritation was very evident to the extent that Dr MacAuslan apologised to me on the way to lunch for upsetting Dr Cotes.[69]

The first of the two PRU commissions was accepted, but the one on lung function in women was subjected to criticism. Indeed, the ill-fated study was beset with difficulties from its inception. At that first difficult meeting with the HSE (represented by MacAuslan), Faulkner (a senior figure in the MRC and the wife of Sir Richard Doll) remarked, 'I could see that Dr MacAuslan wasn't over enthusiastic about this project but he accepted it as some of the others that had been suggested seemed to have even less relevance ... from the HSE point of view.'[70] Even (female!) researchers working at the PRU derided its utility, and Dr Joan E. Box wrote to Faulkner at the MRC urging *against* stimulating HSE's interest in the study and arguing that it would divert attention away from more important activities.[71] Similarly, Box wrote that 'Dr Leece's immediate reaction is that there is unlikely to be strong concern about this – although the subject of improving standards is of some interest to them.'[72] Most surprisingly, the principal investigator, Cotes, himself was described as uninterested in the project: when pressed for costings over the phone 'he was rather vague and said that he had never been keen on this commission and was much more interested in the exercise project.'[73] Faulkner reflected on these messages and on the general lack of enthusiasm for the project, and noted that 'several people make the point that it is probably necessary but dull'.[74] MacAuslan at the HSE even wrote to the MRC specifically to reiterate that the HSE did 'not set a very high priority on this piece of work'.[75]

Yet other researchers working on lung function at the PRU defended its utility against such attacks. For example, Faulkner was puzzled about Cotes's reputed lack of interest in the project and recorded that this seemed 'to be in conflict with what he told me when I visited him last year with Dr MacAuslan – namely that there was a great need for reference values in healthy British women'.[76] Dr J. C. Gilson similarly stressed that 'John Cotes emphasises that there is a great need for prospective studies in women. Nearly all the published data of prospective investigations relate to males.'[77]

Adding to this internal division, the project was then subjected to further criticisms from the HSE statistician, who highlighted several problems with the research application. Namely, he felt that the study proposed was not extensive enough to answer the main research question and argued that the groups (totalling 150 subjects) were too small to show significant differences and were neither representative of regional variation in the UK nor reflective of the targeted working population. For instance, he pointed out that 'there are no women in the 16–25 year interval in any of the groups, which is a surprising omission as this group will be evident very much in industrial working populations'.[78] He also argued that it was unclear what constituted a 'healthy woman' and contended that 'the chosen groups are by no means necessarily representative of healthy women, especially the group whose members all had iron deficiency anaemia'.[79] The statistician used to review this project was apparently new and his comments were not received well by the MRC or the PRU, who variously argued his analysis was 'somewhat inappropriate', based on a 'misunderstanding of the purpose of the work' and that he had 'rather "gone to town" on this commission'.[80] The letter conveying his criticisms was dated 1 April 1976, and the MRC may well have wished that it had been written as a seasonal joke. It was referred to as 'rather embarrassing' and the London MRC headquarters branch considered whether they should simply conceal these criticisms from the directors of the PRU in south Wales by 'sweeping them under the carpet'. However, on further reflection they decided against such a course of action, as Faulkner (working from headquarters in London) explained:

> I don't think we can evade the questions the statistician has raised and on reflection I think it would be best if you would send these down to the unit. It may well be that the best thing to do is to drop this commission, but it perhaps may be no bad thing for Unit directors to learn gradually a little more about the facts of life. We have protected them to a very great extent so far.[81]

As a result of the statistician's criticisms the commission was eventually dropped entirely, and Faulkner wrote to convey the news to the HSE, while reiterating the intrinsic value of the project:

Dr Gilson and Dr Cotes accept your statisticians' comments as justified: they would like to stress, however, that the basic concept behind their work on establishing indices of lung function in women is a valid one. They both emphasise in particular the great need for prospective studies in women, in view of the fact that nearly all the published data of prospective investigations relate to men.[82]

In 1979, just three years after this letter was written, *Thorax* published an article with the title 'Lung Function in Healthy British women', which provided reference values for healthy British women for the first time. This study was identical to the proposal pitched to the HSE (even down to the title), indicating that the statistician's comments had perhaps not been so readily accepted after all.

The standards given in this study were replaced just four years later by the first European standardisation document pertaining to spirometry, which was issued by the European Coal and Steel Community in 1983, then updated in 1993.[83] However, by 1997, there was some concern that the impact of cohort effects (changes to people due to things like improved nutrition and decreased passive smoking) and period effects (changes to techniques, instruments and apparatus) meant that the data used for these reference values, as another *Thorax* article explained, 'derived from 20 unrelated studies performed between 1960 and 1980 with varying apparatus, measurement conditions, and techniques' would no longer be valid.[84] In 2010, an article in the *European Respiratory Journal* bemoaned the constant changes to the so-called 'standard' reference equations, and pointed out that 'the overwhelming number of published reference equations, with at least 15 published for spirometry alone in the past 3 years, complicated the selection of an appropriate reference'.[85]

Historians of technology have long emphasised the fact that technical standards underwrite their own opacity and through doing so becoming increasingly invisible.[86] Standards create conformations of both instruments and people. Such conformations have often been used to objectify and enforce group differences while at the same time perpetuating their invisibility.[87] These constructions are then reified as though they represent objective measurement. As J. C. Gilson and P. Hugh-Jones reflected in their MRC Special Report, 'we must be able to measure breathlessness, either by attempting a quantitative estimate of the symptom ... or by arbitrarily selecting a particular physiological test as the best index and relating other test results to this standard'.[88]

Indeed, the 'will to standardise' in order to attain objectivity has been strong within the MRC and has been remarked upon by historians researching its standardisation of audiometry, depression and Alzheimer's assessment guidelines.[89] Far from being unproblematic and objective, the standardization of disease diagnoses is an inherently political project. For example, the diverse national medical positions on the aetiology of silicosis has been shown to have been directly linked to the social insurance systems present in each different country.[90] Measurement instruments are crucial in promoting standards that allow for easy replication and easy comparison across different disciplines and locations. Standards are especially powerful because they self-perpetuate and, as Timmermans and Berg have demonstrated, standards can function as political tools. For instance, amidst the Covid19 global pandemic, divergent standards between countries in the manner of calculating death rates have been linked to political expediency. Thus, 'standards are inherently political because their construction and application transform the practices in which they become embedded'.[91]

The fight for recognition of and compensation for 'miner's lung' is a clear example of the way in which politics and objective standards can conflict with testimony.

Normal breathing for miners

The Life of Breath Project principal investigators Carel and Macnaughton have explained that the psychological experience of breathlessness has an important effect on the personal perception of respiratory illness.[92] This assessment has been reinforced by recent neuroimaging studies which have identified how variable psychological workings affect the way people experience the bodily sensation of breathlessness.[93] Such testimony concerning the personal perception of illness was provided in 1923 by a miner who wrote to the Somerset Miners' Association's agent to question the compensation available for his illness. He wrote:

> Dear Sir, I am writing a few lines hoping you don't mind as I guess you are pretty busy now with election, but I seen [sic] an announcement to the effect that all amendments regarding workman's compensation bill was passed. I should like for you to let me know if I am likely to get anything as every time I've wrote to the home secretary or the clergyman at my home wrote him, he's always given me so little hope. I cannot see that I shall be doing any work for some months yet although I'm trying my best to get over it but I can't get breath to walk very far and I don't think this place is any good for this complaint. There's an old man here got the same, but I don't expect him to last very long as he's no strength to battle against it.

The strength that the miner believes he has means that he feels he can battle his illness from a better position than the older man. In the same letter he gives more details about the progressive nature of his disability:

> I didn't know I was so bad before I started work so I had to finish. I've seen my Dr today and he said he was in Bath last night and Dr Thomson told I ought to have compensation for it as he said I was as good as done for … it's a clear case. Seeing as I've seen the x rays and they don't tell lies any way.[94]

The miner's assertion that X-rays 'don't tell lies' demonstrates not only faith in the apparently objective physical image, but also pre-emptively responds to potential accusations of malingering that constantly dogged the miner's claims of ill health.[95] As his illness progressed without compensation he kept writing, describing his symptoms on one occasion by saying: 'I have not breath enough to blow a candle out.'[96] The writer was not diagnosed as suffering from silicosis until 1929, and he collapsed and died in July 1930, at the age of forty-five.[97] Historian Joseph Melling has identified that his inquest was pivotal in motivating the subsequent legislative and scientific debates about pulmonary illness in the 1930s.[98]

Moreover, from the miner's letter we can see that the use of historically situated and highly specific metaphors supports the claim that a contextual understanding of breathlessness is vital.[99] Oxley and Macnaughton have demonstrated that the language we use to demonstrate breathlessness is highly variable, and subject to difference between cultures and contexts.[100] While instrumentation is ideally designed to transcend such socio-cultural contexts, the following section will demonstrate that the clinical investigation of respiratory disease in mining communities was impacted by the normalisation of disability within these communities.

That pulmonary disease disproportionately affected mine-workers had been recognised from the early nineteenth century. However, by the end of that century, the orthodox medical position held that tuberculosis due to overcrowding was more likely to be the cause of miners' respiratory distress than the levels of dust.[101] Historian Michael Bloor has attributed the resultant shift in attention from dust in the air to germs in the air to developments in bacteriology.[102] Melling has added that subsequent commitment to this stance was partially fuelled by medics' reluctance to be associated with old-fashioned Victorian fears about coal dust.[103] Moreover, following the work of John Scott Haldane (1860–1936), there was some adherence to the notion that coal dust functioned as a prophylactic. That is, coal dust was beneficial: 'a little dust was good for you'.[104] Indeed, miner D. C. Davies, who worked in Ffaldau colliery in 1930, described inhalation of coal dust being used in Llandough hospital in the late 1930s as a treatment for silicosis.[105] Notable amongst adherents to this view were the Home Office's medical factory inspector, Dr Edgar Collis, and the 1927 medical inspector of mines, Dr Sydney Fisher, both of whom have been identified by historians Perchard and Gildart as key 'merchant[s] of doubt'.[106]

In what follows, I set out a brief outline of the legislative changes relating to coalmining which preceded the MRC investigation. These changes were variously resisted or advocated by a number of important bodies, including: the mine owners (represented by the Mining Association of Great Britain), the South Wales Mining Federation and other trade unions, medical specialists, the Home Office, the Mines Department, the MRC and the labouring communities. Historians disagree about which of these bodies were responsible for the 'stuttering' advances in occupational legislation although there is consensus that complex social, cultural, economic, and political forces interrelated with the contested aetiology of miners' lung.[107]

Compensation for industrial disease was first offered to UK industrial workers in 1906 through the Workmen's Compensation Act, although its extension had been strongly resisted by coal owners.[108] This in turn followed a domestic government investigation into occupational disease, which resulted in diseases being added alongside injuries as eligible for compensation for the first time.[109] This was despite the fact, as Bufton and Melling have noted, that the Home Office remained adamant throughout the interwar years that the state would not provide any funding for industrial compensation.[110] Silicosis-specific compensation (for those exposed to silica dust) was introduced in 1918 but was only for quarrymen and workmen in other silica-based industries – it specifically excluded coal miners.[111] The situation for coal miners improved marginally in 1929 thanks to the Various Industries (Silicosis) Scheme of 1928, but this scheme had strict eligibility criteria and only cases of death or cases of total disability that precluded future work were compensated.[112] This was largely due to the difficulty of assessing partial disability, and also of diagnosing silicosis or pneumoconiosis in its early stage as a disease distinct from tuberculosis.[113] For the medico-legal bureaucracies involved with miners' compensation, this meant that while the presence of illness was not disputed, the causation was highly contested.

In 1930 the MRC Committee on Industrial Pulmonary Disease was appointed and in 1931, the Various Industries Scheme was extended to cover more workers and include partial disability.[114] This may have been precipitated by Britain's substantial involvement in the 1930 International Labour Office Conference on silicosis in Johannesburg. Although the global transfer of silicosis knowledge was important in the development of consensus on mining disease aetiology, historian Arthur McIvor has argued that the conference policies were unsuccessful in practically improving the situation for disabled workers with respiratory disease in Britain.[115] The disabled worker had to obtain medical certificates from his own doctor before applying to the Medical Board, where his case was usually presented by his trade union, as the financial cost for individuals applying directly to the board was prohibitively high.[116] The introduction of partial disability posed new challenges to the medical community in their ability to accurately and convincingly assess its boundaries, which Braun argues was due to 'the lack of correlation between the degree of tissue damage and the severity of breathlessness'.[117] Assessing breathlessness as a symptom of disability was especially difficult and presented further challenges because of the need to correlate reported breathlessness to X-ray images. For instance, the MRC noted that symptoms of respiratory disability manifesting as coughs and breathlessness generally ran in parallel with X-ray changes but often could not be connected to any clinical evidence.[118]

Notwithstanding the condition of their lungs, if miners could not prove that they had been exposed to silica dust from working on rock containing at least 50 per cent silica, then their case could be overturned. Bufton and Melling have argued that this resulted in the prioritisation of geological expertise over clinical criteria.[119] This stipulation also reinforces one of the central claims of this chapter, that socially useful numbers were crucial in negotiating the boundaries of contested disability and compensation. The subsequent lack of concordance between geological and pathological measures was reflected in the realisation that 'the relationship between geological conditions and the onset of disease could not be precisely measured'.[120]

For example, in the pivotal 1935 appeal case of *Wragg v. Samuel Fox & Co. Ltd (Sheffield)*, the county judge ruled that:

> I am satisfied that the applicant was constantly exposed to dust. For the last few years of his life the applicant experienced what he called 'tightness' and finally ceased work on April 19, 1935. He was examined by the medical board appointed for the purpose, and on June 21, 1935, was duly certified as suffering from silicosis and totally incapacitated. The commencement of the disablement was certified as April 19, 1935. After hearing Dr. Platt I was satisfied that the applicant was still totally incapacitated, further that the silicosis was due to the nature of his employment with the respondents, and that the disease could not have been contracted in any other way.[121]

Despite this seemingly damning testimony, when employers Samuel Fox & Co. appealed the decision, Lord Justice Greer took their side because of the proviso in the Act which stated that the employer should not be liable if they could prove that the employee was not exposed to the silica rock.[122] The ability to do this rested on the applicant having the means to secure (expensive) expert testimony from geologists to back their claim and such support was sought by both miners' unions and the mine owners.[123] *Wragg* v. *Fox* proved to be critical in delaying any practical implementation of the 1931 Scheme and influenced miners' leaders in their lobbying for clear diagnostic criteria.[124] The Various Industries (Silicosis) Scheme was thus amended in 1934 to extend to miners working underground, but partial disability would only be granted if 'the nodular features of silica dust were detected on microscopy and X-ray'.[125]

Although both local doctors and miners were convinced of the existence of a disease due to coal dust, this belief did not correlate with the diagnostic criteria for compensation.[126] Furthermore, there was increasing concern that coal miners were suffering from respiratory disability that could not be traced to silica exposure.[127] In 1936 the Chief Medical Officer of the Silicosis Medical Board asserted that the claims for compensation made by coal miners in south Wales were rising. Refusal rates were also increasing, with up to 52 per cent of certificates refused in 1935.[128]

It was at this point in 1936 that the MRC was asked by the Home Office and the Mines Department to try and solve the problem of the disparity between visible tissue damage and subjective reports of illness. It was charged with investigating chronic pulmonary disease among coal miners, with a particular focus on the south Wales coalfields. As I explained in Chapter 1, the MRC had been funded by government to instigate medical and biological research since 1911, and during the interwar years it was divided into numerous subsections which were endowed with significant freedom in their organisation and research.[129] The medical surveys undertaken from 1936 to 1942 were led by Dr Phillip D'Arcy Hart and Dr Edward Aslett, assisted by a large team of engineers, inspectors and pathologists.[130] Retrospectively, D'Arcy Hart attributed government intervention to the rise of compensation costs, concern for the health of the miners and the fact that 'there was a war round the corner and they certainly did not want a dissatisfied coal-producing force'.[131]

The MRC selected an anthracite colliery for detailed investigation, and examined 560 of the men there, both radiologically and clinically.[132] The clinical tests involved included examination of sputum, tuberculin tests and spirometric measurements of lung volume.[133] These lung volume determinations were supplemented by an exercise tolerance test, which categorised levels of 'respiratory embarrassment' under four possible subheadings.[134] These groupings were then further categorised as either normal (class A) or abnormal (further divided by severity into class B or C).[135] The degree of respiratory embarrassment was then measured against the medical history of the miner, which was provided by the mining inspector. The surveyors were satisfied that there was concordance between these two separately obtained measures of breathlessness.

The MRC created further standardised and standardising measures in their classification of X-rays, dividing them into strictly defined categories: (a) normal; (b) reticulation; (c) nodulation; (d) coalescent nodulation; (e) massive shadows; (f) multiple fluffy shadows; and (g–h) indefinite.[136] The identification of the category of reticulation was particularly important because it identified the early stage of disease which resulted in disability in older miners.[137] As Dr Gwent Jones (a GP working in Gower) explained in his 1943 report on silicosis, 'Reticulation describes the X-Ray appearance of the fibrosis as it is first seen – it looks like the first snow on a window'.[138] The MRC reports (published 1942–45) were critical in that they proved that there was a link between length of exposure to coal dust and respiratory disability.[139] This meant that there was now widespread medical acceptance of a disease due to coal dust that was entirely distinct from silicosis. Finally, in 1943, a disease due to coal dust was both legally recognised and duly compensated.[140] The recognition of coalworkers' pneumoconiosis resulted in an exponential rise in certifications under the Act, which overwhelmed the bodies responsible for their administration – the miners' union and the Ministry of Fuel and Power.[141]

Calculations of partial disability levels were based primarily on assessing the functionality of the body in relation to continuing work: could the miner be disabled if he was still working? The MRC assessed the changes that X-ray investigation revealed on the miners' bodies and concluded in its report that 'the X-ray changes might be compatible at first with ability to work, but they were considered to represent a definite impairment of lung structure and to involve an increasing respiratory disability, manifested, for example, by shortness of breath'.[142] The authors of the MRC Medical Survey pondered the seriousness of this disability amongst the working population in the report and questioned whether hidden pulmonary abnormalities 'among *men still at work*' were of any consequence.[143] However, Dr Gwent Jones argued that: 'If the sufferer was only partially incapacitated and obtains a certificate for partial compensation, he is to the labour marker only a part of a man, and being unskilled in any other trade he cannot compete with fit men in new occupations.'[144]

Such disputes regarding the potential for the disabled man to work permeated the MRC's investigations. As disability historians Turner and Blackie have recently explored, this kind of attitude reflected the reality for coal miners in the Victorian period, who would often continue to work while disabled.[145] Jones's criticism of the compensation system highlighted how many men continued to work after certification, 'whether he is a caretaker, or a part-time gardener, or just nothing, the "partial" is fortunate compared to the "full" who may be too short of breath to even lace his own boots'.[146] Evaluating the relationship between work and disability was crucial to the new process of assessing disability and loss of function in the medico-legal field. Adjudicating disability was complex and involved new sets of standardised classifications for what changes constituted disability in relation to respiratory disease.[147] Melling has confirmed that it was very difficult to arrive firmly at any kind of diagnosis using X-ray examination at this time: professional scepticism abounded and techniques and interpretations were not standardised until nearer 1950.[148] In this politically loaded context, in which new X-ray technology could not be fully trusted, the spirometer represented secure evidence of respiratory disease in numerical terms which could be utilised in the complex compensation network. As Braun has demonstrated, the spirometer offered 'an objective marker of disability to industrial medicine'.[149]

However, using spirometry to diagnose pneumoconiosis necessitated a definition of normal with which to make the comparison. Gilson and Hugh-Jones explained in their MRC report on lung function in coalworkers' pneumoconiosis:

> The assessment of the effect of silicosis or pneumoconiosis on lung function implies a definition of normal with which to make the comparison. This is far more difficult than the scant reference [sic] in the literature would suggest.[150]

The MRC's original clinical investigation used normal lung function values separately determined by Aslett, Hart and McMichael. However, the normal adult male subjects used as controls for these determinations were in fact taken from sixty-four members of 'the normal members of the working population of an anthracite colliery in Carmarthenshire, the great majority being of Welsh parentage'.[151] The data sets used a normal standard set by apparently healthy miners rather than a non-mining control group. This would not have necessarily mattered if the investigation involved a longitudinal study – investigating the changing health of the same miners over a number of years. However, part of the point of this investigation was to work out if the environment was causing pulmonary disease and so used a cross-sectional method which compared the health of miners in different geographical areas (see Figure 5.2).

Only one mine was subjected to a full clinical investigation and the spirometry test there was clearly flawed, as it took its measure of normalcy from the very population in which abnormality was already apparent. This analysis is supported by Smith's study of 'Black Lung' in West Virginia, which has demonstrated that pathology in coal miners was considered normal for coal miners and that patient testimony as to their own condition was considered secondary to diagnosis. 'What was "normal" for miners, including even a

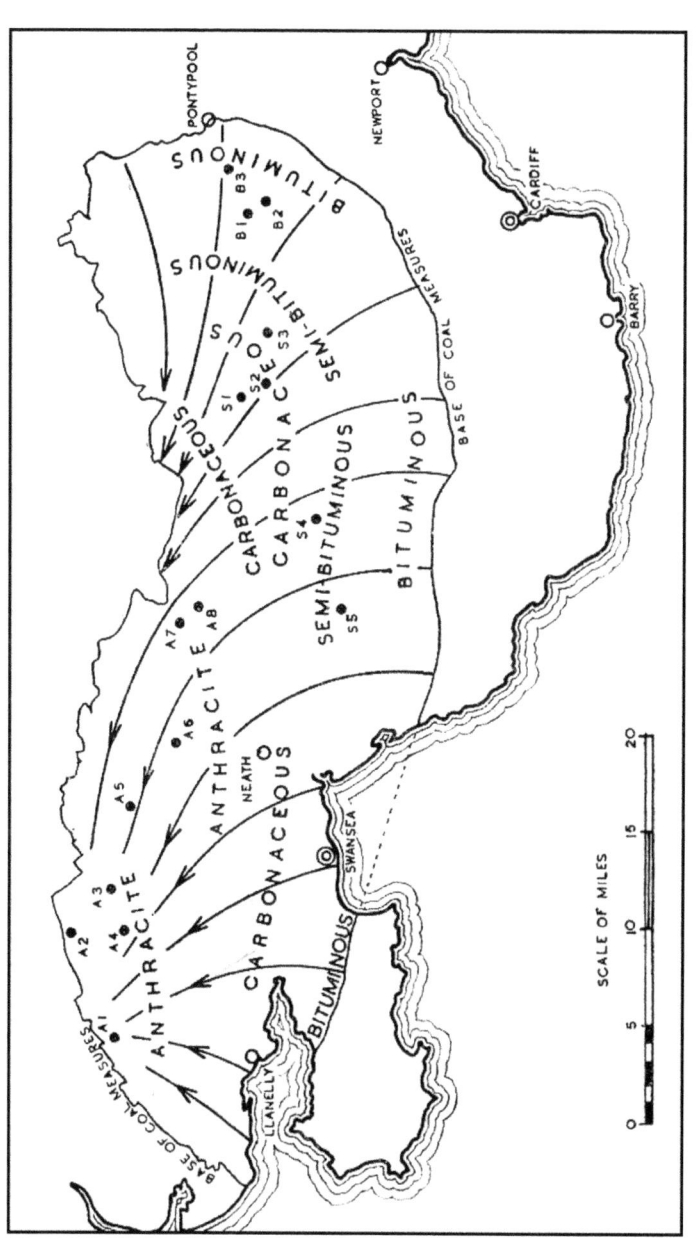

Figure 5.2 Map of the south Wales coalfield marking the positions of the sixteen collieries of the MRC chronic pulmonary disease inquiry, 1942

chronic respiratory condition, was by no means normal for the company doctor – to the extent that [if] their X-rays revealed the pathological changes now associated with coalworkers' pneumoconiosis, these too were considered normal – for coal miners.'[152] Reluctance to attribute diminished lung capacity to the effect of mining work was to continue. For example, in their 1955 report for the MRC, Gilson and Hugh-Jones compared Hart and Aslett's use of working miners as controls to a later (1950) study that used men who had never worked in dusty conditions as controls. The 1950 study 'found a big difference in the maximum breathing capacity compared with men applying for compensation who had no evidence of silicosis on the radiography'.[153] That is, men who had never worked in dusty conditions had greater lung capacity than those who had worked in dusty conditions, even though these men would not have been diagnosed with any respiratory disease. This difference was largely attributed to the constitutions of the men involved rather than their working conditions. Gilson and Hugh-Jones explained that 'They concluded that the difference was psychogenic but it is possible that it was partly due to the effect of mining.'[154]

Thus, if causation from dust or disease could not be established, then it followed that the problem must be related to the essential constitution of the miner. Similarly, attempts to clarify normal reference values were marked by attempts to explain variability in lung function through racial and ethnic difference.[155] The MRC's original investigation reported considerations of whether or not the Welsh were actually a separate racial group, and if so, whether that could account for their abnormalities in stature and high levels of lung disease, commenting 'It is relevant here to mention the suggestion that the high incidence of pneumoconiosis in western Wales is associated in part with the racial composition of its inhabitants.'[156] This idea was rejected not because of environmental considerations but because a number of men at the colliery they examined had English parentage. Thus, we see that innate biological causes and potential ethnic differences were sought in order to supersede social or environmental factors. Similarly, in the lung volume determinations compiled by Aslett, Hart and McMichael, there was consideration of the fact that the vital capacity mean was lower in the normal subjects taken from the mines than it was in 'previous series of normal males' but this difference was attributed to the smaller height and weight of the miners, 'probably due to the Welsh racial characteristics'.[157] Indeed, the idea of a Welsh racial factor had long been used to argue against environmental causes of difference, For example in 1883 Galton compared the stature and weight of Scottish miners favourably against Welsh miners to demonstrate 'an example of the predominance of race over occupation'.[158] Attributing variability in lung function to racial difference was eventually enshrined in spirometric measurements by the MRC PRU in south Wales in its standards for 'Average Normal Values for the Forced Expiratory Volume in White Caucasian Males'.[159] By 1974, the MRC had refined their measurements to allow them to 'correct' for racial difference using a scaling or correction factor of 13 per cent. This reinforced the idea that white lung function was normal lung function and, as Braun has established, this had far-reaching effects in both the compensation system and in the promotion of the thesis that inequality between the races was biological rather than environmental.[160]

Conclusion: ways of breathing

In 1963, *The British Medical Journal* published a letter on 'the sensation of dyspnoea' which argued that 'a respiratory physiologist offering a unitary explanation of breathlessness should arouse the same suspicions as a tattooed Archbishop offering a free ticket to heaven'.[161] To demonstrate the impossibility of replicating the feeling of shortness of breath, the author described an approach to imitate 'the mechanical disadvantages under which patients with asthma and emphysema suffer'.[162] Individuals who were identified as 'normal' were secured with a broad band placed tightly around their chest 'arranged to hinder expiration'.[163] Spirometric readings and assessments of dyspnoea during heavy work were then taken of the individuals with the band on, and then compared to their previous 'normal state'. This experiment indicated to the researchers that the *feeling* of breathlessness was not connected to gas exchange within the lungs or any other quantifiable measurement.

As this experiment signals, medical clinicians throughout the twentieth century were aware of and keenly frustrated by the fact that lung function measurements did not map onto the experience of breathlessness. And today the experience of breathlessness still eludes clinical attempts to capture and quantify it, as 'one of the difficulties in an experimental approach to breathlessness is how to reproduce the sensation in the laboratory and study it quantitatively'.[164] Attempts to reproduce the sensation in the laboratory are problematic because such experimental work needs to be carried out on 'normal subjects whose bodies and minds have not been subjected to years of chronic breathlessness' and the effects that may have on physiology and neural mechanisms.[165] As a result, we are unable to replicate the long-term physiological and neural effects of living with breathlessness. This disability data gap is unavoidable because those living with long-term respiratory conditions are unable to 'spend time lying flat in the enclosed tunnel of an MRI scanner'.[166] Moreover, it is impossible to replicate or standardise the emotions attached to feeling breathless, as 'laboratory dyspnoea does not cause the existential fears dyspnoea sufferers encounter in daily life'.[167]

To address the ongoing complications around reference classes in spirometry, in 2012, the Global Lung Function Initiative was sponsored by the European Respiratory Society to tabulate new 'standard' reference values for spirometry.[168] Of concern to the European Respiratory Society was the way in which the different reference equations available for measuring lung function impacted on the classification of patients as 'normal' or 'abnormal'. One 1999 study found that 'up to 40% of spirometric tests may change their clinical category (from normal to abnormal) simply by changing the equation used'.[169] Such misclassification, the authors noted, had important implications for the assessment of disability, and this phenomenon was exacerbated in the elderly and in women.[170] This analysis adds to the claims made in this book about the classification of disability as dependent on, and variable according to, certain measurements. Interlinked with the problem of appropriate reference equations is the difficulty of defining and assessing normalcy to represent a healthy population in the first place. Not only, as we saw in Chapter 2, is health difficult to define, the reference classes used in lung function complicate matters further, 'height, age, sex and, ideally, ethnic/racial group must be taken into consideration when defining the normal range for lung function. The selection of "healthy" subjects who comprise the reference population is of paramount importance.'[171] The creation of standards, then, is a powerful way of categorising disability and of defining relevant reference classes in an apparently objective manner.

Certainly, current research does demonstrate incontestable sex differences (on average) between men and women, including lower lung function and lower respiratory muscle strength in women compared to men.[172] And there are gender differences, too, for instance in the pattern of COPD diagnosis between men and women: 'never smokers' with COPD are predominantly women (perhaps due to higher exposure to indoor air pollutants); women wait longer to be diagnosed with COPD than men and are more likely to have airflow obstruction left unidentified than men.[173] Beyond these differences, there is a great deal of anecdotal evidence suggesting that current standards of desirability dictate that women ought to be slim with a demonstrably flat stomach, meaning that women in public often attempt to hold their stomachs 'in', consequently impairing their ability to breathe diaphragmatically. How can we be sure to separate out the differences arising from such social pressures as distinct from the biological?

The American folk singer Townes Van Zandt once sang: 'Well, won't you lend your lungs to me, mine are collapsing'. The hopelessness of his plea to breathe in someone else's air is suggestive of the impossibility of ever truly understanding and experiencing another individual's way of breathing. As well as frustrating laboratory studies, the unique individuality attached to breathing impacts on user responses to breath prosthetics, the technologies which are the foci of the following chapter.

Notes

1. See Booth et al., 'The Brain and Breathlessness' and Spathis et al., 'The Breathing, Thinking, Functioning Clinical Model'.
2. Carel et al., 'Invisible Suffering', p. 278.
3. Williams and Carel, 'Breathlessness'.
4. See www.lifeofbreath.org and Macnaughton and Carel, 'Breathing and Breathlessness'.
5. Today vital capacity is measured through total lung capacity minus residual volume.
6. Braun, *Breathing Race into the Machine*, p. 8.
7. Young, I. M., *On Female Body Experience: 'Throwing Like a Girl' and Other Essays* (Oxford: Oxford University Press, 2005), p. 29.
8. Shim, *Heart-Sick*, p. 146 and p. 194.
9. Ibid., p. 146.
10. Ibid., p. 156.
11. Ibid., pp. 156–157.
12. Braun, *Breathing Race into the Machine*, p. 205.
13. Nerbovik, L. T., Kirkengen, A. L., and Hetlevik, I., 'Might a Systematic Reading of the Thickest GP Patient Medical Records Improve our Understandings of Functional Disorders', *La Prensa Medica Argentina*, 101:5 (2015), 1–5, p. 3. For more on Kirkengen's work linking childhood trauma with adult ill health see Kirkingen, A. L., *Inscribed Bodies: Health Impact of Childhood Sexual Abuse* (Dordrecht: Springer, 2010).
14. Hutchinson, J., *Contributions to Vital Statistics, Obtained by Means of a Pneumatic Apparatus for Valuing the Respiratory Power with Relation to Health* (London: Statistical Society of London, 1844). p. 2. Emphasis in original.
15. Hutchinson had previously worked for life insurance companies.
16. Pepys, J., and Bernstein, L., 'Historical Aspects of Occupational Asthma', in M. Chang-Yeung and J. L. Malo (eds), *Asthma in the Workplace* (New York: Marcel Dekker Inc., 1999), pp. 1–28, p. 7.
17. Hutchinson, *Contributions to Vital Statistics*, p. 2.
18. Ibid.
19. His inclusion of 'attitude' is notable and likely was meant to indicate the extent to which cooperation of the patient was necessary for the measurement.
20. To say that a kind is natural is to say that it corresponds to a grouping that reflects the natural world rather than the interests of humans. See Chapter 2 for more on this.
21. Braun, *Breathing Race into the Machine*.
22. Bowker and Star, *Sorting Things Out*.

23 Porter, 'Measurement, Objectivity, and Trust' and Hacking, 'Biopower and the Avalanche of Printed Numbers'.
24 Dreyer, G., 'Investigations on the Normal Vital Capacity in Man and Its Relation to the Size of the Body', *The Lancet*, 194:5006 (1919), 227–234.
25 Smith, D., and Horrocks, S., 'Defining Perfect and Not-So-Perfect Bodies: The Rise and Fall of the "Dreyer Method" for the Assessment of Physique and Fitness, 1918–26', in J. Sobal and D. Maurer (eds), *Weighty Issues: Fatness and Thinness as Social Problems* (London: Routledge, 1999), pp. 74–94.
26 Courtwright, D. T., *Sky as Frontier: Adventure, Aviation, and Empire* (College Station: Texas A&M University Press, 2004), p. 41.
27 Ibid. Statistically, Deaf people are very safe drivers, and there is some evidence suggesting this in linked to superior peripheral vision. See Codina, C., Pascalis, O., Mody, C., Toomey, P., et al., 'Visual Advantage in Deaf Adults Linked to Retinal Changes', *PLoS ONE*, 6:6 (2011), 1–8.
28 Dreyer, 'Investigations on the Normal Vital Capacity', p. 227.
29 Dreyer, G., *The Assessment of Physical Fitness: By Correlation of Vital Capacity and Certain Measurements of the Body* (London: Cassell and Company, 1920), p. 3.
30 Dreyer, 'Investigations on the Normal Vital Capacity'.
31 Dreyer, *The Assessment of Physical Fitness*, pp. 17–18.
32 Smith and Horrocks, 'Defining Perfect and Not-So-Perfect Bodies', p. 78.
33 Dreyer, *The Assessment of Physical Fitness*, p. 18.
34 Smith and Horrocks, 'Defining Perfect and Not-So-Perfect Bodies', p. 78.
35 Heald, C. B., 'The Value and Interpretation of Some Physical Measurements', *The Lancet*, 196:5067 (1920), 736–741.
36 Balfour, T. G., 'Contribution to the Study of Spirometry', *Medico-Chirurgical Transactions*, 43 (1860), 263–269.
37 Cameron, C., 'The Vital Capacity in Pulmonary Tuberculosis', *Tubercle*, 3 (1922), 385–399.
38 Flack, M., 'The Milroy Lectures on Respiratory Efficiency in Relation to Health and Disease', *The Lancet*, 198 (1924), 693–696.
39 For example, see Aslett, E., D'Arcy Hart, P., and McMichael, J., 'The Lung Volume and Its Subdivisions in Normal Males', *Proceedings of the Royal Society of London Series B: Biological Sciences*, 126:845 (1939), 502–528, p. 506.
40 Smith, B. E., 'Black Lung: The Social Production of Disease', *International Journal of Health Services*, 11:3 (1981), 343–359, p. 346.
41 Smith and Horrocks, 'Defining Perfect and Not-So-Perfect Bodies', p. 75.
42 Moncrieff, A., 'Tests for Respiratory Efficiency', *The Lancet*, 220:5696 (1932), 665–669, p. 665.
43 Ibid., p. 668.
44 Ibid., p. 667.
45 Hutchinson, J., *The Spirometer, the Stethoscope, and Scale-Balance: Their Use in Discriminating Diseases of the Chest, and Their Value in Life Offices; With Remarks on the Selection of Lives for Life Assurance Companies* (London: Churchill, 1852), p. 6.

46 Ibid., pp. 6–7.
47 Ibid., p. 66.
48 Galton, F., 'The Final Report of the Anthropometric Committee', *Report of the British Association for the Advancement of Science* (1883), p. 298.
49 He measured their breathing capacities, as well as eyesight, colour-sense, highest audible note, strength, swiftness, arm-span, height and weight. See Galton, F., 'On the Anthropometric Laboratory at the Late International Health Exhibition', *Journal of the Anthropological Institute of Great Britain and Ireland*, 14 (1885), 205–221, p. 210.
50 Ellis, H., *Man and Woman: A Study of Human Secondary Sexual Characters* (London: Walter Scott, 1904), p. 202.
51 Ibid.
52 Ibid., p. 203.
53 Hutchinson, J., 'On the Capacity of the Lungs, and on the Respiratory Movements, with the View of Establishing a Precise and Easy Method of Detecting Disease by the Spirometer', *Medico- Chirurgical Transactions*, 29 (1846), 137–252.
54 Ellis, *Man and Woman*, p. 204.
55 Ibid., pp. 207–208.
56 Ibid.
57 Ibid., p. 210.
58 Ibid., p. 211.
59 Behnke and Browne, *Voice, Song, and Speech*, p. 97.
60 Ibid. Emil Behnke also used the spirometer in his work with deaf children as a tool for promoting oralism, see ibid., p. 96.
61 Ibid., p. 85.
62 Ibid., p. 94.
63 Ellis, *Man and Woman*, p. 203.
64 Ibid., p. 204.
65 The HSE was formed in 1975 and the first HSE advisory committees were set up in that year to promote research expertise on industry and specialist organisations and improve occupational health and safety. It was this call that the PRU was responding to: see www.hse.gov.uk/aboutus/timeline/index.htm and Joan Faulkner, 'Note on Visit with Dr MacAuslan to the Pneumoconiosis Unit', 14 May 1975. Potential Commissions from the Department of Employment: Lung Function in Healthy Women. TNA, FD 9/4168.
66 Commission draft MRC/HSE/182, 'Lung Function in Healthy Women 1. Preamble', 12 February 1976. Potential Commissions from the Department of Employment: Lung Function in Healthy Women. TNA, FD 9/4168.
67 A. Heeson, 'The Coal Mines Act of 1842, Social Reform, and Social Control', *Historical Journal*, 24:1 (1981), 69–88.
68 Campaign groups working for more recognition of these women argue that the incidence of throat and lung infections and later life health problems for these workers has been overlooked. See www.bbc.co.uk/news/uk-england-hereford-worcester-27685286. Accessed July 2019.

69 The HSE had not supported a potential commission on small airways obstruction. Faulkner, 'Note on Visit with Dr MacAuslan'.
70 Ibid.
71 Letter from Dr Box to Dr Faulkner, 26 July 1976. TNA, FD 9/4168. Dr Joan Faulkner (1914–2001) worked at MRC headquarters from 1945 and in 1979 became a Senior Principal Medical Officer. She married Richard Doll in 1949 (she was initially his supervisor) and became Lady Doll when he was knighted in 1971 for his epidemiological work demonstrating a link between smoking and cancer. See Keating, *Smoking Kills* for more on Faulkner.
72 Note to Dr Chapman scribbled in the margin following handwritten notes on the end of a letter from Dr Joan Faulkner to Dr Chapman and Dr Box, 13 April 1976. TNA, FD 9/4168.
73 Note for file 'Costing of Commission 182: Lung Function in Healthy Women', 24 September 1975, Anne Dalton. TNA, FD 9/4168.
74 Letter from Dr Joan Faulkner to Dr Box, 29 July 1976. TNA, FD 9/4168.
75 Letter from Dr Alan MacAuslan to Dr Joan Faulkner, 9 September 1976. TNA, FD 9/4168.
76 It should be noted that Dr Cotes was dealing with a tragic family situation during these years, which may explain some of his inconsistent behaviour. Letter from Dr Joan Faulkner to Dr Box, 29 July 1976, TNA, FD 9/4168.
77 Letter from Dr J. C. Gilson to Dr Joan Faulkner, 'Lung Function in Healthy Women' (No. 182), 30 April 1976. TNA, FD 9/4168.
78 Letter from A. MacAuslan of EMAS (Branch H1 of HSE) detailing comments from the statistician to Dr J. Faulkner, MRC, London, 1 April 1976. TNA, FD 9/4168.
79 Ibid.
80 Letter from Dr J. E. Box, MRC, London, to Dr J. C. Gilson at MRC Pneumoconiosis Unit, 30 April 1976, and letter from Dr Joan Faulkner to Dr Chapman and Dr Box, 13 April 1976. TNA, FD 9/4168.
81 Letter from Dr Joan Faulkner to Dr Chapman and Dr Box, 13 April 1976. TNA, FD 9/4168.
82 Letter from Dr Joan Faulkner to Dr Alan MacAuslan, 9 June 1976. TNA, FD 9/4168.
83 Quanjer, Ph. H., Tammeling, G. J., Cotes, J. E., Pedersen, O. F., et al., 'Lung Volumes and Forced Ventilatory Flows: Report Working Party Standardization of Lung Function Tests, European Community for Steel and Coal', *European Respiratory Journal Supplement*, 6 (1993), 5–40.
84 Kerstjens, H. A., Rijcken, B., Schouten, J. P., and Postma, D. S., 'Decline of FEV1 by Age and Smoking Status: Facts, Figures, and Fallacies', *Thorax*, 52 (1997), 820–827, p. 822. In 2012, the Global Lung Function Initiative was sponsored by the European Respiratory Society to tabulate new reference values for spirometry. See Backman, H., Lindberg, A., Sovijarvi, A., Larsson, K., et al., 'Evaluation of the

Global Lung Function Initiative 2012 Reference Values in a Swedish Population Sample', *BMC Pulmonary Medicine*, 15:26 (2015), 1602–1611.
85 Stanojevic, S., Wade, A., and Stocks, J., 'Reference Values for Lung Function: Past, Present and Future', *European Respiratory Journal*, 36:1 (2010), 12–19.
86 Sumner, J., and Gooday, G., 'Introduction: Does Standardization Make Things Standard?', *History of Technology*, 28 (2008), 1–13. For example, a British person driving would not notice that the designs of cars, roads, roundabouts, signage and so forth are all embedded and constructed to conform with the arbitrary standard of agreed driving on the left, but these standards become very visible when attempting to drive in the USA.
87 Clarke, A. E., Shim, J. K., Mamo, L., Fosket, J. R., et al., 'Biomedicalization: Technoscientific Transformations of Health, Illness, and U.S. Biomedicine', *American Sociological Association*, 68:2 (2003), 161–194, p. 174.
88 Gilson, J. C., and Hugh-Jones, P., *Lung Function in Coalworkers' Pneumoconiosis*. (Medical Research Council Special Report Series No. 290) (London: Her Majesty's Stationery Office, 1955), p. 132.
89 The phrase 'will to standardise' is Timmermans and Berg's, and they use it in reference to the 'Gold Standard' in healthcare. See Timmermans, C., and Berg, M., *The Gold Standard: The Challenge of Evidence-Based Medicine and Standardization in Health Care* (Philadelphia: Temple University Press, 2003). For a discussion of the MRC's standardised assessment of Alzheimer's disease diagnosis see Wilson, D., 'Calculable People? Standardising Assessment Guidelines for Alzheimer's Disease in 1980s Britain', *Medical History*, 61:4 (2017), 500–525. For a discussion of the standardisation of audiometric testing within the MRC see Virdi and McGuire, 'Phyllis M. Tookey Kerridge'. Michael Worboys points out that the MRC invented a new 'MRC scale' instead of using the HRSD or Hamilton scale in its study of depression between 1964 and 1965, which supports the claim that the organisation places a high value on standardised scales. See Worboys, M., 'The Hamilton Rating Scale for Depression: The Making of a "Gold Standard" and the Unmaking of a Chronic Illness, 1960–1980', *Chronic Illness*, 9:3 (2012), 202–219, p. 210.
90 Cayet, T., Rosental, P. A., and Thebaud-Sorger, M., 'How International Organisations Compete: Occupational Safety and Health at the ILO, a Diplomacy of Expertise', *Journal of Modern European History*, 7:2 (2009), 174–196, p. 177.
91 Timmermans and Berg, *The Gold Standard*, p. 22.
92 Macnaughton and Carel, 'Breathing and Breathlessness'.
93 Faull et al., 'Breathlessness and the Body'.
94 Edgar King to Fred Swift, 20 November 1923. Somerset Miners' Association, Bristol University Library Special Collections, DM 443, Box 6.
95 For my original analysis of this case see McGuire, C., '"X-Rays Don't Tell Lies": The Medical Research Council and the Measurement of Respiratory Disability, 1936–1945', *British Journal for the History of Science* 52:3 (2019), 447–465.

96 Ibid.
97 Melling, J., 'Beyond a Shadow of a Doubt? Experts, Lay Knowledge, and the Role of Radiography in the Diagnosis of Silicosis in Britain, c. 1919–1945', *Bulletin of the History of Medicine*, 84:3 (2010), 424–466.
98 Ibid., p. 427.
99 Oxley, R., and Macnaughton, J., 'Inspiring Change: Humanities and Social Science Insights into the Experience and Management of Breathlessness', *Current Opinion in Supportive & Palliative Care*, 10:3 (2017), 256–261, p. 257.
100 Ibid. This is also true of the subjective and invisible experience of pain, which Joanna Bourke has examined by analysing the metaphors that are used for describing pain, which differ according to time period and participant identity (i.e. their gender, ethnicity and religion). See Bourke, *The Story of Pain*.
101 Bloor, M., 'The South Wales Miners Federation, Miners' Lung and the Instrumental Use of Expertise, 1900–1950', *Social Studies of Science* 30:1 (2000), 125–140, p. 129.
102 Ibid.
103 Melling, 'Beyond a Shadow of a Doubt?', p. 428.
104 This expression is attributed to an address on 'The Effects of Dust Inhalation in Mines' that J. S. Haldane delivered to the South Wales Institute of Engineers in 1923 and is quoted in Cotes, J. E., 'The Medical Research Council Pneumoconiosis Research Unit, 1945–1985: A Short History and Tribute', *History of Occupational Medicine*, 50:6 (2000), 440–449, p. 440. For a more thorough discussion of this remark in the context of the 1930 controversy about miners' silicosis see Meiklejohn, A., 'History of Lung Diseases of Coal Miners in Great Britain: Part 3, 1930–1952', *British Journal of Industrial Medicine*, 9 (1952), 208–220, p. 211.
105 Interview, D. C. Davies, 1930–1976. South Wales Miners' Library, Swansea, transcript reference AUD 387, p. 2. The theory was that the irritation in the lungs would cause the men to spit up the silicosis dust.
106 Perchard, A., and Gildart, K., ' "Buying Brains and Experts": British Coal Owners, Regulatory Capture and Miners' Health', *Labor History*, 56:4 (2015), 459–480, p. 464.
107 'Stuttering' is aptly used in Melling, 'Beyond a Shadow of a Doubt?', p. 430.
108 Perchard and Gildart, ' "Buying Brains and Experts" ', p. 462.
109 McIvor, A., 'Miners, Silica and Disability: The Bi-National Interplay between South Africa and the United Kingdom, c. 1900–1930s', *American Journal of Industrial Medicine*, 5:S1 (2015), 523–530, p. 525.
110 Bufton, M., and Melling, J., ' "A Mere Matter of Rock": Organised Labour, Scientific Evidence and British Government Schemes for Compensation of Silicosis and Pneumoconiosis among Coalminers, 1926–1940', *Medical History*, 49:2 (2005), 155–178, p. 157.
111 Bloor, 'The South Wales Miners Federation', p. 129.
112 See Bufton and Melling, ' "A Mere Matter of Rock" ' and McIvor, 'Miners, Silica and Disability', p. 526.

113 McIvor, 'Miners, Silica and Disability', p. 525.
114 Braun, *Breathing Race into the Machine*, p. 143.
115 McIvor, 'Miners, Silica and Disability', p. 528.
116 The Silicosis Medical Board in Wales was based in Cardiff. See Dr Gwent Jones, draft report, 'A Survey on Silicosis in Wales' (1943). Richard Burton Archives, Swansea University, SWCC, MNC/PP/15/1, p. 19. Henceforth Jones, 'A Survey on Silicosis in Wales', SWCC, MNC/PP/15/1.
117 Braun, *Breathing Race into the Machine*, p. 143 and p. 144.
118 *Chronic Pulmonary Disease in South Wales Coalminers: Report by the Committee* (Medical Research Council Special Report Series No. 243) (London: His Majesty's Stationery Office, 1942), Introduction, p. ix. TNA, FD 41243. Henceforth MRC Special Report 243, TNA, FD 41243.
119 Bufton, M., and Melling, J., 'Coming Up for Air: Experts, Employers, and Workers in Campaigns to Compensate Silicosis Sufferers in Britain, 1918–1939', *Social History of Medicine*, 18:1 (2005), 63–86, p. 75.
120 Bufton and Melling, ' "A Mere Matter of Rock" ', p. 161.
121 'Report of Court of Appeal Decision Upholding Employers Appeal against Compensation Award'. Various Industries Scheme – Extension to Coal Mines, 1934. TNA, PIN 12/72.
122 Newspaper clipping, 'Appeals against Compensation Won. Employers' Protection under Silicosis Scheme'. Various Industries Scheme – Extension to Coal Mines, 1934. TNA, PIN 12/72.
123 Bufton and Melling, ' "A Mere Matter of Rock" ', p. 164.
124 Ibid., p. 167.
125 Braun, *Breathing Race into the Machine*, p. 143.
126 MRC Special Report 243, TNA, FD 41243, Introduction, p. vi.
127 D'Arcy Hart, P., 'Chronic Pulmonary Disease in South Wales Coal Mines: An Eye-Witness Account of the MRC Surveys (1937–1942)', *Social History of Medicine*, 11:3 (1998), 459–468, p. 462.
128 MRC Special Report 243, TNA, FD 41243, Introduction, p. v.
129 Valier, H., and Timmermans, C., 'Clinical Trials and the Reorganization of Medical Research in Post-Second World War Britain', *Medical History*, 52 (2008), 493–510.
130 D'Arcy Hart, 'Chronic Pulmonary Disease', p. 462; MRC Special Report 243, TNA, FD 41243, Introduction, p. v, which states that the medical survey was undertaken by Hart and Aslett with contributions from Hicks and Yates and the pathological report was made by T. H. Belt with assistance from A. A. Ferris.
131 D'Arcy Hart, 'Chronic Pulmonary Disease', p. 462.
132 MRC Special Report 243, TNA, FD 41243, Preface.
133 See ibid., Medical Survey, p. 35 and Preface, p. vii.
134 The four categories were scaled from 'no, or only slight, respiratory embarrassment' to 'breathless at rest' and included intermediate points. Ibid., Medical Survey, p. 47.

135 Ibid.
136 It is worth noting that these categories are described as 'convenient' and there were some initial restrictions of this compensation. See 'Summary of Chapter 5', ibid., Introduction, p. v.
137 Braun, *Breathing Race into the Machine*, p. 145.
138 Jones, 'A Survey on Silicosis in Wales', SWCC, MNC/PP/15/1, p. 12.
139 Braun, *Breathing Race into the Machine*, p. 145.
140 Bloor, 'The South Wales Miners Federation'.
141 Braun, *Breathing Race into the Machine*, p. 146.
142 MRC Special Report 243, TNA, FD 41243, Medical Survey, p. 143.
143 Ibid., Medical Survey (ii) Incidence of X-ray Changes in Different Mining Occupations, p. 168. Emphasis in original.
144 Jones, 'A Survey on Silicosis in Wales', SWCC, MNC/PP/15/1, p. 17.
145 Turner, D., and Blackie, D., *Disability in the Industrial Revolution: Physical Impairment in British Coalmining, 1780–1880* (Manchester: Manchester University Press, 2018).
146 Jones, 'A Survey on Silicosis in Wales', SWCC, MNC/PP/15/1, p. 17.
147 Braun, *Breathing Race into the Machine*, p. 144.
148 Melling, 'Beyond a Shadow of a Doubt?', pp. 446–448.
149 Braun, *Breathing Race into the Machine*, p. 143.
150 Gilson and Hugh-Jones, *Lung Function in Coalworkers' Pneumoconiosis*, p. 27.
151 Aslett et al., 'Lung Volume', p. 504.
152 Smith, 'Black Lung', pp. 347–348.
153 Gilson and Hugh-Jones, *Lung Function in Coalworkers' Pneumoconiosis*, p. 27.
154 Ibid.
155 Braun, *Breathing Race into the Machine*, p. 160.
156 MRC Special Report 243, TNA, FD 41243, pp. 109–111.
157 Aslett et al., 'Lung Volume', p. 505.
158 Galton, 'The Final Report of the Anthropometric Committee', p. 20.
159 Braun, *Breathing Race into the Machine*, p. 162.
160 Ibid., p. 160 and p. 164.
161 Campbell, E. J. M., and Howell, J. B. L., 'The Sensation of Dyspnoea', *British Medical Journal*, 2:5361 (1963), 868, later referenced in a letter to *The Lancet*: 'Breathlessness', *The Lancet*, 287:7447 (1966), 1140.
162 'Shortness of Breath', *The Lancet*, 220:5693 (1932), 798–799.
163 Ibid.
164 'Breathlessness', p. 1140.
165 Malpass, A., McGuire, C., and Macnaughton, J., 'The Body Says It: The Difficulty of Measuring and Communicating Sensations of Breathlessness', *Medical Humanities* (under review).
166 Johnson, M. J., Kanaan, M., Richardson, G., Nabb, S., et al., 'A Randomised Controlled Trial of Three or One Breathing Technique Training Sessions for Breathlessness in People with Malignant Lung Disease', *BMC Medicine*, 13:1 (2015), 213.

167 Hayen, A., Herigstad, M., and Pattinson, K. T. S., 'Understanding Dyspnoea as a Complex Individual Experience', *Maturitas*, 76:1 (2013), 45–50.
168 Backman et al., 'Evaluation of the Global Lung Function Initiative', p. 2.
169 Quadrelli, S., Roncoroni, A., and Montiel, G., 'Assessment of Respiratory Function: Influence of Spirometric Reference Values and Normality Criteria Selection', *Respiratory Medicine*, 93 (1999), 523–535, p. 529.
170 Ibid., p. 534.
171 Stanojevic et al., 'Reference Values for Lung Function', p. 13.
172 Aslan, S. C., McKay, W. B., Singh, G., and Ovechkin, A. V., 'Respiratory Muscle Activation Patterns during Maximum Airway Pressure Efforts Are Different in Women and Men', *Respiratory Physiology and Neurobiology*, 259 (2019), 143–148.
173 For gender differences in COPD diagnosis see Raghavan, D., Varkey, A., and Bartter, T., 'Chronic Obstructive Pulmonary Disease: The Impact of Gender', *Current Opinion in Pulmonary Medicine*, 23:2 (2017), 117–123. For airway obstruction see Miller, M. R., 'Chronic Obstructive Pulmonary Disease: Missed Diagnosis versus Misdiagnosis', *British Medical Journal*, 351:3021 (2015), 1–5, p. 2. For more on indoor air pollution's disproportionate impact on women in the developing world and the lack of attention paid to these health effects see Olopade, C. O., Frank, E., Bartlett, E., Alexander, D., et al., 'Effect of a Clean Stove Intervention on Inflammatory Biomarkers in Pregnant Women in Ibadan, Nigeria: A Randomised Controlled Study', *Environment International*, 98 (2017), 181–190.

6

THE RESPIRATOR AND THE MECHANISATION OF NORMAL BREATHING

Breath prosthetics

In 1937, a physician led nine patients down to the basement of the Brompton hospital and into a compressed air chamber called an 'air bath'. It must have been an eerie experience. Air baths had fallen out of fashion years before, and were situated in the basement of the hospital, near the engine room and adjacent to three Turkish baths. Even when such machines had been in regular use in the nineteenth century, historian Jen Wallis notes that the Brompton ones were remarkably 'medicalised and industrialised' and, once inside, the patient was entirely isolated and disconnected from the outside world.[1] The two air baths at the Brompton hospital were purchased between 1879 and 1880 and were originally designed to prevent the advancement of consumption for patients in the early stages of the disease.[2] Since their usage had fallen into disrepute in the intervening fifty-seven years, it must have felt very strange for the patients to be led into these dark, unfamiliar and no doubt dusty old machines.[3] However, the consulting physician, George Ernest Beaumont (1888–1974), had a theory that the compressed air baths could work to bring 'into use previously dormant alveoli' by opening them up through the 'pressure of oxygen in the atmospheric air'.[4] Before undergoing this experimental treatment, the nine chosen patients had their vital capacity measured by Beaumont, and this was done again upon their exit from the machine. Beaumont explained that, 'the VC readings did not improve so did not support the idea that they opened up the alveoli'.[5] For Beaumont, this confirmed the limited value of the treatment. The patients, however, did find value in the experience. Beaumont noted that 'Eight patients stated that while in the bath they experienced sensations described as "comfort" "looseness" or "freedom". Two patients considered that they were constantly less short of breath than they had been before the treatment was started.'[6] However, because their spirometric readings did not indicate improvement, the patients' assessment of the value of the air bath was entirely disregarded. Their testimony was noted – but downgraded against the superior numerical data provided by the spirometer. This vignette provides another example of mechanical epistemic injustice and highlights the tension inherent to assessing individual experience of technologies designed to assist breathing.

The previous chapter highlighted the difficulties of classifying individual respiratory disability. In this chapter I explore how those so classified lived with this disability in the interwar period. To do so, I examine the ways in which various institutional and individual bodies engaged with technologies to extend, adapt and supplement their breath. As the last chapter emphasised, the invisibility and individuality of normal breathing made it a particularly difficult phenomenon to measure as standard. These difficulties similarly permeated attempts to design assistive respiratory technologies.

The possibility of using technology to facilitate breathing was advanced during the early twentieth century partly because of the prevalence of seasonal polio epidemics which could leave victims with paralysed respiratory muscles. However, as in the case of the hearing-assistive technologies discussed in Chapter 4, there were debates during the interwar period about which bodies ought to be responsible for providing and perfecting such technologies. Should respiratory technologies be designed by engineers or by medical men? Or by those using the technologies themselves? In this debate, there were parallels between the development of assistive technologies designed for hearing loss and breathlessness. By utilising such assistive technology, the user makes visible a previously invisible disability, and in doing so, can become subject to increased stigmatisation.[7] Both technologies are also notable for high levels of user innovation and, as I explain in the section below on the origins of pneumatic medicine, individual experimentation was incorporated into its beginnings. User modification of respiratory technologies is explored further in the section that follows, which analyses an early 'breathing machine' called the Bragg–Paul pulsator, originally designed in collaboration between a user and an engineer.[8] Yet the embodied knowledge that was used to create this mechanical respirator was not accepted by the medical establishment. Physiotherapists disputed its viability and questioned the health benefits of the principles by which the pulsator operated, and we will see in the section on 'Patient experiences in the machine' that this dispute led to the MRC leading an intervention to decide on a 'standard' breathing machine. However, these inimitable breathing machines proved to be remarkably difficult to standardise.

Technologies designed to enable breathing are unique in their association with life, death and voice.[9] As I have previously discussed with philosopher Havi Carel and healthcare professional Kate Binnie, 'technologies bringing oxygen into the body have a special symbolic resonance related to fundamental meanings associated with breath (e.g. life, spirit, inspiration). These meanings and the experience of their antonyms (death, struggle, expiration) contribute to a gripping and pervasive anxiety that cannot necessarily be ameliorated by technology alone'.[10] Here I recover historical experiences with respiratory technologies by prioritising users' voices. In doing so, I outline (in the section 'From home to hospital') the extent to which user experiences and voices were prioritised or not as respiratory technology moved from the home to the hospital during the interwar period. The lack of recognition of the individuality of breathing meant these individuals were inspired to adapt and 'tinker' with respiratory assistive technology in order to make them work for them. It is important to note, however, that certain of the respiratory technologies in this chapter were designed to manually stimulate the lungs, facilitating the breath by literally forcing compression of the chest. This kind of respiratory-assistive technology does the breathing for the user (like a modern-day ventilator) and thus differs from the kind of ambulatory oxygen which gives auxiliary oxygen to its user, which we might now more commonly associate with the term 'breath prosthetic'. However, using oxygen in this way does have important historical precedent in the field of pneumatic medicine, which I explore in the next section to set up the connections between measurement, individuality and oxygen, a theme I return to in the conclusion to this chapter.

The origins of pneumatic medicine

The radical individualism that characterised Enlightenment thinking was central to the eighteenth-century race to identify oxygen as a discrete substance distinct from the surrounding air.[11] In the process of his experiments with mice trapped in bell jars Joseph Priestley (1733–1804) initially termed the unknown air he had isolated 'dephlogisticated air' in line with the then dominant understanding of combustion as resulting from phlogiston. This was, of course, replaced by the 'fragile' oxygen theory 'crafted by Lavoisier', as Hasok Chang has put it.[12] But before the so-called 'chemical revolution' Priestley had generated 'oxygen' by placing powdered mercuric oxide (previously burnt mercury) in a bell jar so that the gas it generated would be captured in a bottle above.[13] When he put a candle in the bottle containing the gas, the flame burnt more strongly. Priestley therefore surmised that this was a 'new' kind of pure air, which could be important for processes including combustion, calcination and respiration.[14] He experimented with mice, showing that they could live and prosper in this newly isolated gas, whereas they would die rapidly in a sealed container filled with 'common air'.[15] Following the mice trials he immediately experimented on himself, and after he inhaled the unidentified air, mused: 'I fancied that my breath felt peculiarly light and easy for some time afterwar. Who can tell but that in time this pure air may become a fashionable article in luxury.'[16]

Such emphasis on the individual sensory experience of breathing marked initial experiments with oxygen as a health substance. David Phillip Miller and Trevor H. Levere have argued that the initial development of pneumatic medicine can be encapsulated in the phrase 'inhale it and see'.[17] Individual experience was crucial to the pneumatic medicine project, and sensory experience was integral to the production of knowledge about breathing. Thus, we can see that the individual body has at various points played an important part in developing knowledge about respiration technologies.

There was great initial optimism about using such 'airs' to treat disease, evident from the creation of institutions like the Pneumatic Institution, founded by Thomas Beddoes (1760–1808) in Hotwells, Bristol, in 1799.[18] Beddoes was assisted by Humphrey Davy (1778–1829) and was joined by James Watt (1736–1819) in 1794. Their collaborations between 1792 and 1798 focused on devising apparatus that could deliver various airs to patients.[19] The typical treatment at the institution was 'a pint of oxygen air in a bagful of common air'.[20] This bagful of air was literally a *bag full of air*. Usually the bag was made of oiled silk material and the air would ideally be inhaled directly from the bag into the mouth.[21] Mouthpieces were developed for users who found this difficult, initially comprised of two valves of silk and a small pipe. Eventually, mouthpieces were created from materials including vulcanite, glass, metal, ivory, velveteen and leather.[22]

Beddoes and Watt's ideas about the medical uses of airs were published in *Considerations on the Medicinal Use and Production of Factitious Airs* in 1795.[23] Included in this book were reports from individual users experimenting with oxygen as well as case notes from physicians using oxygen on their patients. Beddoes made notes under each of the cases, which are rich in idiosyncratic personal details. Take the 1795 case of Mr Danby, who relates that he got drunk on port wine at an inn near Lymington before he fell into sickness which threatened his life for five months until he was able to 'make trial of the vital air'. Upon acquiring some from a Dr Thornton, he reported that 'A week has not passed from the time of my first inhaling the vital air, before my appetite returned, and my nights were rendered so comfortable and refreshing that my wife could scarce get me up at a reasonable hour in the morning.'[24]

The movement of oxygen therapy machines from chemistry to medicine during this period mirrored the uptake of electric therapy. In both cases, there was initial optimism and a sense of harnessing the power of nature to heal, as well as conflict around how to quantify sensorial knowledge.[25] Historian Vanessa Heggie has argued that there have been long historical tensions around bodily knowledge versus laboratory knowledge in the design of artificial respiration. For example, she has shown that by the middle of the twentieth century, physiological 'facts' related to technologies of artificial respiration used in mountaineering could not be created in laboratories and were only accepted if they had been established through field observations made by individuals on the mountain.[26]

Medicinal use of oxygen fell out of favour in mainstream medicine during the 1800s and was largely abandoned before becoming specialised and reinstitutionalised within hospital medicine.[27] Oxygen use was revived during the First World War, when portable oxygen was used to treat the victims of poison gas in 1917.[28] The work of John Scott Haldane helped to demonstrate and standardise the use of oxygen therapy for those affected by poison gas, but opinions differed concerning its efficacy in the treatment of respiratory disease, and there were concerns over whether it should be given continuously or intermittently. The Haldane Oxygen Administration Apparatus was developed for treating poison gas victims, and this took the form of a metal gas mask. It was then brought into use in general medicine and described in 1921 as the most 'efficient, convenient, and economical method for oxygen administration', but a drawback to its usage was the fact that the mask could be 'strongly resented' by patients and was not tolerated in some cases.[29] In the post-war period, one can imagine that the use of an apparatus which so closely resembled a gas mask may have caused particular discomfort and disorientation, especially in children. If the mask was rejected, the nasal catheter method (which involved inserting the tube directly into the nose) could be used, but this was often criticised for its inefficiency. In an emergency, Dr Whitridge Davies recommended in 1922 that a cardboard hat box could be appropriated.[30]

Between 1920 and 1940 there were disputes about whether oxygen should be given at all, and if so, for what conditions, under what circumstances and in what form? In 1921, for example, William C. Stadie (1886–1959) described an oxygen chamber used for pneumonia treatment at the hospital of the Rockefeller Institute for Medical Research. This oxygen chamber was built just off the main ward and included a 'food lock' for passing food and small items without opening the door. The patients enclosed within could communicate with the outside world by telephone.[31] This was the method of oxygen administration carried out in the Cambridge Physiological Laboratory to treat men gassed in the First World War.[32]

However, the more traditional means of administrating oxygen at that time was still by 'means of a rubber tube and glass funnel'.[33] This funnel was described in 1924 by Dr G. D. Laing as commonly used but expensive and ineffective.[34] Laing also felt that the various masks available were not appropriate for nervous patients or children, describing them as 'cumbersome, uncomfortable, and distressing to the patient'.[35] He advocated instead for the catheter to go into the mouth. It could then be fixed to the cheek or chin by a plaster, or for children the tube could be dipped into sugar and water flavoured with peppermint.[36] His criticism appeared in the context of a debate in the *British Medical Journal* in 1924 about the best way to administer oxygen. The funnel-style methods were criticised in the *Edinburgh Medical Journal* in 1922 by Dr Whittington Davies as faulty and ineffective and were blamed for oxygen's usage falling into disrepute.[37] Like Laing, Davies argued that it was a mistake to administer oxygen only as a last resort before death, and that it should instead be considered as type of drug treatment which should be given early, ideally through encasement in an oxygen chamber. The other alternative Laing considered better than mask administration was the oxygen tent. Measurement of oxygen level in the individual body was not yet feasible and administration of oxygen at a level above 40–60 per cent was considered dangerous because it had been shown to cause fatal pneumonia when trialled on animals.[38]

However, technologies designed by individuals for individuals could succeed in a way that confounded the expectations of the medical establishment. This is especially evident in analysis of the Bragg–Paul pulsator, which was originally invented by Nobel prize-winning physicist William H. Bragg (1862–1942) in collaboration with its user, his neighbour Samuel Crosby Halahan (1869–1936).[39]

The Bragg–Paul pulsator

Captain Samuel Crosby Halahan lived in West Sussex and had what Bragg described as a 'terrible wasting of the muscles'.[40] Not much is known about Halahan's life other than he served in the military and that his friendship with Bragg resulted in the design of a new home-made 'breathing machine'. Beginning in 1926, Halahan began progressively losing all 'power of moving his limbs' until he was unable to drive a car or write, and he gradually lost weight. Halahan was unable to breathe without assistance for over a year, eventually employing two nurses:

For a long time two nurses were employed giving artificial respiration continually: the wife felt very much the disability of being unable to speak to him except in the presence of a nurse because her strength had considerably diminished due to the strain of her husband's illness, and she was unable therefore to give artificial respiration herself.[41]

Halahan's respiratory paralysis, which first began in 1931, was diagnosed as resulting from progressive muscular atrophy; continuous artificial respiration was necessary to keep him alive from the onset of paralysis until his death in 1936 at the age of sixty-six.[42] Given the strain continuous artificial respiration placed on Halahan's relationship with his wife, Bragg 'had the idea that [he] could ease matters by a simple system of india [sic] rubber bladders, football bladders in fact' to substitute the human effort. To devise this automated system, he bandaged one of the bladders under a binder on Halahan's chest and the other to a pair of hinged boards on the ground, then connected the two with a long tube. This bellows device applied rhythmic pressure directly to the chest, forcing the diaphragm to contract and air to enter and leave the lungs. Bragg's invention used positive pressure (unlike the iron lung, which used negative pressure) to enforce expiration of air by forcing the ribs in.

Despite the mechanical improvement, the labour remained arduous for the nurses and Maud (his wife), so Bragg asked instrument maker Robert W. Paul (1869–1943) to construct a small hydraulic machine which could be connected to the main water supply.[43] This new design worked effectively – except on occasions when the water pipes froze or the water supply was shut off for repairs without notice – and was estimated to have caused 15 million involuntary respirations in Halahan's lifetime.[44] It was discreet, as the hollow bandage that replaced the football bladder could be hidden by the bedcovers.[45] Furthermore, it made Halahan's relationships easier, as Maud could 'give artificial respiration while she sits and reads to her husband' and only one nurse was required to assist.[46] He wore the device for up to seventeen hours at a time, as he could not 'bear the constriction of the bandage' all day; the remaining hours were filled with manual respiration.[47] Bragg's portable system offered Halahan more mobility, privacy and control over his own breathing. The system was adjusted to fit to Halahan's body, leaving him 'free to do as much as he could have done if it had not been applied'.[48] It was even allegedly modified so that it could be used while driving.[49]

As I have previously argued alongside Carel, the elements of co-production in its design origins involved engagement with the patient's needs beyond the strictly medical.[50] For example, it was inconspicuous and could be easily disguised so 'that there was no evidence of anything unusual except the quiet click-clack of the pulsator in another part of the room'.[51] The pulsator method was a relatively cheap and portable respirator which offered its users a relatively high degree of mobility and independence. Such considerations were set up in comparison to the so called 'iron-lung'-style respirators which developed concurrently with the pulsator. The first 'iron lungs' were designed in the USA at Harvard University by Philip Drinker (1894–1972) and Louis Agassiz Shaw, Jr (1886–1940), and used (negative) vacuum pressure to mechanically force a patient's diaphragm to expand and contract to exert alternating pressure through a push-pull motion.[52] By regulating the rate and depth of respiration, the device allowed for prolonged artificial respiration, either until the patient recovered muscle strength or until an alternative method of treatment became available.

The Drinker device, as it became known, was first used in the UK in 1930.[53] However, it was expensive, bulky and heavy, and so difficult to transport. It was eventually superseded by Australian inventor Edward T. Both's (1908–87) plywood-based iron lung, which was presented as a more affordable alternative.[54] Like the Drinker device, the Both iron lung required the patient to be entirely encased in a cabinet with only the head protruding and with only the capacity to eat, drink and sleep.[55] However, the depth and rate of their breathing was controlled by an attendant, not by the patient.[56] One user described the challenge of moderating eating and breathing patterns to the machine:

> You can eat in the iron lung because your head is outside but the rest of your body is inside, although since you are flat on your back you really need to be careful when you swallow; you have to swallow in rhythm with the machine because it's pulling your diaphragm in and then pushing it out again. You just wait until it's breathing out and then you swallow. Coughing was a bit more difficult because you don't cough in rhythm with the iron lung. It was something you had to work around.[57]

By comparison, through using positive pressure to force expiration of air, the Bragg–Paul pulsator represented a cheap and *portable* alternative to the iron-lung respirators, designed such that it could be carried by a single porter for use in a private home or a hospital ward.[58] Bragg's initial iteration worked through manual rhythmical manipulation of the pump, and Paul ensured that the bellows could be actuated by hand as well if necessary. Yet, even though their design provided greater agency to the patient by freeing them from completely mechanised enclosure, the breathing was still controlled by an attendant. This reliance and the need to protect the pulsator against any unforeseen complications (such as electrical or water failures) meant that Halahan was never left alone. He was also to use his tongue and teeth without breath to sound an alarm danger signal 'resembling that of a bird' to alert the attendant.[59] This technique is similar to 'frog breathing', which involved patients with paralysed chests utilising the muscles of the neck to breathe in a gulping fashion 'like a frog'.[60]

The benefits of a portable, semi-mechanical respirator being widely available were not lost on Bragg and Paul. In 1933, Bragg contacted several hospitals to inquire whether there was any medical interest in the pulsator. One reply, from K. N. Knapp of Swindon and North Wilts Victoria Hospital, agreed that it would be beneficial to have the device in the hospital, arguing that such 'a semi-mechanical respirator would often be most useful, and would save labour and Staff'.[61] Knapp also advised Bragg to contact physiologists to improve the mechanisation of the device and so Paul contacted Dr Edward Poulton at the London School of Hygiene and Tropical Medicine, to help work out how to standardise the measurements of ventilation efficiency needed for different patients.[62] This was a necessary step for allowing large-scale usage of the respirator and for its incorporation into a hospital setting.[63]

To ensure the pulsator was available to hospitals, and to popularise it as an alternative to iron lungs, Paul took upon himself the financial responsibility to order six devices for hospitals using his limited personal funds. Both Bragg and Paul explained that they were not 'financially interested' in their machine and thus chose not to patent it or request royalties.[64] The machine was manufactured by the firm Siebe Gorman and Co. (who had made the aforementioned Haldane gas masks) at a cost of £30.[65] They also substituted steel for brass in certain parts to 'strengthen the design of the apparatus'.[66] By this stage the pulsator was electrically driven and Bragg emphasised that this meant it was 'practically noiseless' – especially when compared with the Drinker machine, which was notoriously loud.[67] Its externally audible noisiness was amplified further for users in the iron lung, who could also feel the pump vibrations. Thirteen pulsators were installed in British hospitals by 1937 (a further six were sent overseas), and another sixteen were on order.[68] Even more were placed on backorder, perhaps because in 1938 there were several polio outbreaks and an increased number of diphtheria cases requiring ventilators.

The pulsator's highest-profile promotion was given by the BBC on a Friday night on 8 July 1938. The BBC sent out an emergency SOS for a Bragg–Paul pulsator needed at an Ipswich hospital to save the life of a child.[69] One was immediately sent by car from a London hospital, but the patient died while it was in transit.[70] On 14 July 1938, this case was discussed in the House of Commons and the Minister of Health was asked whether he could provide more pulsators to hospitals throughout Britain to extend coverage from the eighteen already in use.[71] Similarly, on 24 July 1938, a fifty-eight-year-old man died in the Royal Infirmary in Liverpool after a plane was sent to rush a Bragg–Paul pulsator from Ipswich to Liverpool.[72] Presumably the respirator had been in Ipswich since it had earlier been sent from London, and it was immediately sent back by train for another ill patient. Such well-publicised crises led to huge media interest but there was some initial confusion in the British press between the Drinker apparatus and the pulsator. Paul hastened to write to Dr Sommerville Hastings following the broadcast to explain the advantages of the pulsator, explaining 'I, personally, find it hard to imagine the continuous use of the other type for three years on a patient.'[73] However, Hasting replied that the Drinker machine was thought by physiologists to be better because it used negative pressure (creating a vacuum), which more closely imitated natural breathing.[74]

Head- and chest-only machines (like the Bragg–Paul) meant that the user was less restricted and more independent. Yet its manner of working (using positive pressure) was of concern to some medics, who highlighted the increased risk of cardiovascular problems resulting from reduced circulation and blood pressure.[75] Its unusual invention and the involvement of an engineer was also considered suspect by certain medical professionals.

A film made in the 1940s to demonstrate the different mechanical methods of artificial respiration shows how different the Bragg–Paul pulsator looks in use compared to the fully enclosed machines.[76] The film begins with the opening intertitle '1. The Paul–Bragg pulsator. The chest is rhythmically subjected to positive pressure.' After showing the working of the machine the camera focuses in on a white-coated doctor wrapping the waistcoat around a bare-chested man and securing it before plugging him into the pulsator beside the bed. The man's chest moves up and down dramatically in a wave-like motion and it almost seems as if there is something trying to escape from under his skin. This method seems almost animalistic compared with the other artificial methods shown. When the doctor covers the patient with a shirt and leaves the waistcoat on underneath it is clearly much less obtrusive. The way that it made visible so clearly the process of *forced* breathing, without the apparent security and concealment offered by the more technologised devices, was uncomfortable to watch. For me, it gave quite a different impression of the Bragg–Paul pulsator compared to the textual primary sources I had so far been reliant on and it made me feel more sympathy with the physiologists who argued against its use as 'unnatural'. I found myself unconsciously holding my breath while watching it and becoming increasingly conscious of my own breathing.

Patient experiences in the machine

The debate over negative versus positive pressure led to the MRC appointing a committee to investigate the best mechanical apparatus for 'preventing asphyxia due to respiratory paralysis'.[77] This MRC intervention was designed to fix on a standard machine for artificial respiration. This intervention was facilitated by a 'Respirators (Poliomyelitis) Committee' which comprised eight medical professionals who planned to compare the advantages of the different mechanical respirators then available.[78] The committee was especially interested in whether negative or positive pressure was preferable for artificial respiration and considered a wide variety of what they termed, 'breathing machines'. As well as considering the division between negative and positive pressure, the committee was also concerned with whether full body enclosure machines or head- and chest-only enclosure-style devices were preferable. This subject demanded immediate attention, as a serious polio epidemic had hit England and Wales in 1938.[79] Patients and users were explicitly not considered as possible members of this committee, which was convened to 'examine the various forms of machine available and to consider the problem from the physiological point of view'.[80] Initially, the committee aimed to evaluate whether negative or positive pressure was best for artificial respiration and therefore conclude whether the Bragg–Paul pulsator or the iron lung device should be recommended as standard. However, the variability of respiratory conditions under consideration and the complexities of individual cases meant that the report expanded to consider a wide variety of respiratory conditions and a wide variety of so-called 'breathing machines'. This section will argue that the heterogeneity of the conditions that required such machines, combined with the individual nature of breathing, conflicted with the MRC's remit to standardise breathing machine usage.

The committee divided power-driven machines into three categories: first, machines that enclosed the full body of the patient; second, machines that enclosed the body and head; and finally machines that did not involve total enclosure of the body. These categories suggest how bodily autonomy and movement of the patient was factored into consideration of the usefulness and effectiveness of the machines. The Barospirator was invented in 1906 and was the only device that enclosed both the body and the head. It worked like the aforementioned oxygen rooms, through strict atmospheric controls applied to a large chamber which the patient and up to two others could remain in. The control of carbon dioxide this necessitated was considered by the committee to be too onerous and so this invention was not given detailed consideration.

Thus, the main debate was over full body enclosure or not. Full-body enclosure devices included: the Drinker respirator, the Drinker–Collins respirator, the Emerson respirator, the Henderson respirator, the Siebe–Gorman 'Drinker' respirator and the Both respirator. Devices that worked without full body enclosure included: the 'Biomotor' of Dr Eisenmenger, the Bragg–Paul pulsator, the Burstall jacket respirator, the London County Council Cuirass respirator, the Turner jacket respirator, the Laffer-Lewis apparatus and Eve's Motor Rocking Bed. The latter worked on a different principle from the others: rather than using negative or positive pressure, it used gravity and the weight of the patient to force their diaphragm to move in and out. Such rocking beds were used regularly in the US on partially paralysed polio patients, but this one was presumably included under power-driven machines because it used an electronic motor to rock the bed.[81] Historian Dora Vargha has vividly explained how full-body enclosure-style devices worked in practice.

> The patient lay on her back, her whole body inside the machine, with only her head on the outside. The machine created a vacuum inside the tank, which made the patient's chest rise, resulting in inhalation. The pressure then changed in the tank, letting the chest fall and creating exhalation.[82]

The MRC report contains a section devoted to 'preparing the patient for the machine', which indicated what kind of clothes the patient should wear in this kind of device (see Figure 6.1). Only pyjama trousers and an undervest were allowed until the patient was secured inside the machine and then the pyjama jacket was put on back to front to avoid skin irritation from the rubber neck-hole rubbing against the neck.[83] The boxes used in Britain were typically made of plywood ('iron lung' was technically a misnomer) and so a thin layer of cotton wool was applied (and held in place with a bandage) to avoid skin irritation. It was crucial that 'bedsocks' were worn to avoid chilled feet from the air that rushed in from the suction hole at the end of the machine, and blankets were strategically placed to prevent patient complaints of 'cold spots' and to avoid bed sores. Careful consideration of clothing and the handling of the patient was important because of patient complaints of extreme tenderness and 'hyperaesthesia' (excessive skin sensitivity), which could make any handling very painful and distressing.[84] Adjusting the temperature of the patient within the machine was clearly an issue of some concern, and heated lamps within the cabinet were utilised alongside hot-water bottles and bellows (for cooling). Learning to eat and drink also required adjustment, as users had to learn how to adjust their swallowing to fit with the rhythms of the machine.[85] This was memorably described by home ventilation user David Brooks in 1990. Though Brook's assessment came much later than the MRC report, it

PLATE I

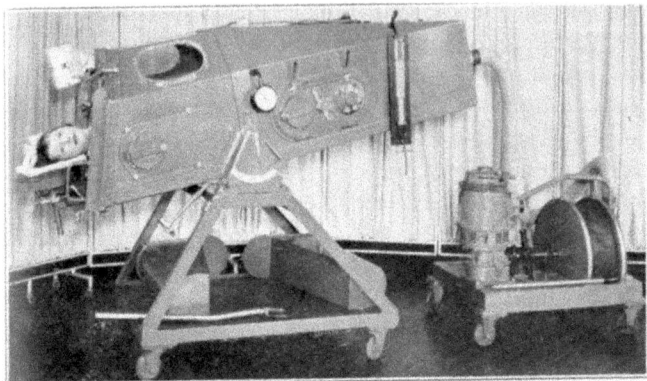

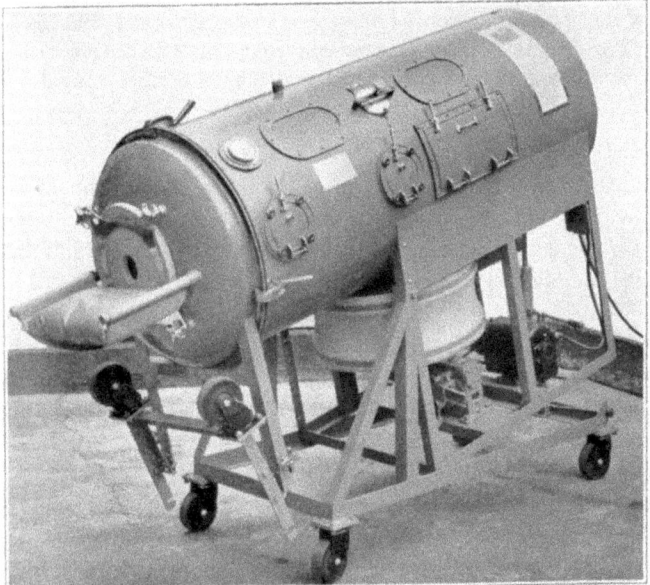

Figure 6.1 Drinker respirator and Drinker–Collins respirator

vividly portrays the difficulties associated with returning to normal activities while on breathing support.

In addition to breathing, body movements, walking and talking, the most energy sapping activity is surprisingly eating. Having lost so much weight following lung cancer, the removal of my right lung and radiotherapy, it rather added insult to injury to find that the mechanics of eating, swallowing and digesting so intimately involved the respiratory system. Exhausted swallowing muscles and pain filled chest muscles convulse along with my uselessly flapping diaphragm. They are my accompaniments to meal times, a constant battle ground between the requirements of nutrition and the insistent distress of respiratory despair.[86]

The MRC report also highlighted significant concerns about how best to synchronise an individual's breathing with the rhythm of the machine. If conscious, patients could 'frequently' indicate what pressure felt most comfortable and best matched their personal breathing rate.[87] This did not always lead to a perfect fit, as:

> The Patient's breathing will usually be, for a short time, irregular and 'out of step' with the regular breathing of the machine, but cases with respiratory insufficiency readily adapt themselves to the rate of the machine. If the patient's breathing persistently fails to synchronise, it means that he has an adequate power of natural breathing and does not require treatment in the machine.[88]

This quotation reveals the difficulty inherent to standardising measures for a process as individual and variable as breathing. Moreover, the suggestion that users adapt themselves to the machine suggests that users were required to modify themselves to fit the technology, rather than the other way around. If patients were continually unable to adapt themselves in this way or were apprehensive of doing so, their breathing rate was adjusted slowly and without their knowledge.[89] Similar tactics were used to wean 'nervous' patients off the machines by tricking them into believing the machine was still working: 'the pressure can, without their knowledge, be gradually reduced until finally the motor is running but no negative pressure is being produced'.[90] More resistant patients were simply given a sedative to force their cooperation: 'sedatives are not required for long, as most patients soon learn to co-operate with the machine'.[91] Clearly, there was awareness of how distressing these breathing machines could be for users. However, the report insisted that for seriously ill patients, 'the relief afforded is so great and so sudden that any psychological stress is quickly banished'.[92] Perhaps surprisingly given Bragg's reference to noise as a problem, the rhythmical noise of the motor was suggested in the report to be soothing and conducive to deep sleeping. This assessment was a marked contrast to Brooks's (admittedly much later) description of sleeping in an assisted ventilation unit: 'the noise at night of all these pumps, huffing and puffing, inevitably at different tempos, was rather like a poorly syncopated orchestra with a demented wind section'.[93]

Moreover, the MRC's optimistic analysis was not wholly supported by the details provided in the appendix to the report, which provided quantitative and qualitative details in relation to individual case reports from across the

UK involving use of the Drinker respirator and the Bragg–Paul pulsator.[94] There were repeated instances of user rejection in these tables. For instance, one patient survived treatment with the 'Both'-type machine but 'objected strongly to being put in it'.[95] One patient used the Bragg–Paul pulsator but 'tended to breathe against it' and died after a day of its use. Similarly, another user of the pulsator had difficulty adjusting to its breathing rate: 'Difficulty in synchronisation of artificial and natural respiration caused discomfort and led to cessation of treatment.'[96] Many patients simply refused to use the machines, and though some survived, in other cases this refusal was noted as contributing to their death. In certain cases, the patient is simply noted as finding the machine either a source of 'relief' or as 'uncomfortable', though one specific case noted 'discomfort in machine so severe that patient's removal from it was ordered'.[97] Another patient was described as 'so terror-stricken by machine that he had to be removed'.[98] Comparing the images from the report (shown here as Figure 6.1 and Figure 6.2) might provide clues to explain this reaction. While the Burstall jacket respirator and the Bragg–Paul pulsator do look strange, with the latter resembling diving apparatus (unsurprising given that the manufacturing company Siebe–Gorman specialised in diving apparatus), they clearly allow for movement and control; on the other hand, the Both-style iron lung resembles, more than anything else, a coffin. Overall, the impression of user experience of these 'breathing machines' was highly variable. And, crucially, the user's inability or unwillingness to use the machines was a repeated motif and clearly affected the viability of this kind of treatment.

One key appeal of the pulsator was that while wearing it, the patient was not hindered or inconvenienced by its movements. With an attachment, it could also be used by two patients at the same time, forcing them to literally conspire together.[99] However, there was concern that positive pressure respiration could depress circulation and reduce cardiac output and blood pressure, a concern which was heightened for bulbar polio patients suffering from circulatory damage.[100] It was crucial then, the MRC decided, for patients using an artificial respirator to be under the expert management of doctors, nurses and other attendants who were 'acquainted with certain points and difficulties which arise during the use of mechanical aids to respiration', especially when repair was required.[101] The MRC report emphasised that those using such machines must only do so under the supervision of medical professionals.[102] Care was also necessary to ensure that infections, bed sores, vomiting and constipation were managed so as not to cause serious complications, especially in patients with respiratory paralysis.

The MRC report on 'Breathing Machines and their Use in Treatment' was published in 1939, just as William Morris, later Lord Nuffield (1877–1963),

THE RESPIRATOR AND MECHANISATION 189

Plate III

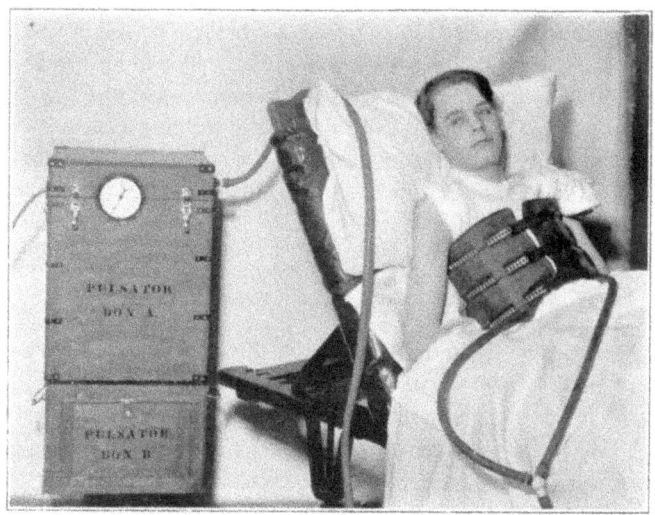

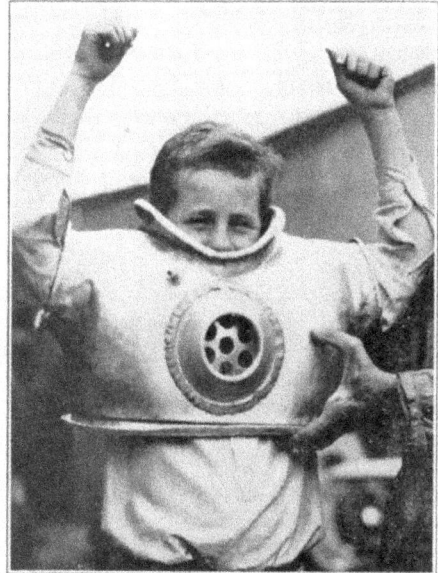

Figure 6.2 Bragg–Paul pulsator and Burstall jacket respirator

announced his intent to widely distribute 800 Both-style respirators around Britain, free of charge. Morris manufactured the iron lungs in his car factories and eventually donated more than 5,000 of these devices.[103] The donation of iron lungs to hospitals throughout Britain allowed for free and easy institutional usage, especially as the MRC recommended that it was more beneficial to bring patients to the hospital than to bring equipment to the home. By the end of March 1939, there were just over 1,000 respirators in the British Isles: 965 Both respirators, 43 Bragg–Paul pulsators and 30 Drinker machines.[104]

From home to hospital

Bringing patients to the hospital and placing them in these machines became standard practice after the Second World War. However, this solution (while medically and economically advisable) could lead to added distress to families, who lost the ability to communicate with their loved ones. Not only were patients quarantined (physically isolated), it was also difficult for them to communicate with the medical team as a result of their encasement and reduced visibility in the iron lung. Literally, this encasement impeded patient voice, as they could only talk on the out-breath of the machine. We can determine the practical consequences of such isolation from cases like that of sixteen-year-old Dorothy, who woke in the night of 28 September 1950 with severe back pain.[105] Over the next two days her pain worsened, until she was vomiting from agony and forced to go to hospital. The attending doctor noted that she had widespread paralysis and diagnosed APM (acute poliomyelitis). Her subsequent isolation caused severe anxiety to her mother, who wrote to the hospital to explain:

> [W]hen Dorothy was taken away I had 2 shocks first was to be told by her own Dr, that Dorothy was 10 weeks pregnant, second was to hear she had Polio, this has drove me nearly crazy [sic] with worry, as Dorothy was in such awful pain I decided not to say anything to her about being pregnant until she was better, but instead she got worse and was taken away.[106]

The physician treating Dorothy replied somewhat caustically that 'I can hardly doubt but that Dorothy knows quite well that she is pregnant', but reassured her mother that the paralysis was improving, and that Dorothy had not lost the baby. However, by the end of November he decided that it was necessary to terminate the pregnancy to save the patient. After this, Dorothy's condition rapidly improved, she was able to undergo physiotherapy and after ninety-four days in hospital, she was discharged. Although her experience was undoubtedly traumatic for her and her family – she was described twice in the notes as hysterical – Dorothy's case at least ended with recovery.

By contrast, twenty-nine-year-old polio patient Rose was admitted to the same hospital on 16 October 1950 and was immediately placed in a mechanical respirator.[107] Her abdominal reflexes were described as 'absent' and she had 'little movement' in her diaphragm. Her distress was such that she was only partially examined before being placed straight into the respirator. Once in the respirator, she was given physiotherapy 'in so far as can be managed with patient in respirator'.[108] By December, she could be taken out of the respirator for controlled periods, only initially managing two to three minutes but up to four to five minutes by the end of the month. On 31 December 1950 there was an electricity failure in the hospital which meant Rose 'almost died' before it was possible to get the 'manual operation working'. This may be the reason that six days later she was transferred from the Drinker respirator to the Both respirator – a change which made her both more cheerful and comfortable. However, over the following month she contracted pneumonia and, despite rallying towards the end of January, she had a 'sudden attack of dyspnoea' (breathlessness) at midnight on 1 February 1951, became unconscious, was briefly revived and described as 'terrified', before she subsequently died.[109]

The practice of gradually building up the time the patient spent breathing unaided outside the respirator was a standard treatment for polio patients with respiratory paralysis, especially as it allowed them to participate in physiotherapy. Patients using the respirator were encouraged to stay out for longer periods and once they could remain out for forty-five minutes, they started taking their meals outside the machine. Although adult patients were relatively isolated and relied on epistolary correspondence to communicate with the outside world, parents were able to visit younger children living in the iron lungs, often for extended periods. One such child patient spent 218 days in this hospital in the Drinker machine. When he died, the attending physician described it as a 'welcome event', noting that he 'would never have lived independent of respirator' but that he was 'quite cheerful up to end. Parents helped a great deal by visiting daily without fail.'[110] The child's GP agreed with this assessment and wrote to the hospital physician to thank him for his care, noting 'I agree with you that it was the best thing that could have happened to the poor child, under the unhappy circumstances.'[111] These notes illuminate the changing conception of the respirator, from a prosthetic enabling the user to continue life at home, to emergency hospital equipment in which life was considered untenable. Even though these patients were described as cheerful, the iron lung was not being used in the hospital as a prosthetic in the way that Halahan had used his pulsator at home. However, there is evidence that some contemporary users were using iron lungs to live full and productive lives in this period, as in the case of Mr Fred Suite, who lived in an iron lung when he was married in 1939 and went on honeymoon in a specially weight-adapted trailer.[112]

Furthermore, there are accounts of users of iron lungs and their family members designing home-made personalised machines during this period in Britain. For instance, in 1949 Mr A. F. Evans, a motor engineer in Coventry, designed a specific style of iron lung for his daughter which would allow her to live at home. He explained that he had built the device in his garage with some assistance from his employees and his daughter's friend, and emphasised that 'This new lung I have made covers only the abdomen and chest. It keeps Ann breathing and allows the physiotherapist to give massage and to exercise the limbs to bring fresh life into them.'[113] A twenty-six-year-old man in Essex who had virtually no movement except of his head and neck lived at home and was reported to 'frog-breathe for up to three hours but otherwise needs a Tunnicliffe respirator and pump'.[114] In a letter to the editor of *The Lancet*, his doctor detailed the different organisations involved in his care, which included the installation of a Post Office telephone; the doctor explained that 'The County Health Department provide a special nurse; the local council have altered the house; the GPO installed a telephone within 24 hours; the next-door neighbour services the pump; and the Association for the Physically Handicapped have helped in many ways.'[115] Bess Williamson has explored similar instances of users of respiratory technology appropriating medical prothesis to their own designs, by altering 'familiar technologies to work for their own disabled bodies'.[116] In Williamson's analysis of post-1950s magazines for self-nominalised 'respos', she finds that the equipment that disabled users ordered from hospitals often failed to integrate into their users' lives and required individual adaptation and 'tinkering'. Despite the wide acknowledgement of this tinkering in the disabled community in the US, respiratory technology designers did not advertise to users and the medical establishment ignored patient input in this arena.[117]

In part, such individualistic 'tinkering' may have stemmed from the specific nature of individuals' breathing preferences. While some users emphasised the greater portability and independence that chest-only devices offered, others preferred the all-encompassing relief offered by the standard iron lung's negative pressure. For example, Marshall Barr developed polio in Britain in 1949 and began using an iron lung in 1971. He described the experience of encasement as a 'relief' and highlighted the relaxing qualities of its sounds and vibrations, 'like: ... breathing, bump; breathing, bump ... It was not quite like a smooth breath.'[118] Paul Alexander, who started using an iron lung in 1952, used it in his university dorm in the US to pursue a successful career as a lawyer and remains in the machine at the time of writing.[119] In 2017, Martha Lillard, one of three people still using iron lungs in the US described how the lung provided relief by taking away the effort of breathing for her: 'Imagine if you were real tired of breathing, how good that would feel – if you were struggling to take a breath.'[120] For Martha and others still reliant on these older technologies, one of the main challenges is finding technicians willing to repair the iron lungs, as the private companies which originally designed them no longer take responsibility for maintaining them.[121]

As this chapter has emphasised, the heterogeneity of respiratory disability experiences proved challenging for the development of standardised treatments. This historical analysis highlights the importance of prioritising patient voices today, especially when making judgements about quality of life. Caution in this respect is highlighted by 'the disability paradox' explored in Chapter 2. That is, the fact that many disabled people rate their quality of life as good or excellent although external observers imagine them to have an 'undesirable daily existence'.[122] When asked to imagine the well-being of disabled people, non-disabled people tend to imagine it to be far worse than it is, and this error is exacerbated if the non-disabled person is a healthcare professional and corrected if they have spent time with disabled people. Given these findings, this historical episode highlights the crucial importance of making patient voices central, and especially disabled voices, in all discussions about prosthetic technology.

Conclusion: the ergodic switch

In the late 1800s, physicists working with gases encountered a measurement problem that is especially pertinent to the concerns of this chapter and the overall message of this book. While these physicists could easily measure the *collective* qualities of a group of gas molecules, identifying the specific features of each individual molecule proved challenging. To meet this challenge, the measurers decided to 'use the average behaviour of a group of gas molecules to predict the average behaviour of a single gas molecule'.[123] In doing so, they invoked a set of mathematical principles known as ergodic theory. As Todd Rose explains: 'According to ergodic theory, you are allowed to use a group average to make predictions about individuals if two conditions are true: (1) every member of the group is identical, and (2) every member of the group will remain the same in the future.'[124] As it turned out, most gas molecules did not conform to these rules, and, as this chapter has outlined, neither do most people. Yet using group averages to measure and assess individuals as though they are ergodic is precisely how we have calculated the thresholds of normalcy in a variety of statistical studies about human abilities. The idea that people can be ranked as though identical and immutable has been dubbed 'the ergodic assumption' by Peter Molenaar, who explains that 'using a group average to evaluate individuals would only be valid if human beings were frozen clones, identical and unchanging'.[125] As this chapter has outlined, using the measurements of a group to standardise technologies for individuals that are part of that group has led to user modification and rejection of assistive technology.

The nine patients of Brompton hospital that we discussed in the introduction to this chapter believed that they *felt better* as a result of their experience in the air baths. Fundamental to knowledge of health and illness is this precise question: how do you feel? But how do you know how you feel? Bodily intuition was traditionally relied upon, but over the course of the twentieth century, the veneration of numerical data as a guide to our bodies has superseded embodied knowledge. Such a position suggests that numbers and quantified data are understood to be neutral, objective and valid in a way that lived experience is not. Many have criticised this suppression and dismissal of bodily intuition as inherently reductionist, arguing that important personal perspectives are being discounted. I have argued here that this can also create mechanical epistemic injustice, which has especially deleterious impacts on the disabled.

This is an issue that is exacerbated in cases of invisible disability and further intensified by the multidimensional nature of breath, which resists reductive measurement approaches. As I have shown in this chapter, attempts to establish a standard 'breathing machine' eluded the MRC as it struggled to catch the breath of the idiosyncratic individuals under their investigation. In contrast, by working closely with a user, William Bragg and Robert Paul's design prioritised the goals and priorities of the intended consumer. Yet this meant that their design needed essential modifications (made by medical professional Dr Phyllis Kerridge) before it could be standardised for a variety of bodies in a hospital setting. Yet as standardised respiratory technologies moved from the home to the hospital and back out again, individual users made modifications to their design to suit themselves. As I argue here and elsewhere in this book, the distinctive kind of embodied knowledge that the disabled have about their own bodies resulted in innovation and invention during the interwar period. Technologies designed by individuals for individuals could be surprisingly successful. Ironically, the individual nature of this insight can work as a barrier to standardised usage (as we see in the case of the pulsator versus the iron lung). The kind of standardised usage that is necessary for institutional use in hospital settings meant that patients had to increasingly adapt to the machines they were placed in. Yet users often resisted this kind of technological intervention.

Such experiences have not been entirely relegated to the domain of history, as the kind of mechanical ventilation commonly used in intensive care units can now be done while patients are still conscious, and the experience of being unable to control one's own breathing or to speak has been recently found to result in panic, fear and enduring anxiety.[126] Moreover, original embodied knowledge often becomes invisible when embedded in technological designs or is lost with the individual or with the end of company involvement – a situation which points to the danger of privatising life-saving devices. If the insights of intended users were embedded at the start of the design process through co-production efforts then the inevitable user rejection and modification of assistive technology could be avoided and the end product would, no doubt, be much improved.

Notes

1 Wallis, J., 'A Machine in the Garden: The Compressed Air Bath and the Nineteenth-Century Health Resort', in J. Agar and J. Ward (eds), *Histories of Technology, the Environment and Modern Britain* (London: UCL Press, 2018), pp. 76–100, p. 83.
2 Ibid.
3 G. E. Beaumont, 'The Effect of Compressed Air Baths upon the Vital Capacity in Emphysema', in Brompton Hospital Reports, vol. 6, 1937. Royal London Hospital Archives, London, RLBH/A/13/63, p. 118.
4 Ibid.
5 Ibid., p. 120.
6 Ibid.
7 McGuire and Carel, 'The Visible and the Invisible'.
8 For a full explanation of the building of the Bragg–Paul pulsator see McGuire, C., Virdi, J., and Hutton, J., 'Respiratory Technologies and the Co-Production of Breathing in the Twentieth Century', in A. Hanley and J. Meyer (eds), *Patient Voices* (Manchester: Manchester University Press, forthcoming). Some of the material in the sections on 'The origins of pneumatic medicine' and 'The Bragg–Paul pulsator' originally appeared in that chapter and is reproduced here with permission.
9 Binnie, K., McGuire, C., and Carel, H., 'Objects of Safety and Imprisonment', *Journal of Material Culture* (under review).
10 Ibid.
11 For an earlier history of artificial respiration, see Barrington, A. B., 'Artificial Respiration, the History of an Idea', *Medical History*, 15:4 (1971), 336–351.
12 Chang, H., 'The Hidden History of Phlogiston: How Philosophical Failure Can Generate Historiographical Refinement', *HYLE: International Journal for Philosophy of Chemistry*, 16:2 (2010), 47–79, p. 71.
13 Jackson, J., *A World on Fire: A Heretic, an Aristocrat, and the Race to Discover Oxygen* (New York: Viking, 2005), p. 126.

14 McEvoy, J. G., 'Gases, God and the Balance of Nature: A Commentary on Priestley (1772) "Observations on Different Kinds of Air"', *Philosophical Transactions of the Royal Society A: Mathematical, Physical and Engineering Sciences*, 373:2039 (2015), 1–11, p. 4.
15 Jackson, *A World on Fire*, pp. 169–170.
16 Joseph Priestley, quoted ibid., p. 172.
17 Miller, D. P., and Levere, T. H., '"Inhale It and See?": The Collaboration between Thomas Beddoes and James Watt in Pneumatic Medicine', *Ambix*, 55:1 (2008), 5–28.
18 Grainge, C., 'Breath of Life: The Evolution of Oxygen Therapy', *Journal of the Royal Society of Medicine*, 97:10 (2004), 489–493.
19 Miller and Levere, '"Inhale It and See?"', pp. 7–8.
20 Ibid.
21 Leigh, J. M., 'The Evolution of Oxygen Therapy Apparatus', *Anaesthesia*, 29 (1974), 462–485.
22 However, use of a mouthpiece required willing cooperation and when oxygen began to be used as an anesthetic from the 1840s, face masks were developed to fully cover the mouth and nose. See ibid.
23 Beddoes, T., and Watt, J., *Considerations on the Medicinal Use and Production of Factitious Airs*, part 3 (Bristol: Bulgin and Rosser, for J. Johnson, London, 1795), University of Bristol Library Special Collections.
24 Ibid., p. 30.
25 Ueyama, T., *Health in the Marketplace: Professionalism, Therapeutic Desires, and Medical Commodification in Late Victorian London* (Palo Alto, CA: Society for the Promotion of Science and Scholarship, 2010). From 1868, compressed oxygen gas could be stored in cylinders and this removed the need for the physician to manufacture oxygen on an individual basis. See Leigh, 'The Evolution of Oxygen Therapy Apparatus'.
26 Heggie, V., 'Experimental Physiology, Everest and Oxygen: From the Ghastly Kitchens to the Gasping Lung', *British Journal for the History of Science*, 46:1 (2013), 123–147.
27 Except in home remedies and 'quack medicine'. See Ueyama, *Health in the Marketplace*.
28 'Editorial: The Therapeutic Use of Oxygen', *Canadian Medical Association Journal*, 16:6 (1926), 696–697, and Grainge, 'Breath of Life', p. 491.
29 It was manufactured by Messrs Siebe, Gorman & Co. in London. See Davies, H. W., 'Methods for the Therapeutic Administration of Oxygen', *Edinburgh Medical Journal*, 29:5 (1922), 161–168, p. 166.
30 This method was described as follows: 'the patient's head is enclosed in a cardboard hat box of suitable size, a suitable opening being cut for the neck, and the stream of oxygen being directed into the box'. See Davies, 'Methods for the Therapeutic Administration of Oxygen'.
31 Stadie, W. C., 'Construction of an Oxygen Chamber for the Treatment of Pneumonia', *Journal of Experimental Medicine*, 35:3 (1922), 323–335, p. 326.

32 Barcroft, J., 'Discussion of the Therapeutic Uses of Oxygen', *Proceedings of the Royal Society of Medicine, Section of Therapeutics and Pharmacology*, 13 (1920), 59–68.
33 Davies, 'Methods for the Therapeutic Administration of Oxygen'.
34 Laing, G. D., 'The Administration of Oxygen', *British Medical Journal*, 1:3311 (1924), 1074–1075.
35 Ibid.
36 Ibid.
37 Ibid.
38 Bert's experiments on sparrows first demonstrated this; see Heggie, 'Experimental Physiology, Everest and Oxygen'; and cf. Binger, C. J., Faulkner, J. M., and Moore, R. L., 'Oxygen Poisoning in Mammals', *Journal of Experimental Medicine*, 35:5 (1927), 849–864, and Evans, J. H., 'The Inhalation of Pure Oxygen in the Treatment of Disease', *Canadian Medical Association Journal*, 22:4 (1930), 518–522.
39 For a full discussion of the process of the Bragg–Paul pulsator's invention see McGuire et al., 'Respiratory Technologies'.
40 Bragg described Halahan as his friend and 'neighbour in the country'. Bragg was working in London at this time but may have had a second home/main base in West Sussex. Letter from W. H. Bragg to Leonard Hill, 4 January 1934. Royal Institution of Great Britain, London, William Henry Bragg RI Admin. Correspondence 1933–39 (hereafter WHB), RI MS WHB/27E/5. Information on Samuel Crosby Halahan was retrieved from GENi. www.geni.com/people/Samuel-Halahan/6000000015282798567. Accessed June 2019.
41 Letter from Bragg to Hill, 4 January 1934.
42 Kerridge, P. M. T., 'Artificial Respiration for Three and a Half Years', *The Lancet*, 227:5870 (1936), p. 504. The discussion of the nurses' continuous artificial respiration is discussed in a newspaper clipping titled 'Iron Lungs'. Royal Institution of Great Britain, William H. Bragg Miscellaneous Correspondence (hereafter WHBMC), Bragg–Paul Pulsator (15 March–15 August), RI MS WHB/8B/9. See also: Blackwell, U., 'Mechanical Respiration', *The Lancet*, 254:6568 (1949), 99–102.
43 Paul was internationally renowned for his scientific instruments, including the galvanometer, early wireless telegraphy sets and devices for submarine warfare; he is also famous today as a pioneer of British film, devising cameras and projectors for motion pictures.
44 'Iron Lungs'. WHBMC.
45 Bragg, W. H., 'Bragg–Paul Pulsator', *British Medical Journal*, 10:1136 (1938), 254.
46 Letter from Bragg to Hill, 4 January 1934.
47 Bragg, 'Bragg–Paul Pulsator'.
48 Copy of letter from William H. Bragg to Secretary of the British Red Cross Society, addressed to Colonel Day, 11 July 1938. WHBMC, WHB/8B/4–5. The Red Cross was also interested in Bragg's creation, especially since that organisation helped to commercialise oxygen tents, as indicated by a letter of 17 July 1938 from Sir Harold B. Facus, the Director-General of the British Red Cross Society to Bragg. WHBMC, WHB/8B/6.

49 'Iron Lungs'. WHBMC.
50 McGuire and Carel, 'The Visible and the Invisible'.
51 Bragg, 'Bragg–Paul Pulsator'.
52 Oshinsk, D. M., *Polio: An American Story* (Oxford: Oxford University Press, 2006), p. 61.
53 Ibid.
54 The device was originally requested by the South Australian Government in 1938 to combat a devastating poliomyelitis epidemic.
55 Drinker, P., 'Prolonged Administration of Artificial Respiration', *The Lancet*, 217:5622 (1931), 1186–1188.
56 The attendant was also essential for enabling toilet function, through bedpans and enemas. Ibid.
57 Barr, M., 'The Iron Lung: A Polio Patient's Story', *Journal of the Royal Society of Medicine*, 103:6 (2010), 256–259, p. 256.
58 'Iron Lungs'. WHBMC.
59 Kerridge, 'Artificial Respiration for Three and a Half Years'.
60 This technique is called glossopharyngeal breathing. See Wilson, D. J., *Living with Polio: The Epidemic and Its Survivors* (Chicago: University of Chicago Press, 2005), p. 91.
61 Letter from K. N. Knapp to William Bragg, 18 September 1933. WHB 27E/4.
62 Poulton also invited Bragg and Paul to present their device to the Therapeutic and Pharmaceutical Section of the Royal Society of Medicine.
63 For more on the development of the pulsator and the role Dr Phyllis Kerridge played in its development see McGuire et al., 'Respiratory Technologies'.
64 Letter from Bragg to Secretary of British Red Cross Society.
65 Letter from William Bragg to S. C. Dyke, 7 June 1934. WHB 27E/20.
66 Letter from Siebe–Gorman & Co. Ltd to Robert W. Paul, 21 May 1936. WHB 27E/29.
67 The same company that designed the oxygen mask equipment. Bragg, 'Bragg–Paul Pulsator', p. 254. On the noisiness of the Drinker machine see Gilbertson, A. A., 'Before Intensive Therapy?', *Journal of the Royal Society of Medicine*, 88:8 (1995), 459–463, p. 461.
68 Letter from Robert Paul to Dr J. R. Hutchinson, Deputy Senior Medical Officer, Ministry of Health, 12 August 1938. WHB 8B/24–26. Pulsators were distributed to hospitals in Manchester, Birmingham, London, Norwich, Ipswich, and Liverpool.
69 'Bragg Paul Respirator', HC Deb 14 July 1938, vol. 338, cc. 1517–1518. https://api.parliament.uk/historic-hansard/commons/1938/jul/14/bragg-paul-respirator. Accessed July 2019.
70 Letter from Robert Paul to C. J. McSweeny, 17 July 1938. WHBMC, WHB/8B/8.
71 'Bragg Paul Respirator', HC Deb 14 July 1938.
72 'Plane's Vain Dash with Respirator', *The Scotsman*, 25 July 1939. British Newspaper Archive, BL 0000540/19380725/107/0012.

73 Letter from Paul to Dr Somerville Hastings, 2 January 1938 (re. BBC broadcast). Paul was sent the transcript by Bragg. WHB 27E/66.
74 Letter from Dr Somerville Hastings to Paul. WHB 27E/66.
75 Wilson, J. G., 'A Continuing Battle against the Virus of Polio', *Municipal Journal*, 59 (6 July 1951), 1577–1581, p. 1577 and p. 1581.
76 This film was made by Oxford University's newly instated (1937) Department of Anaesthetics and has been made available by Wellcome on YouTube. See www.youtube.com/watch?v=21PEC3ppStc and http://catalogue.wellcomelibrary.org/record=b1677731~S3. Accessed July 2019. It was probably designed to accompany Lord Nuffield's iron lung donation and the film is referenced in a letter explaining the donation of the iron lung to St Bart's hospital. See 'Gift of a Mechanical Respirator from the Nuffield Trust', 1939. St Bartholomew's Hospital Archives, London, SBHB MR/32/4.
77 Medical Research Council, *'Breathing Machines' and Their Use in Treatment: Report of the Respirators (Poliomyelitis) Committee* (Medical Research Council Special Report Series, No. 237) (London: His Majesty's Stationery Office, 1939). TNA, FD 4/237 (henceforth MRC, *'Breathing Machines'*), p. 3.
78 Ibid.
79 'Review: Medical Research Council. Special Report Series no. 237', *Indian Medical Gazette* (1940).
80 MRC, *'Breathing Machines'*, p. 2.
81 Wilson, *Living with Polio*.
82 Vargha, D., *Polio across the Iron Curtain: Hungary's Cold War with an Epidemic* (Cambridge: Cambridge University Press, 2018), p. 60.
83 MRC, *'Breathing Machines'*, p. 46.
84 Ibid., p. 47.
85 Ibid., p. 51.
86 Brooks, D. H. M., 'Living with Ventilation: Confessions of an Addict', *Care of the Critically Ill*, 8:5 (1992), 205–207; cf. Brooks, D. H. M., 'The Route to Home Ventilation: A Patient's Perspective', *Care of the Critically Ill*, 6:3 (1990), 96–97.
87 MRC, *'Breathing Machines'*, p. 48.
88 Ibid.
89 Ibid., p. 52.
90 Ibid.
91 Ibid., p. 49.
92 Ibid.
93 Brooks, 'Living with Ventilation', p. 207.
94 That these were the only two machines that this kind of data was available for indicates that they were two most widely used machines in Britain at the time of the report's compilation.
95 MRC, *'Breathing Machines'*, Appendix, 'Table A – Continued', p. 76.
96 Ibid., p. 90.
97 MRC, *'Breathing Machines'*, Appendix, 'Table E – Continued', p. 88.

98 Ibid., p. 89.
99 'Iron Lungs Will Help Save Midland Kiddies', *Birmingham Gazette*, 4 November 1938. British Newspaper Archive, BL 0000669/19381104/057/0004. Note that although the headline refers to iron lungs, it was a Bragg–Paul pulsator which was gifted. 'Iron lung' was often used in the popular press to refer to a variety of styles of respirators. Children could also be attached in groups to the iron lung. 'Conspire' as from the Latin *conspirare*, *com* (with, together) and *spirare* (to breathe) See entry for 'conspire' in Online Etymology Dictionary. www.etymonline.com/word/conspire?ref=etymonline_crossreference. Accessed June 2019.
100 Wilson, 'A Continuing Battle'.
101 MRC, '*Breathing Machines*', p. 43.
102 Ibid.
103 Hurley, S., 'The Man behind the Motor: William Morris and the Iron Lung', *Science Museum Blog*, 7 March 2013. https://blog.sciencemuseum.org.uk/the-man-behind-the-motor-william-morris-and-the-iron-lung/. Accessed June 2019.
104 Gilbertson, 'Before Intensive Therapy?', p. 462.
105 All patient names have been changed to preserve anonymity.
106 Ham Green Hospital, Bristol, Records of Poliomyelitis, Chicken Pox, Herpes, Zoster, Rubella, Mumps, 1951. Patient Reg No. 1236/50, letter to resident physician James Macrae inserted into patient records 10 January 1950 to 1 January 1951.
107 Ham Green Hospital, Bristol, Records of Poliomyelitis, Chicken Pox, Herpes, Zoster, Rubella, Mumps, 1951. Patient Reg. No. 1298/50, patient records 16 October 1950 to 2 February 1951.
108 Ibid.
109 Ibid.
110 Ham Green Hospital, Bristol, Records of Poliomyelitis, Chicken Pox, Herpes, Zoster, Rubella, Mumps, 1951. Patient Reg. No. 1360/50, patient records 30 October 1950 to 3 June 1951.
111 Ibid., Patient Reg. No. 1360/50, letter inserted from Gloucester Road surgery, 7 June 1951.
112 'Iron Lung Man Wed', *Telegraph and Independent*, Sheffield, 11 August 1939. British Newspaper Archive, BL 0000702/19390811/007/0001.
113 'Home-Made Iron Lung Speeds Girl's Recovery', *Coventry Evening Telegraph*, August 24 1949. British Newspaper Archive, BL 0000769/19490824/256/0017.
114 Graves, J. C., Letter to the Editor, 'Domiciliary Rehabilitation of the Respiratory Cripple', *The Lancet*, 274:7110 (1959), 1033.
115 Ibid.
116 Williamson, B., 'Electric Moms and Quad Drivers: People with Disabilities Buying, Making, and Using Technology in Postwar America', *American Studies*, 52:1 (2012), 5–30, p. 23.
117 Ibid., p. 11.
118 Barr, 'The Iron Lung', p. 256.

119 Brown, J., 'The Last of the Iron Lungs', *Gizmodo*, 20 November 2017. https://gizmodo.com/the-last-of-the-iron-lungs-1819079169. Accessed June 2019.
120 Ibid.
121 Ibid.
122 Albrecht and Devlieger, 'The Disability Paradox', p. 977.
123 Rose, *The End of Average*, p. 63.
124 Ibid. See also, Molenaar, P. C. M., 'On the Implications of the Classical Ergodic Theorems: Analysis of Developmental Processes Has to Focus on Individual Variation', *Developmental Psychobiology*, 50:1 (2007), 60–69.
125 Interview, Peter Molenaar and Todd Rose, quoted in Rose, *The End of Average*, p. 63.
126 I am grateful to historian Oriana Walker, who made this point in her presentation at the recent History of Science Society meeting in Utrecht and pointed out the accompanying source, Karlsson, V., Bergbom, I., and Forsberg, A., 'The Lived Experiences of Adult Intensive Care Patients Who Were Conscious during Mechanical Ventilation: A Phenomenological-Hermeneutic Study', *Intensive and Critical Care Nursing*, 28 (2012), 6–15.

7

MEASURING OURSELVES

The interwar years made the previously invisible limits of the body visible and measurable. In the eighteenth century, there had been interest in and attempts at measuring the boundaries of human capabilities. In the nineteenth century, these attempts took on eugenic imperatives as disability was increasingly defined as abnormality. However, the First World War changed the way we thought about disability through greater recognition and awareness that disability could be acquired and could affect anyone. Furthermore, the war marked the start of strong connections between both the Post Office and the MRC with the state, which allowed them to interact as and with the wider British government. Ameliorating the impact of disability on society thus became a concern of national importance as the post-war years were marked by growing state intervention into welfare and increased recognition of government's duty to moderate societal health. Further state explorations of disability were motivated by the incentive to generate national anthropometric standards to measure and halt the progress of perceived interwar degeneration. The idea of degeneration inspired stricter definitions of disability that could be utilised in the military/industrial complex to test potential employees and moderate subsequent compensation.

How relevant are these classification systems today? Deaf activist Chrissy provoked a conversation on this topic when she asked why people with only 50 db loss were identifying as deaf. She believed 90 db was the threshold point that counted as deafness and queried 'all these "deaf" people who can easily talk on the phone and have all this privilege.'[1] In response to her inquiry, people hotly debated this issue and explained why they identified as deaf or hard of hearing in different contexts and situations and discussed the extent to which this decision related to the associated number on their audiogram. The ensuing discussion showed that the kinds of single-number measurements discussed in this book are not only important to medical classification systems and compensation frameworks; they are significant markers of identity and meaning for us. How we are classified matters to us. Numbers are elevated on an individual level, as well as a bureaucratic level.

As a result, in this conclusion, I move from focusing on clinical measurement to ask what it means to turn these tools onto ourselves in the form of self-tracking. Self-tracking typically involves regular recording of personal data, such as information about bodily function, diet or activity. But such devices are not always used positively: users sometimes fixate on their data to the point that they develop conditions like anxiety, anorexia, orthorexia, obsession with perfect sleep (orthosomnia), or even use their wearables to enable dangerous drug use. We have almost no understanding of how usage of such devices impacts on individual interoception, embodiment, anxiety or cognition of sensation. Related concerns are growing about how the data these devices generate will be stored and used in the future, especially by the state. The kind of data embedded in spirometric standards and in the artificial ear was recoverable and available in archives, but this is unlikely to be the case in the context of private commercial companies used in nationalised contexts. Indeed, an influential think tank has proposed that fitness trackers should be prescribed on the NHS to help tackle health inequality and ensure the poor and the disabled are not left out of this 'technological revolution in medicine'.[2] However, it is unclear what cost or benefit this move would bring to healthcare outcomes. Moreover, it is an assumption that these devices – which are calibrated to healthy bodies – will work effectively on disabled bodies. Furthermore, it is becoming apparent that the increased potential for measurement associated with these tools may shift our understanding of normalcy, for example in the consistent and systematic measurements of glucose enabled by self-trackers, which has changed the standard for 'normal' blood-sugar ranges.[3]

The control and management of our health data is emerging as a key site for future conflict between citizens, corporations and healthcare authorities. This conclusion will therefore pose a series of questions about big data and health to ask: how does self-tracking relate to the longer history of measurement as a normative force outlined in this volume? Can we use our knowledge of the past to look to the future and use self-tracking to mitigate against the kinds of mechanical epistemic injustice explored in Chapter 2? In other words, can this kind of technology be a good thing?

As Crawford et al. point out, 'The already tired binary of big data – is it good or bad? – neglects a far more complex reality that is developing.'[4] In particular, we need to consider how self-tracking might enable clearer expression of embodied knowledge and how this might help individuals to assert their lived experience. Self-tracking may offer a way out of these binary dichotomies by offering a way for people to more clearly correlate their sensations to 'objective' evidence and thus demonstrate the validity of their experiences. However, this possibility is likely to depend on what exactly is being measured. How we measure the more ineffable sensations of health and illness is a key focus here. Whether there is a conflict between self-tracking and embodiment may depend on what is being measured and whether the experience of it holds the essence of the sensation. As Chow-White and Green argue, data are treated as synonymous with facts without consideration of how they have been represented and *made to mean*: 'data are representations, cultural objects that stand in for stimuli and mediate relations'.[5] As I have shown in this book, data which is made to 'stand in' as a proxy measurement for that which is usually individual, inaccessible and subjective, like hearing and breathing, is particularly vulnerable to error or abuse, and we need more awareness and consideration of this in the context of disability and big data.

As I outlined in Chapter 1, health measurements are prioritised if they are easily calculable and capable of producing single-number proxies. The decision to use certain group categories (reference classes) and the process of selecting people to represent the ideal standards of health within these classes have impacted on our understanding of disability. As Chapter 2 elucidated, decisions about which groups are important have historically interrelated with the prioritisation of certain groups as valuable. Against this selective valorisation of certain bodies as normal, other bodies were defined as abnormal. Exploring these processes of disablement has been necessarily intersectional, as gender, class and race variously intersected with this decision-making process through the choice of suitable reference classes. Considering the changing historical usage of reference classes not only indicates the ways in which they can interact with and modify disability levels, but also highlights the difficulty of attributing disease to either biological or environmental/social factors. This focus thus draws attention to the biopower associated with systems, which has emerged as a central area of concern for modern healthcare in the second decade of the twenty-first century.

Professor Philip Alston (UN Special Rapporteur on extreme poverty and human rights) recently visited the UK and reported on the impact that the austerity measures implemented since 2010 had had on the disabled. One of the aspects of these measures that he repeatedly emphasised was the extent to which the system for claiming employment and support benefits (ESA) had been designed *to be difficult*. This was facilitated by the system's 'digital by default' design, which he argued had been purposefully intended to work as a 'digital barrier' to put off applicants and to help ensure application failure.[6] He argued:

> There is nothing inherent in Artificial Intelligence and other technologies that enable automation that threatens human rights and the rule of law. The reality is that governments simply seek to operationalize their political preferences through technology; the outcomes may be good or bad.[7]

As I have made clear in this book, technologies can and do feature innate political preferences. For example, biases are embedded through the choices of inclusion in data set compilation. We are becoming more aware of the potential ramifications of this in machine-learning software, which actively amplifies the stereotypes and biases embedded in data sets.[8] As Chapter 2 detailed, the reference classes utilised in categorisation systems can also work to obscure the social determinants of health inequalities. Reference classes may serve to essentialise inappropriate social classes, and through this process conceal causes of health inequality. Alston further emphasised that one of the reasons why it was difficult to assess poverty in the UK is the way it measures poverty – utilising four separate measures which 'allows it to pick and choose which numbers to use'.[9] Alston's insights are reflected in the findings of this book, which has shown how bureaucracies and measurement systems can be powerfully utilised to control access to compensation. As I discussed particularly in Chapter 5 of this book, using proxy or 'surrogate' measurements in this way has historically been used to promote such systemic manipulation.[10]

Moreover, while it is important to look at these measures and how they may be manipulated, this book has also shown that we need to look at the numbers that are missing. As I demonstrated in Chapter 3, such measures may include a disability data gap. We saw this in the case of the artificial ear, which allowed the Post Office to manage the variability of hearing and standardise the norms of human hearing while simultaneously distorting it to reflect an idealised average. As Amundson emphasises, these decisions are practical ones that have epistemological consequences: 'If medical textbooks emphasize average or typical cases, there may well be pragmatic reasons to do so. It would be a mistake to infer from this that diversity constitutes abnormality.'[11] Such diversity has been a key concern of this book, as individuals' inherent variance has repeatedly been at odds with the movement for standardisation driving institutions like the Post Office and the MRC. The main project of this book has been to outline the complex historical circumstances and contingencies which have led to the prioritisation of measurements of particular kinds. Through this analysis, we can see that the statistical promotion of the average has often worked in opposition to individual variance and that this has been especially problematic in attempts to quantify breathing and hearing. Tools like the audiometer and the spirometer defined disability as measurable pathology within a naturalistic paradigm, which linked trusted instruments with objectivity and accuracy. This determination to consider body processes as quantifiable was driven by the need to compensate for hearing loss and respiratory disability occasioned by warfare or industry. Audiometry and spirometry were therefore embraced as objective ways of testing, which could confound malingerers and allow for testing of large groups of people. The resulting disconnect between objective and subjective measures has emerged as a crucial theme in this book.

Biomedicine demands quantitative data, and yet there is growing realisation that testing procedures fail to measure breathlessness or capture the rich realm of feeling associated with it. Despite the multidimensional aspects of hearing and breathing, hearing loss and breathlessness that were not obviously biological were misinterpreted in the absence of clinical evidence as 'hysterical', as I demonstrated in Chapter 3 and Chapter 5. In Chapter 2 I introduced the concept of 'mechanical epistemic injustice' to better elucidate this specific kind of instrument-based discrimination. This, as might be anticipated, is paralleled in illnesses that do not clearly map onto signs of physiological function, a phenomenon associated with conditions like chronic fatigue or MUS (medically unexplained symptoms). As the discussion about what decibel threshold level 'counts' as deafness demonstrated, diagnostic tools can be very meaningful and helpful, not only in identity formation. They are critical in enabling access to adequate and appropriate healthcare. However, lack of concordance between subjective symptom reports and physiological change has been found in a long list of conditions more commonly assumed to be somatic, including diabetes, gastro-oesophageal reflux disease, heart disease and a wide variety of respiratory conditions.[12]

Highlighting these issues is not intended to undermine or call into question the necessary procedures of biomedicine without offering any kind of solution – an oft-repeated criticism of medical humanities researches. Nonetheless, the prevalent assumption in the clinic is that patients' sensory experience of a symptom is directly related to measurable physiological disease. Indeed, the paradigm of symptom assessment following through consequent diagnosis depends on our faith that the relationship between symptom experience and measurement is accurate.[13] While I am not advocating for an enduring state of pessimistic meta-induction in which we are unable to trust in scientific progress because of awareness of past error, it is clear that historically our faith in this accurate relationship has been misguided. As I have demonstrated, this is especially true in cases where disease causation was linked to the biological traits of a group rather than associated with specific ways of living as a member of that group. The choice of certain subjects to create a standard of normalcy worked as a powerful way to categorise disability as well as obscuring its true causes. Whose bodies mattered for these measurements mattered.

The instrumental measurement of disability is not only an epistemologically significant issue, it has been embraced by the military/industrial nexus to control and moderate compensation claims and to avoid corporate responsibility for health. Responsibility has been a recurring theme within this book, with repeated discussion over who was responsible for the design of prosthetics and their distribution – whether prosthetics were products for engineering or for medicine to design was debated while they were variously rejected or appropriated by users creating devices for themselves. My discussion of the Post Office also highlights the extent to which nationalisation worked as a positive force to ensure extensive state support for those with hearing loss – a positive consequence of nationalisation that has remained largely invisible to posterity. On the other hand, while this book has highlighted innovation within the state, it has equally demonstrated the innovation of disabled users. Moreover, the embodied knowledge gained through disability has been consistently undervalued and obscured. We saw in Chapter 4 that individuals' lived experience of hearing conflicted with the Post Office's desire for standardisation. And as the example of the Bragg–Paul pulsator in Chapter 6 made especially clear, technologies designed by individuals for individuals were not trusted or easily standardised, and patients were increasingly encouraged to adapt themselves to machines rather than the other way around.

Diversity of user experiences of these hearing and breathing machines recurred not only between 'kinds' of disability but between individuals classified in the same way. The apparent dichotomy between visible and invisible is thus problematised through consideration of the lived experience of individuals. Bringing together connections between hearing and breathing, and sound and breath reveals some of the conceptual difficulties in using disability as a catch-all term. Indeed, I argue that the heterogeneity and uniqueness of individual bodies has often been at odds with the standardisation of biomedicine. In Chapter 2 I raised the question of whether disability could be a reference class of its own. Steven Epstein has argued that the likelihood of groups being considered as medically relevant distinct classes is reduced when 'the group is not so well mobilized; when it articulates demands in relation to a form of social difference that is not already institutionalized in state policies;

and when its frames do not resonate with the public of policymakers, perhaps because of the difficulty of advancing a biological difference argument'.[14] If we consider disability, as Elizabeth Barnes does, as primarily a social phenomenon, then we could indeed argue that there are good health-related reasons to consider disability to be a reference class. Against this, we should perhaps be cautious of essentialising disease as natural to that class. Some have used this worry to argue against using class instead of race (in opposition to those who decry that race is being used as a proxy for class) in lung function measurements. And yet using class as a relevant categorisation may well allow us to make the social and political causes of ill health clearer and so drive political campaigns to improve societal health. What is clear is that these are difficult questions that require an intersectional approach. As I pointed out in Chapter 2, approaches that only consider one category (such as gender) miss the powerful complexities of these categorisation processes. Insisting on considering disadvantaged groups as different has, as this book has demonstrated, been historically used to their disadvantage. Despite these caveats, I argue that we need to prioritise further research to answer these questions. In particular, more work is needed to answer how equating the average with the normal has impacted on our understanding of disability.

In making this argument I offer a new contribution to disability history, using a multidisciplinary approach to understand multisensorial phenomena. My approach here is especially salient to the social model of disability as it shows how the naturalist approach to disability is undermined through consideration of relevant data sets and instrumental measurements. The classification of disability has been dependent on, and variable according to, certain measurements. Technology perceived as 'objective' has been utilised to control the messy variability of human bodies.

Measurement has shaped disability. Measurements, and their manipulation, have been underestimated as crucial historical forces motivating and guiding the way we think about disability. The standards embedded in instrumentation created strict, but ultimately arbitrary thresholds of normalcy and abnormalcy. Considering these standards from a long historical perspective reveals how these dividing lines shifted when pushed. The necessary pressure was brought to bear by diverse and varied impacts: different data sets, newly created categorisation systems, updated technologies, and through the conscious and unconscious manipulation of political actors working to negotiate compensation frameworks. This history leads us to a heightened awareness of the importance of prioritising disabled actors' voices as we work to facilitate ongoing resolution between lived experience and the clinical view.

Notes

1 Chrissy @life_laughter_, 'I Identified as HoH for a Long Time with 80 db Loss ...'. Twitter thread, 18 July 2019. https://twitter.com/life_laughter_/status/1151976942108889099. Accessed July 2019.
2 Savage, M., 'Call for Poor and Disabled to Be Given NHS Fitness Trackers', *The Observer*, 5 May 2019. www.theguardian.com/inequality/2019/may/04/fitbits-nhs-reduce-inequality-health-disability-poverty. Accessed July 2019.
3 Fiore-Gartland, B., and Neff, G., 'Communication, Mediation, and the Expectations of Data: Data Valances across Health and Wellness Communities', *International Journal of Communication*, 9 (2015), 1466–1484, p. 1469.
4 Crawford, K., Miltner, K., and Gray, M. L., 'Critiquing Big Data: Politics, Ethics, Epistemology', *International Journal of Communication*, 8 (2014), 1663–1672.
5 Chow-White and Green, 'Data Mining Differences', p. 562.
6 Alston, P., 'Statement on Visit to the United Kingdom, London, 16 November 2018', p. 9. www.ohchr.org/Documents/Issues/Poverty/EOM_GB_16Nov2018.pdf. Accessed July 2019.
7 Ibid., p. 11.
8 Bolukbasi, T., Chang, K.-W., Zou, J., Seligrama, V., and Kalai, A., 'Man Is to Computer Programmer as Woman Is to Homemaker? Debiasing Word Embeddings'. Boston University and Microsoft Research Paper, submitted 21 July 2018. https://arxiv.org/abs/1607.06520. Accessed July 2019.
9 Ibid., pp. 15–16.
10 We might ask where whether the growing self-tracking movement is a naïve attempt to 'manipulate back' but this is a question for future research.
11 Amundson, 'Against Normal Function', p. 45.
12 Van den Bergh, O., Witthoft, M., Petersen, S., and Brown, R. J., 'Symptoms and the Body: Taking the Inferential Leap', *Neuroscience and Behavioral Reviews*, 74 (2017), 1–79, pp. 15–16.
13 Malpass et al., 'The Body Says It'.
14 Epstein, *Inclusion*, pp. 142–143.

Bibliography

Primary sources

Archives
British Newspaper Archive, online
British Postal Museum Archive, London (BPMA)
British Telecom Archives, London (BTA)
Ham Green Hospital, Bristol
Hansard
The National Archives, Kew, London (TNA)
Richard Burton Archives, Swansea University, Swansea
Royal Institution of Great Britain, London (WHB)
Royal London Hospital Archives, London
St Bartholomew's Hospital Archives, London
South Wales Miners' Library, Swansea
Thackray Medical Museum, Leeds
UCL Ear Institute and Action on Hearing Loss Library, London (AOHL)
University of Bristol Library Special Collections, Bristol
University of Glasgow Special Collections, Glasgow
Wellcome Library Archives, London

Published works
Anon., 'War Injuries and Neuroses of the Ear', *The Lancet*, 189:4878 (1917), 304.
Anon., 'The Problem of the Deaf', *The Lancet*, 220:5703 (1932), 1347–1349 [summary of report by Dr A. Eichholz CBE to the Ministry of Health and the Board of Education].
Anon., 'The Hearing Power of School-Children', *The Lancet*, 222:5754 (1933), 1328.
Anon., 'Hearing-Aids: A Report to the Medical Research Council', *The Lancet*, 229:5919 (1937), 340–341.
Anon., 'The Limitations of Hearing-Aids', *The Lancet*, 229:5920 (1937), 395–396.
Aslett, E., D'Arcy Hart, P., and McMichael, J., 'The Lung Volume and Its Subdivisions in Normal Males', *Proceedings of the Royal Society of London Series B: Biological Sciences*, 126:845 (1939), 502–528.
Balbi, C. M. R., 'The Audiometer and Its Application to Medical Research', *The Lancet*, 205:5305 (1925), 954–956.
Balfour, T. G., 'Contribution to the Study of Spirometry', *Medico-Chirurgical Transactions*, 43 (1860), 263–269.
Barcroft, J., 'Discussion of the Therapeutic Uses of Oxygen', *Proceedings of the Royal Society of Medicine: Section of Therapeutics and Pharmacology*, 13 (1920), 59–68.
Behnke, E., and Browne, L., *Voice, Song, and Speech: A Practical guide for Singers and Speakers* (London: Sampson Low, Marston and Company, 1891).

Binger, C. J., Faulkner, J. M., and Moore, R. L., 'Oxygen Poisoning in Mammals', *Journal of Experimental Medicine*, 35:5 (1927), 849–864.
Blackwell, U., 'Mechanical Respiration', *The Lancet*, 254:6568 (1949), 99–102.
Bragg, W. H., 'Bragg–Paul Pulsator', *British Medical Journal*, 10:1136 (1938), 254.
'Breathlessness', *The Lancet*, 287:7447 (1966), 1140.
Bunch, C. C., 'Methods of Testing the Hearing in Infants and Young Children', *Journal of Paediatrics*, 5:4 (1934), 535–544.
Cameron, C., 'The Vital Capacity in Pulmonary Tuberculosis', *Tubercle*, 3 (1922), 385–399.
Campbell, E. J. M., and Howell, J. B. L., 'The Sensation of Dyspnoea', *British Medical Journal*, 2:5361 (1963), 868.
Crowden, G. P., 'Measurement of Deafness in School-Children', *The Lancet*, 218:5650 (1931), 1324–1325.
Cruikshank, W., 'Editorial Notes and Comments', *Post Office Electrical Engineers' Journal*, 12 (1919), 173–178.
Cruikshank, W., 'Editorial Notes and Comments', *Post Office Electrical Engineers' Journal*, 13 (1920), 76–80.
D'Arcy Hart, P., 'Chronic Pulmonary Disease in South Wales Coal Mines: An Eye-Witness Account of the MRC Surveys (1937–1942)', *Social History of Medicine*, 11:3 (1998), 459–468.
Davies, H. W., 'Methods for the Therapeutic Administration of Oxygen', *Edinburgh Medical Journal*, 29:5 (1922), 161–168.
Dreyer, G., 'Investigations on the Normal Vital Capacity in Man and Its Relation to the Size of the Body', *The Lancet*, 194:5006 (1919), 227–234.
Dreyer, G., *The Assessment of Physical Fitness: By Correlation of Vital Capacity and Certain Measurements of the Body* (London: Cassell and Company, 1920).
Drinker, P., 'Prolonged Administration of Artificial Respiration', *The Lancet*, 217:5622 (1931), 1186–1188.
'Editorial: The Telephone Repeater', *Post Office Electrical Engineers' Journal*, 12 (1919), 7–8.
'Editorial: The Therapeutic Use of Oxygen', *Canadian Medical Association Journal*, 16:6 (1926), 696–697.
Ellis, H., *Man and Woman: A Study of Human Secondary Sexual Characters* (London: Walter Scott, 1904).
Evans, J. H., 'The Inhalation of Pure Oxygen in the Treatment of Disease', *Canadian Medical Association Journal*, 22:4 (1930), 518–522.
Flack, M., 'The Milroy Lectures on Respiratory Efficiency in Relation to Health and Disease', *The Lancet*, 198 (1924), 693–696.
Fletcher, H., 'Physical Measurements of Audition and Their Bearing on the Theory of Hearing', *Journal of the Franklin Institute*, 196:3 (1923), 289–326.
Fraser-Harris, D. F., 'The Treatment of Deafness', *The Lancet*, 224:5792 (1934), 481–483.
Fry, D. B., and Kerridge. P. M. T., 'Tests for the Hearing of Speech by Deaf People', *The Lancet*, 233:6020 (1939), 106–109.

Galton, F., 'The Final Report of the Anthropometric Committee', *Report of the British Association for the Advancement of Science* (1883), 253–308.

Galton, F., 'On the Anthropometric Laboratory at the Late International Health Exhibition', *Journal of the Anthropological Institute of Great Britain and Ireland*, 14 (1885), 205–221.

Gilson, J. C., and Hugh-Jones, P., *Lung Function in Coalworkers' Pneumoconiosis* (Medical Research Council Special Report Series No. 290) (London: Her Majesty's Stationery Office, 1955).

Graves, J. C., Letter to the Editor, 'Domiciliary Rehabilitation of the Respiratory Cripple', *The Lancet*, 274:7110 (1959), 1033.

Hays, H., 'The Social and Economic Importance of Deafness', *Volta Review*, 15:7 (1913), 301–311.

Heald, C. B., 'The Value and Interpretation of Some Physical Measurements', *The Lancet*, 196:5067 (1920), 736–741.

Hughes, D. E., 'On an Induction-Currents Balance, and Experimental Researches Made Therewith', *Proceedings of the Royal Society of London*, 29:196–199 (1879), 56–65.

Hurst, A. F., Letter to the Editor, 'War Deafness', *The Lancet*, 192:4955 (1918), 218–219.

Hurst, A. F., and Peters, E. A., 'A Report on the Pathology, Diagnosis and Treatment of Absolute Hysterical Deafness in Soldiers', *The Lancet*, 190:4910 (1917), 517–519.

Hutchinson, J., *Contributions to Vital Statistics, Obtained by Means of a Pneumatic Apparatus for Valuing the Respiratory Power with Relation to Health* (London: Statistical Society of London, 1844).

Hutchinson, J., 'On the Capacity of the Lungs, and on the Respiratory Movements, with the View of Establishing a Precise and Easy Method of Detecting Disease by the Spirometer', *Medico-Chirurgical Transactions*, 29 (1846), 137–252.

Hutchinson, J., *The Spirometer, the Stethoscope, and Scale-Balance: Their Use in Discriminating Diseases of the Chest, and Their Value in Life Offices; With Remarks on the Selection of Lives for Life Assurance Companies* (London: Churchill, 1852).

Kelvin, W. T., 'Electrical Units of Measurement: A Lecture Delivered at the Institution of Civil Engineers on May 3, 1883; Being One of a Series of Six Lectures on "The Practical Applications of Electricity"', *Nature Series: Popular Lectures and Addresses* (London: Macmillan, 1889), 73–136.

Kerridge, P. M. T., 'Aids for the Deaf', *British Medical Journal*, 3886:1 (1935), 1314–1317.

Kerridge, P. M. T., 'Can Physics Help the Deaf Child?', *The Lancet*, 225:5811 (1935), 104–108.

Kerridge, P. M. T., 'Artificial Respiration for Three and a Half Years', *The Lancet*, 227:5870 (1936), 504.

Kerridge, P. M. T., *Hearing and Speech in Deaf Children* (Medical Research Council: Reports of the Hearing Committee, Special Report Series No. 221) (London: His Majesty's Stationery Office, 1937).

Laing, G. D., 'The Administration of Oxygen', *British Medical Journal*, 1:3311 (1924), 1074–1075.

McBride, P., and Turner, A. L., 'War Deafness, with Special Reference to the Value of Vestibular Tests', *The Lancet*, 192:4951 (1918), 73–74.

Medical Research Council, *Hearing Aids and Audiometers* (Special Report Series No. 261) (London: His Majesty's Stationery Office, 1949).

Moncrieff, A., 'Tests for Respiratory Efficiency', *The Lancet*, 220:5696 (1932), 665–669.

Ogilvie, A., 'Reply: Complimentary Dinner to Sir Andrew Ogilvie', *Post Office Electrical Engineers' Journal*, 12 (1920), 70–81.

Report of Societies, 'Tests and Classifications of Hearing', *British Medical Journal*, 10:2/3540 (1928), 845–848.

'Review: Medical Research Council. Special Report Series no. 237', *Indian Medical Gazette* (1940).

Richardson, B. W., 'Some Researches with Professor Hughes' New Instrument for the Measurement of Hearing: The Audiometer', *Proceedings of the Royal Society of London*, 29:196–199 (1879), 65–66.

'Shortness of Breath', *The Lancet*, 220:5693 (1932), 798–799.

Stadie, W. C., 'Construction of an Oxygen Chamber for the Treatment of Pneumonia', *Journal of Experimental Medicine*, 35:3 (1922), 323–335.

Stevens, A. E., Letter to the Editor, 'Hearing Aids for Deafness', *The Lancet*, 231:5988 (1938), 1307.

Tallents, S., *Post Office Publicity* (Post Office Green Paper No. 8) (London: His Majesty's Stationery Office, 1935).

Turner, W. A., 'Remarks on Cases of Nervous and Mental Shock: Observed in the Base Hospital in France', *British Medical Journal*, 1:2837 (1915), 833–835.

West, W., *Room Noise and Reverberation* (Post Office Green Paper No. 2) (London: His Majesty's Stationery Office, 1934).

Wharry, H. M., and Crowden, G. P., 'Correction of Hearing Defects', *British Medical Journal*, 1:3727 (1932), 1189.

Wilson, J. G., 'A Continuing Battle against the Virus of Polio', *Municipal Journal*, 59 (6 July 1951), 1577–1581.

Yearsley, M., Letter to the Editor, 'Hearing Aids for Deafness', *The Lancet*, 231:5981 (1938), 914.

Secondary sources

Agar, J., *Constant Touch: A Global History of the Mobile Phone* (Cambridge: Icon Books, 2003).

Ahrens, K. A., Rossen, L. M., and Simon, A. E., 'Relationship between Mean Leucocyte Telomere Length and Measures of Allostatic Load in US Reproductive-Aged Women, NHNES 1999–2002', *Paediatric and Perinatal Epidemiology*, 30:4 (2016), 325–335.

Albrecht, G. L., and Devlieger, P. J., 'The Disability Paradox: High Quality of Life against All Odds', *Social Science and Medicine*, 48:8 (1999), 977–988.

Alston, P., 'Statement on Visit to the United Kingdom, London, 16 November 2018'. https://www.ohchr.org/EN/pages/home.aspx. Accessed July 2019.

Amundson, R., 'Against Normal Function', *Studies in History and Philosophy of Biological and Biomedical Sciences*, 31:1 (2000), 33–53.

Amundson, R., 'Quality of Life, Disability, and Hedonic Psychology', *Journal for the Theory of Social Behaviour*, 40:4 (2010), 374–392.

Anderson, J., *War, Disability and Rehabilitation in Britain* (Manchester: Manchester University Press, 2011).

Arapostathis, S., and Gooday, G., *Patently Contestable: Electrical Technologies and Inventor Identities on Trial in Britain* (Cambridge, MA: MIT Press, 2013).

Armstrong, D., 'The Rise of Surveillance Medicine', *Sociology of Health and Illness*, 17:3 (1995), 393–404.

Aslan, S. C., McKay, W. B., Singh, G., and Ovechkin, A. V., 'Respiratory Muscle Activation Patterns during Maximum Airway Pressure Efforts Are Different in Women and Men', *Respiratory Physiology and Neurobiology*, 259 (2019), 143–148.

Austoker, J., and Bryder, L., 'The National Institute for Medical Research and Related Activities of the MRC', in J. Austoker and L. Bryder (eds), *Historical Perspectives on the Role of the MRC: Essays in the History of the Medical Research Council of the United Kingdom and Its Predecessor, the Medical Research Committee, 1913–1953* (Oxford: Oxford University Press, 1989), pp. 35–57.

Backman, H., Lindberg, A., Sovijarvi, A., Larsson, K., Lundback, B., and Ronmark, E., 'Evaluation of the Global Lung Function Initiative 2012 Reference Values in a Swedish Population Sample', *BMC Pulmonary Medicine*, 15:26 (2015), 1602–1611.

Bajorek, J. P., 'Voice Recognition Still Has Significant Race and Gender Biases', *Harvard Business Review: Technology* (10 May 2019). https://hbr.org/2019/05/voicerecognition-still-has-significant-race-and-gender-biases. Accessed July 2019.

Barham, P., *Forgotten Lunatics of the Great War* (New Haven, CT: Yale University Press, 2004).

Barnes, E., *The Minority Body* (Oxford: Oxford University Press, 2016).

Barr, M., 'The Iron Lung: A Polio Patient's Story', *Journal of the Royal Society of Medicine*, 103:6 (2010), 256–259.

Barrington, A. B., 'Artificial Respiration, the History of an Idea', *Medical History*, 15:4 (1971), 336–351.

Bathurst, B., *Sound: Stories of Hearing Lost and Found* (London: Profile Books, 2017).

Baynton, D. C., ' "Savages and Deaf Mutes": Evolutionary Theory and the Campaign against Sign Language in the Nineteenth Century', in J. V. van Cleve (ed.), *Deaf History Unveiled* (Washington, DC: Gallaudet University Press, 1993), pp. 92–112.

Baynton, D. C., *Defectives in the Land: Disability and Immigration in the Age of Eugenics* (Chicago: Chicago University Press, 2016).

Berger, K. W., *The Hearing Aid: Its Operation and Development* (Livonia, MI: National Hearing Aid Society, 1970).

Berger, K. W., 'Genealogy of the Words "Audiology" and "Audiologist"', *Journal of the American Audiology Society*, 2:2 (1976), 38–44.

Bijker, W. E., *Of Bicycles, Bakelite and Bulbs: Towards a Theory of Sociotechnical Change* (Cambridge, MA: MIT Press, 1995).

Binnie, K., McGuire, C., and Carel, H., 'Objects of Safety and Imprisonment', *Journal of Material Culture* (accepted, in press).

Biss, E., 'The Pain Scale', in J. E. Sullivan III (ed.), *Ways of Reading: An Anthology for Writers* (Boston and New York: Bedford/St. Martin's, 2011), pp. 171–182.

Blease, C., Carel, H., and Geraghty, K., 'Epistemic Injustice in Healthcare Encounters: Evidence from Chronic Fatigue Syndrome', *Journal of Medical Ethics*, 43:8 (2016), 549–557.

Bloor, M., 'The South Wales Miners' Federation, Miners' Lung and the Instrumental Use of Expertise, 1900–1950', *Social Studies of Science* 30:1 (2000), 125–140.

Blume, S., *The Artificial Ear: Cochlear Implants and the Culture of Deafness* (London: Rutgers University Press, 2010).

Bolukbasi, T., Chang, K.-W., Zou, J., Seligrama, V., and Kalai, A., 'Man Is to Computer Programmer as Woman Is to Homemaker? Debiasing Word Embeddings'. Boston University and Microsoft Research Paper, submitted 21 July 2018. https://arxiv.org/abs/1607.06520. Accessed July 2019.

Boorse, C., 'Health as a Theoretical Concept', *Philosophy of Science*, 44:4 (1997), 542–573.

Boorse, C., 'Disability and Medical Theory', in D. Ralston and J. Ho (eds), *Philosophical Reflections on Disability* (Dordrecht: Springer, 2010), pp. 55–88.

Boorse, C., 'A Second Rebuttal on Health', *Journal of Medicine and Philosophy*, 39:6 (2014), 683–724.

Booth, S., Chin, C., and Spathis, A., 'The Brain and Breathlessness: Understanding and Disseminating a Palliative Care Approach', *Palliative Medicine*, 29:5 (2015), 396–398.

Bouk, D., *How Our Days Became Numbered: Risk and the Rise of the Statistical Individual* (Chicago: University of Chicago Press, 2015).

Bourke, J., *The Story of Pain: From Prayer to Painkillers* (Oxford: Oxford University Press, 2014).

Bowker, G. C., and Star, S. L., *Sorting Things Out: Classification and Its Consequences* (Cambridge, MA: MIT Press, 2000).

Bramwell, E., 'Rethinking Patent Medicine Culture in Britain, 1909–1949' (PhD dissertation, University of Lancaster, 2020).

Branson, J., and Miller, D., *Damned for Their Difference: The Cultural Construction of Deaf People as Disabled* (Washington, DC: Gallaudet University Press, 2002).

Braun, L., *Breathing Race into the Machine: The Surprising Career of the Spirometer from Plantation to Genetics* (Minneapolis: University of Minnesota Press, 2014).

Braun, L., and Kopinski, H., 'Casual Understandings: Controversy, Social Context, and Mesothelioma Research', *Biosocieties*, 13:3 (2018), 557–579.

Bridge, M., and Pegg, J., *Call to Arms: A History of Military Communications from the Crimean War to the Present Day* (Tavistock: Focus Publishing, 2001).

Brooks, D. H. M., 'The Route to Home Ventilation: A Patient's Perspective', *Care of the Critically Ill*, 6:3 (1990), 96–97.

Brooks, D. H. M., 'Living with Ventilation: Confessions of an Addict', *Care of the Critically Ill*, 8:5 (1992), 205–207.

Brown, J., 'The Last of the Iron Lungs', *Gizmodo*, 20 November 2017. https://gizmodo.com/the-last-of-the-iron-lungs-1819079169. Accessed June 2019.

Brueggemann, B. J., *Lend Me Your Ear: Rhetorical Constructions of Deafness* (Washington, DC: Gallaudet University Press, 1999).

Brune, A., and Wilson, D. J., *Disability and Passing: Blurring the Lines of Identity* (Philadelphia: Temple University Press, 2013).

Bryder, L., 'Tuberculosis and the MRC', in J. Austoker and L. Bryder (eds), *Historical Perspectives on the Role of the MRC: Essays in the History of the Medical Research Council of the United Kingdom and Its Predecessor, the Medical Research Committee, 1913–1953* (Oxford: Oxford University Press, 1989), pp. 1–21.

Bufton, M., and Melling, J., '"A Mere Matter of Rock": Organised Labour, Scientific Evidence and British Government Schemes for Compensation of Silicosis and Pneumoconiosis among Coalminers, 1926–1940', *Medical History*, 49:2 (2005), 155–178.

Bufton, M., and Melling, J., 'Coming Up for Air: Experts, Employers, and Workers in Campaigns to Compensate Silicosis Sufferers in Britain, 1918–1939', *Social History of Medicine*, 18:1 (2005), 63–86.

Campbell-Smith, D., *Masters of the Post: The Authorised History of the Royal Mail* (London: Penguin Books, 2011).

Canguilhem, G., *The Normal and the Pathological* (Cambridge, MA: Zone Books, 3rd edn, 1991).

Carel, H., 'Breathless: Philosophical Lessons from Respiratory Illness', *Journal of Medical Humanities*, 6:1 (2014), 1–6.

Carel, H., 'Ill, but Well: A Phenomenology of Well-Being in Chronic Illness', in J. E. Bickenback, F. Felder and B. Schmitz (eds), *Disability and the Good Human Life* (Cambridge: Cambridge University Press, 2014), pp. 243–270.

Carel, H., and Kidd, I., 'Epistemic Injustice in Healthcare: A Philosophical Analysis', *Medicine, Health Care and Philosophy*, 17:4 (2014), 529–540.

Carel, H., Macnaughton, J., and Dodd, J., 'Invisible Suffering: Breathlessness in and beyond the Clinic', *The Lancet: Respiratory Medicine*, 3:4 (2015), 278–279.

Cayet, T., Rosental, P. A., and Thebaud-Sorger, M., 'How International Organisations Compete: Occupational Safety and Health at the ILO, a Diplomacy of Expertise', *Journal of Modern European History*, 7:2 (2009), 174–196.

Chang, H., 'The Hidden History of Phlogiston: How Philosophical Failure Can Generate Historiographical Refinement', *HYLE: International Journal for Philosophy of Chemistry*, 16:2 (2010), 47–79.

Chapman, R., 'Neurodiversity, Disability, Wellbeing', in N. Chown, A. Stenning and H. Rosquvist (eds), *Neurodiversity Studies: A New Critical Paradigm* (Routledge, forthcoming).

Chin-Yee, B., and Upshur, R. E. G., 'Re-Evaluating Concepts of Biological Function in Clinical Medicine: Towards a New Naturalistic Theory of Disease', *Theoretical Medicine and Bioethics*, 38:4 (2017), 245–264.

Chrissy @life_laughter_, 'I Identified as HoH for a Long Time with 80 db Loss ...', Twitter thread, 18 July 2019. https://twitter.com/EssentialSign_/status/1151976942108889099. Accessed July 2019.

Chow-White, P. A., and Green, J. R., 'Data Mining Differences in the Age of Big Data: Communication and the Social Shaping of Genome Technologies from 1998 to 2007', *International Journal of Communication*, 7 (2013), 556–583.

Clark, B. M. J., 'The Rejection of Psychological Approaches to Mental Disorder in Late Nineteenth-Century Psychiatry', in A. Scull (ed.), *Madhouses, Mad-Doctors, and Madmen: The Social History of Psychiatry in the Victorian Era* (London: Athlone, 1981), pp. 271–312.

Clarke, A. E., Shim, J. K., Mamo, L., Fosket, J. R., and Fishman, J. R., 'Biomedicalization: Technoscientific Transformations of Health, Illness, and U.S. Biomedicine', *American Sociological Association*, 68:2 (2003), 161–194.

Codina, C., Pascalis, O., Mody, C., Toomey, P., Rose, J., Gummer, L., and Buckley, D., 'Visual Advantage in Deaf Adults Linked to Retinal Changes', *PLoS ONE*, 6:6 (2011), 1–8.

Cooper, R., 'Disease', *Studies in History and Philosophy of Biological and Biomedical Sciences*, 22:2 (2002), 263–282.

Cooper, R., 'Are Culture-Bound Syndromes as Real as Universally-Occurring Disorders?', *Studies in History and Philosophy of Biological and Biomedical Sciences*, 41:4 (2010), 325–332.

Cooper, R., 'Shifting Boundaries Between the Normal and the Pathological: The Case of Mild Intellectual Disability', *History of Psychiatry*, 25:2 (2014), 171–186.

Cotes, J. E., 'The Medical Research Council Pneumoconiosis Research Unit, 1945–1985: A Short History and Tribute', *History of Occupational Medicine*, 50:6 (2000), 440–449.

Courtwright, D. T., *Sky as Frontier: Adventure, Aviation, and Empire* (College Station: Texas A&M University Press, 2004).

Crawford, K., Miltner, K., and Gray, M. L., 'Critiquing Big Data: Politics, Ethics, Epistemology', *International Journal of Communication*, 8 (2014), 1663–1672.

Crenshaw, K., 'Mapping the Margins: Intersectionality, Identity, Politics, and Violence against Women of Color', *Stanford Law Review*, 43:6 (1991), 1241–1299.

Crutchley, E. T., *GPO* (Cambridge: Cambridge University Press, 1938).

Cryle, P., and Stephens, E., *Normality: A Critical Genealogy* (Chicago: University of Chicago Press, 2017).

Cureton, A., 'Hiding a Disability and Passing as Non-Disabled', in A. Cureton and T. E. Hill Jnr (eds), *Disability in Practice: Attitudes, Policies and Relationships* (Oxford: Oxford University Press, 2018), pp. 15–32.

Daniels, N., *Just Health Care* (Cambridge: Cambridge University Press, 1985).

Daniels, N., 'Normal Functioning and the Treatment–Enhancement Distinction', *Cambridge Quarterly of Healthcare Ethics*, 9:3 (2000), 314–315.
Daston, L., and Galison, P., *Objectivity* (New York: Zone Books, 2007).
Davis, L. J., *Enforcing Normalcy: Disability, Deafness, and the Body* (London: Verso, 1995).
Dotson, K., 'A Cautionary Tale: On Limiting Epistemic Oppression', *Frontiers: A Journal of Women Studies*, 33:1 (2012), 24–47.
Eknoyan, G., 'Historical Note: Adolphe Quetelet (1796–1874) – The Average Man and the Indices of Obesity', *Nephrology Dialysis Transplantation*, 23:1 (2008), 47–51.
Elster, J., *Sour Grapes: Studies in the Subversion of Rationality* (Cambridge: Cambridge University Press, 2016).
Enke, J., 'War Noises on the Battlefield: On Fighting Underground and Learning to Listen in the Great War', *German Historical Institute London Bulletin*, 37:1 (2015), 7–21.
Enns, A., 'The Human Telephone: Physiology, Neurology, and Sound Technologies', in D. Morat (ed.), *Sounds of Modern History: Auditory Cultures in 19th- and 20th-Century Europe* (New York: Berghahn, 2014), pp. 46–68.
Epstein, S., 'Bodily Differences and Collective Identities: The Politics of Gender and Race in Biomedical Research in the United States', *Body and Society* 10:2–3 (2004), 183–203.
Epstein, S., *Inclusion: The Politics of Difference in Medical Research* (Chicago: University of Chicago Press, 2007).
Eriksson, P., *The History of Deaf People: A Source Book* (Orebro: Daufr, 1991).
Esmail, J., *Reading Victorian Deafness: Signs and Sounds in Victorian Literature and Culture* (Athens: Ohio University Press, 2014).
Faull, O. K., Hayen, A., and Pattinson, K. T. S., 'Breathlessness and the Body: Neuroimaging Clues for the Inferential Leap', *Cortex*, 95 (2017), 211–221.
Faull, O. K., Marlow, L., Finnegan, S. L., and Pattinson, K. T. S., 'Chronic Breathlessness: Re-Thinking the Symptom', *European Respiratory Journal*, 51:1 (2018), 1–5.
Fiore-Gartland, B., and Neff, G., 'Communication, Mediation, and the Expectations of Data: Data Valances across Health and Wellness Communities', *International Journal of Communication*, 9 (2015), 1466–1484.
Flynn, J. R., *What is Intelligence?* (Cambridge: Cambridge University Press, 2007).
Foucault, M., *The History of Sexuality: Volume One* (London: Penguin Books, 1976).
Fourcade, M., 'The Problem of Embodiment in the Sociology of Knowledge: Afterword to the Special Issue on Knowledge in Practice', *Qualitative Sociology*, 33:4 (2010), 569–574.
Fricker, M., *Epistemic Injustice: Power and the Ethics of Knowing* (Oxford: Oxford University Press, 2007).
Gay, R., *Hunger: A Memoir of (My) Body* (London: HarperCollins, 2007).
George, G. F., 'The Federal Communications Commission and the Bell System: Abdication of Regulatory Responsibility', *Indiana Law Journal*, 44:3 (1969), 459–477.
Gerber, D. A., 'Introduction: Finding Disabled Veterans in History', in D. A. Gerber (ed.), *Disabled Veterans in History* (Ann Arbor: University of Michigan Press, 2000), pp. 1–52.

Gilbertson, A. A., 'Before Intensive Therapy?', *Journal of the Royal Society of Medicine*, 88:8 (1995), 459–463.

Glynn, S., and Oxborrow, J., *Interwar Britain: A Social and Economic History* (London: George Allen & Unwin, 1976).

Goldberg, D. S., 'Pain, Objectivity and History: Understanding Pain Stigma', *Medical Humanities*, 42 (2017), 238–243.

Goldstein, J., *Hysteria Complicated by Ecstasy: The Case of Nanette Leroux* (Princeton, NJ: Princeton University Press, 2010).

Gooday, G., *The Morals of Measurement: Accuracy, Irony, and Trust in Late Victorian Electrical Practice* (Cambridge: Cambridge University Press, 2004).

Gooday, G., and Sayer, K., *Managing the Experience of Hearing Loss in Britain, 1830–1930* (London: Palgrave Macmillan, 2017).

Gotzsche, P. C., *Deadly Medicine and Organised Crime: How Big Pharma has Corrupted Healthcare* (London: Radcliffe Publishing, 2013).

Gould, S. J., *The Mismeasure of Man* (New York: Norton & Company, 2nd edn, 1996).

Grainge, C., 'Breath of Life: The Evolution of Oxygen Therapy', *Journal of the Royal Society of Medicine*, 97:10 (2004), 489–493.

Gribenski, F., 'Negotiating the Pitch: For a Diplomatic History of A, at the Crossroads of Politics, Music, Science and Industry', in F. Ramel and C. Prévost-Thomas (eds), *International Relations, Music and Diplomacy: Sounds and Voices on the International Stage* (Cham: Palgrave Macmillan, 2018), pp. 173–192.

Hacking, I., 'Biopower and the Avalanche of Printed Numbers', *Humanities in Society*, 5 (1982), 279–295.

Haigh, A., 'Post Office War Research. "To Strive, To Seek, To Find": Post Office Engineering Research from the Experimenting Room to "Dollis Hill", 1908–1938' (PhD dissertation, University of Leeds, forthcoming).

Hall, B. N., 'The Life-Blood of Command? The British Army, Communications and the Telephone, 1871–1914', *War and Society*, 27:2 (2008), 43–65.

Hayen, A., Herigstad, M., and Pattinson, K. T. S., 'Understanding Dyspnoea as a Complex Individual Experience', *Maturitas*, 76:1 (2013), 45–50.

Heeson, A., 'The Coal Mines Act of 1842, Social Reform, and Social Control', *Historical Journal*, 24:1 (1981), 69–88.

Heggie, V., 'Testing Sex and Gender in Sports: Reinventing, Reimagining and Reconstructing Histories', *Endeavour*, 34:4 (2010), 157–163.

Heggie, V., 'Experimental Physiology, Everest and Oxygen: From the Ghastly Kitchens to the Gasping Lung', *British Journal for the History of Science*, 46:1 (2013), 123–147.

Hendy, D., *Noise: A Human History of Sound and Listening* (London: Profile Books, 2013).

Herzog, M., Sucec, J., Diest, I. V., Chevinesse, C., Davenport, P., Similowski, T., and von Leupoldt, A., 'Observing Dyspnoea in Others Elicits Dyspnoea, Negative Affect and Brain Responses', *European Respiratory Journal*, 51:4 (2018), 1–10.

Hoffman, A. L. 'Data Violence and How Bad Engineering Choices Can Damage Society', *Medium*, 30 April 2018. https://medium.com/s/story/data-violence-and-how-bad-engineering-choices-can-damage-society-39e44150e1d4. Accessed July 2019.

Hong, S., *Wireless: From Marconi's Black-Box to the Audion* (Cambridge, MA: MIT Press, 2001).

Hughes, B., and Paterson, K., 'The Social Model of Disability and the Disappearing Body: Towards a Sociology of Impairment', *Disability and Society*, 12:3 (1997), 324–340.

Hurley, S., 'The Man behind the Motor: William Morris and the Iron Lung', *Science Museum Blog*, 7 March 2013. https://blog.sciencemuseum.org.uk/the-man-behind-the-motor-william-morris-and-the-iron-lung/. Accessed June 2019.

Hutchison, I., 'Oralism: A Sign of the Times? The Contest for Deaf Communication in Education Provision in Late Nineteenth-Century Scotland', *European Review of History*, 14:4 (2007), 481–501.

Jackson, J., *A World on Fire: A Heretic, an Aristocrat, and the Race to Discover Oxygen* (New York: Viking, 2005).

Jewson, N. F., 'The Disappearance of the Sick Man from Medical Cosmology, 1770–1870', *Sociology*, 10:2 (1976), 225–244.

Johnson, M. J., Kanaan, M., Richardson, G., Nabb, S., Torgerson, D., English, A., and Booth, S., 'A Randomised Controlled Trial of Three or One Breathing Technique Training Sessions for Breathlessness in People with Malignant Lung Disease', *BMC Medicine*, 13:1 (2015), 213.

Juniper, D., 'The First World War and Radio Development', *RUSI Journal*, 148:1 (2003), 84–89.

Karlsson, V., Bergbom, I., and Forsberg, A., 'The Lived Experiences of Adult Intensive Care Patients Who Were Conscious during Mechanical Ventilation: A Phenomenological-Hermeneutic Study', *Intensive and Critical Care Nursing*, 28 (2012), 6–15.

Kay, M., 'Inventing Telephone Usage: Debating Ownership, Entitlement and Purpose in Early British Telephony' (PhD dissertation, University of Leeds, 2015).

Keating, C., *Smoking Kills: The Revolutionary Life of Richard Doll* (Oxford: Signal Books, 2014).

Kerstjens, H. A., Rijcken, B., Schouten, J. P., and Postma, D. S., 'Decline of FEV1 by Age and Smoking Status: Facts, Figures, and Fallacies', *Thorax*, 52 (1997), 820–827.

Kingma, E., 'What Is It to Be Healthy?', *Analysis*, 67:294 (2007), 128–133.

Kingma, E., 'Paracetamol, Poison, and Polio: Why Boorse's Account of Function Fails to Distinguish Health and Disease', *British Journal for the Philosophy of Science*, 61:2 (2010), 241–264.

Kingma, E., 'Health and Disease: Social Constructivism as a Combination of Naturalism and Normativism', in H. Carel and R. Cooper (eds), *Health, Illness and Disease: Philosophical Essays* (Durham: Acumen Publishing, 2013), pp. 37–56.

Kirkingen, A. L., *Inscribed Bodies: Health Impact of Childhood Sexual Abuse* (Dordrecht: Springer, 2010).

Kohrman, M., 'Why Am I Not Disabled? Making State Subjects, Making Statistics in Post-Mao China', *Medical Anthropology Quarterly*, 17:1 (2003), 5–24.

Kudlick, C., 'Disability History: Why We Need Another "Other"', *American Historical Review*, 108:3 (2003), 763–793.

Kuhane, G., and Savulescu, J., 'The Welfarist Account of Disability', in K. Brownlee and A. Cureton (eds), *Disability and Disadvantage* (Oxford: Oxford University Press, 2009), pp. 1–37.

Lane, H., *When the Mind Hears: A History of the Deaf* (New York: Random House, 1984).

Lang, H. G., *A Phone of Our Own: The Deaf Insurrection against Ma Bell* (Washington, DC: Gallaudet University Press, 2000).

Latour, B., and Woolgar, S., *Laboratory Life* (Princeton, NJ: Princeton University Press, 1979).

Leigh, J. M., 'The Evolution of Oxygen Therapy Apparatus', *Anaesthesia*, 29 (1974), 462–485.

Lewis, J. E., DeGusta, D., Meyer, M. R., Monge, J. M., Mann, A. E., and Holloway, R. E., 'Correction: The Mismeasure of Science: Stephen Jay Gould versus Samuel George Morton on Skulls and Bias', *PLoS Biology*, 9:7 (2011), 1–6.

Li, X., and Mills, M., 'Vocal Features: From Voice Identification to Speech Recognition by Machine', *Technology and Culture*, 60:2 (2019), 129–160.

Linden, S. C., and Jones, E., '"Shell Shock" Revisited: An Examination of the Case Records of the National Hospital', *Medical History*, 58:4 (2014), 519–545.

Linker, B., 'On the Borderland of Medical and Disability History: A Study of the Fields', *Bulletin of the History of Medicine*, 87:4 (2013), 499–535.

Lock, M., 'The Tempering of Medical Anthropology: Troubling Natural Categories', *Medical Anthropology Quarterly*, 15:4 (2001), 478–492.

McEvoy, J. G., 'Gases, God and the Balance of Nature: A Commentary on Priestley (1772) "Observations on Different Kinds of Air"', *Philosophical Transactions of the Royal Society A: Mathematical, Physical and Engineering Sciences*, 373:2039 (2015), 1–11.

McGuire, C., 'Inventing Amplified Telephony: The Co-Creation of Aural Technology and Disability', in C. Jones (ed.), *Rethinking Modern Prostheses in Anglo-American Commodity Cultures, 1820–1939* (Manchester: Manchester University Press, 2017), pp. 70–90.

McGuire, C., '"X-Rays Don't Tell Lies": The Medical Research Council and the Measurement of Respiratory Disability 1936–1945', *British Journal for the History of Science*, 52:3 (2019), 447–465.

McGuire, C., 'The Categorisation of Hearing Loss in Inter-War Telephony', in G. Balbi and C. Berth (eds), Special Issue: 'A New History of the Telephone', *Journal of History and Technology*, 35:2 (2019), 138–155.

McGuire, C., 'Dust to Dust', *The Lancet*, 7:5 (2019), 383–384.

McGuire, C., and Carel, H., 'The Visible and the Invisible: Disability, Assistive Technology, and Stigma', in D. T. Wasserman and A. Cureton (eds), *The Oxford Handbook of Philosophy and Disability* (Oxford: Oxford University Press, 2019), pp. 598–615.

McGuire, C., Virdi, J., and Hutton, J., 'Respiratory Technologies and the Co-Production of Breathing in the Twentieth Century', in A. Hanley and J. Meyer (eds), *Patient Voices* (Manchester: Manchester University Press, forthcoming).

McIvor, A., 'Miners, Silica and Disability: The Bi-National Interplay between South Africa and the United Kingdom, c. 1900–1930s', *American Journal of Industrial Medicine*, 5:S1 (2015), 523–530.

Macnaughton, J., 'Numbers, Scales, and Qualitative Research', *The Lancet*, 347:9008 (1996), 1099–1100.

Macnaughton, J., and Carel, H., 'Breathing and Breathlessness in Clinic and Culture: Using Critical Medical Humanities to Bridge an Epistemic Gap', in A. Whitehead and A. Woods (gen. eds), *The Edinburgh Companion to the Critical Medical Humanities* (Edinburgh: Edinburgh University Press, 2016), pp. 294–309.

Malpass, A., McGuire, C., and Macnaughton, J., 'The Body Says It: The Difficulty of Measuring and Communicating Sensations of Breathlessness', *Medical Humanities* (under review).

Meiklejohn, A., 'History of Lung Diseases of Coal Miners in Great Britain: Part 3, 1930–1952', *British Journal of Industrial Medicine*, 9 (1952), 208–220.

Melling, J., 'Beyond a Shadow of a Doubt? Experts, Lay Knowledge, and the Role of Radiography in the Diagnosis of Silicosis in Britain, c. 1919–1945', *Bulletin of the History of Medicine*, 84:3 (2010), 424–426.

Meyer, J., 'Not Septimus Now: Wives of Disabled Veterans and Cultural Memory of the First World War in Britain', *Women's History Review*, 13:1 (2004), 117–138.

Miller, D. P., and Levere, T. H., ' "Inhale It and See?": The Collaboration between Thomas Beddoes and James Watt in Pneumatic Medicine', *Ambix*, 55:1 (2008), 5–28.

Miller, M. R., 'Chronic Obstructive Pulmonary Disease: Missed Diagnosis versus Misdiagnosis', *British Medical Journal*, 351:3021 (2015), 1–5.

Mills, M., 'When Mobile Technologies Were New', *Endeavour*, 33:4 (2009), 140–146.

Mills, M., 'Deafening: Noise and the Engineering of Communication in the Telephone System', *Grey Room*, 43 (2011), 118–143.

Mills, M., 'Hearing Aids and the History of Electronics Miniaturization', *IEEE Annals of the History of Computing*, 33:2 (2011), 24–45.

Mjolstad, B. P., Kirkengen, A. L., Getz, L., and Hetlevik, I., 'What Do GPs Actually Know about Their Patients as Persons?', *European Journal for Person Centered Healthcare*, 1:1 (2012), 149–160.

Molenaar, P. C. M., 'On the Implications of the Classical Ergodic Theorems: Analysis of Developmental Processes Has to Focus on Individual Variation', *Developmental Psychobiology*, 50:1 (2007), 60–69.

Neff, G., and Nafus, D., *Self-Tracking* (Cambridge, MA: MIT Press, 2016).

Nerbovik, L. T., Kirkengen, A. L., and Hetlevik, I., 'Might a Systematic Reading of the Thickest GP Patient Medical Records Improve our Understandings of Functional Disorders', *La Prensa Medica Argentina*, 101:5 (2015), 1–5.

Nicholls, D., 'Breathlessness: A Qualitative Model of Meaning', *Physiotherapy*, 86:1 (2000), 23–27.

Noble, S. U., *Algorithms of Oppression: How Search Engines Reinforce Racism* (New York: New York University Press, 2018).

Noble, W. G., *Assessment of Impaired Hearing: A Critique and New Method* (New York: Academic Press, 1978).

Norman, A., *Ask Me about My Uterus* (New York: Nation Books, 2018).

Nuttall, F. W., 'Body Mass Index: Obesity, BMIT, and Health: A Critical Review', *Nutrition Today*, 50:3 (2015), 117–128.

Olopade, C. O., Frank, E., Bartlett, E., Alexander, D., Dutta, A., Ibigbami, T., Adu, D., Olamijulo, J., Arinola, G., Karrison, T., and Ojengbede, O., 'Effect of a Clean Stove Intervention on Inflammatory Biomarkers in Pregnant Women in Ibadan, Nigeria: A Randomised Controlled Study', *Environment International*, 98 (2017), 181–190.

Oshinsk, D. M., *Polio: An American Story* (Oxford: Oxford University Press, 2006).

Oxley, R., and Macnaughton, J., 'Inspiring Change: Humanities and Social Science Insights into the Experience and Management of Breathlessness', *Current Opinion in Supportive & Palliative Care*, 10:3 (2017), 256–261.

Padden, C., and Humphries, T., *Inside Deaf Culture* (Cambridge, MA: Harvard University Press, 2005).

Peden, G. C., *British Rearmament and the Treasury: 1932–1939* (Edinburgh: Scottish Academic Press, 1979).

Pepys, J., and Bernstein, L., 'Historical Aspects of Occupational Asthma', in L. Bernstein, M. Chan-Yeung and J. L. Malo (eds), *Asthma in the Workplace* (New York: Marcel Dekker Inc., 1999), pp. 1–28.

Perchard, A., and Gildart, K., ' "Buying Brains and Experts": British Coal Owners, Regulatory Capture and Miners' Health', *Labor History*, 56:4 (2015), 459–480.

Perez, C. C., *Invisible Women: Exposing Data Bias in a World Designed for Men* (London: Chatto & Windus, 2019).

Perry, C. R., 'The British Experience', in I. D. Pool (ed.), *The Social Impact of the Telephone* (Cambridge, MA: MIT Press, 1977), pp. 69–96.

Petty, C., 'Primary Research and Public Health: The Prioritization of Nutrition Research in Interwar Britain', in J. Austoker and L. Bryder (eds), *Historical Perspectives on the Role of the MRC: Essays in the History of the Medical Research Council of the United Kingdom and Its Predecessor, the Medical Research Committee, 1913–1953* (Oxford: Oxford University Press, 1989), pp. 83–108.

Pinch, T., and Bijker, W. E., 'The Social Construction of Facts and Artifacts: Or How the Sociology of Science and the Sociology of Technology Might Benefit Each Other', *Social Studies of Science*, 14:3 (1984), 399–431.

Pinch, T., and Oudshoorn, N. (eds), *How Users Matter: The Co-Construction of Users and Technology* (Cambridge, MA: MIT Press, 2005).

Porter, T. M., 'Objectivity as Standardization: The Rhetoric of Impersonality in Measurement, Statistics, and Cost-Benefit Analysis', in A. Megill (ed.), *Rethinking Objectivity* (Durham, NC and London: Duke University Press, 1994), pp. 197–237.

Porter, T. M., 'Measurement, Objectivity, and Trust', *Measurement: Interdisciplinary Research and Perspectives*, 1:4 (2003), 241–255.

Prescott, H. M., 'Using the Student Body: College and University Students as Research Subjects in the United States during the Twentieth Century', *Journal of the History of Medicine and Allied Sciences*, 57:1 (2002), 3–38.

Quadrelli, S., Roncoroni, A., and Montiel, G., 'Assessment of Respiratory Function: Influence of Spirometric Reference Values and Normality Criteria Selection', *Respiratory Medicine*, 93 (1999), 523–535.

Quanjer, Ph. H., Tammeling, G. J., Cotes, J. E., Pedersen, O. F., Peslin, R., and Yernault, J. C., 'Lung Volumes and Forced Ventilatory Flows: Report Working Party Standardization of Lung Function Tests, European Community for Steel and Coal', *European Respiratory Journal Supplement*, 6 (1993), 5–40.

Raghavan, D., Varkey, A., and Bartter, T., 'Chronic Obstructive Pulmonary Disease: The Impact of Gender', *Current Opinion in Pulmonary Medicine*, 23:2 (2017), 117–123.

Rasmussen, N., 'Downsizing Obesity: On Ancel Keys, the Origins of BMI, and the Neglect of Excess Weight as a Health Hazard in the United States from the 1950s to 1970s', *The History of the Behavioral Sciences*, 55:4 (2019), 299–318.

Reid, F., *Broken Men: Shell Shock, Treatment and Recovery in Britain 1914–30* (London: Continuum, 2010).

Rose, T., *The End of Average* (London: Allen Lane, 2016).

Rosenberg, N., *Exploring the Black Box: Technology, Economics, and History* (Cambridge: Cambridge University Press, 1994).

Sacks, O., *Seeing Voices: A Journey into the World of the Deaf* (Berkeley and Los Angeles: University of California Press, 1989).

Saini, A., *Inferior: The True Power of Women and the Science that Shows It* (London: HarperCollins, 2017).

Savage, M., 'Call for Poor and Disabled to Be Given NHS Fitness Trackers', *The Observer*, 5 May 2019. https://www.theguardian.com/inequality/2019/may/04/fitbits-nhs-reduce-inequality-health-disability-poverty. Accessed July 2019.

Schwyter, J. R., *Dictating to the Mob: The History of the BBC Advisory Committee on Spoken English* (Oxford: Oxford University Press, 2016).

Scull, A., *Hysteria: The Disturbing History* (Oxford: Oxford University Press, 2009).

Scully, J. L., 'From "She Would Say That, Wouldn't She?" to "Does She Take Sugar?" Epistemic Injustice and Disability', *International Journal of Feminist Approaches to Bioethics*, 11:1 (2018), 106–124.

Shakespeare, T., 'The Social Model of Disability: An Outdated Ideology?', *Research in Social Science and Disability*, 2 (2002), 9–28.

Shakespeare, T., *Disability Rights and Wrongs Revisited* (London: Routledge, 2nd edn, 2013).

Shakespeare, T., 'The Social Model of Disability', in L. J. Davis (ed.), *The Disability Studies Reader* (London: Routledge, 4th edn, 2013), pp. 214–221.
Shakespeare, T., 'Nasty, Brutish, and Short? On the Predicament of Disability and Embodiment', in J. E. Bickenback, F. Felder and B. Schmitz (eds), *Disability and the Good Human Life* (Cambridge: Cambridge University Press, 2014), pp. 93–112.
Shim, J. K., *Heart-Sick: The Politics of Risk, Inequality, and Heart Disease* (New York: New York University Press, 2014).
Showalter, E., *The Female Malady: Women, Madness and English Culture, 1830–1980* (London: Penguin Books, 1987).
Shulman, S., *The Telephone Gambit: Chasing Alexander Graham Bell's Secret* (New York: Norton, 2008).
Smith, B. E., 'Black Lung: The Social Production of Disease', *International Journal of Health Services*, 11:3 (1981), 343–359.
Smith, D., and Horrocks, S., 'Defining Perfect and Not-So-Perfect Bodies: The Rise and Fall of the "Dreyer Method" for the Assessment of Physique and Fitness, 1918–26', in J. Sobal and D. Maurer (eds), *Weighty Issues: Fatness and Thinness as Social Problems* (London: Routledge, 1999), pp. 74–94.
Spathis, A., Booth, S., Moffat, C., Hurst, R., Ryan, R., Chin, C., and Burkin, J., 'The Breathing, Thinking, Functioning Clinical Model: A Proposal to Facilitate Evidence-Based Breathlessness Management in Chronic Respiratory Illness', *NPJ Primary Care Respiratory Medicine*, 27:1 (2017), 1–6.
Spriggs, E. A., 'The History of Spirometry', *British Journal of Diseases of the Chest*, 72 (1978), 165–180.
Stanojevic, S., Wade, A., and Stocks, J., 'Reference Values for Lung Function: Past, Present and Future', *European Respiratory Journal*, 36:1 (2010), 12–19.
Stephens, E., 'The Object of Normality: The Search for Norma Competition', Queer Objects Symposium Paper, October 2014. https://www.academia.edu/8893077/The_Object_of_Normality_The_Search_for_Norma_Competition. Accessed May 2019.
Sterling, B., 'The Hacker Crackdown: Evolution of the US Telephone Network', in N. W. Heap (ed.), *Information Technology and Society* (London: Sage, 1995), pp. 33–40.
Sterne, J., *The Audible Past: Cultural Origins of Sound Reproduction* (Durham, NC: Duke University Press, 2003).
Stokes, M., '"What Does fMRI Measure?" Brain Metrics: How Measuring Brain Biology Can Explain the Phenomena of Mind', *Nature Blog*, 16 May 2019. https://www.nature.com/scitable/blog/brain-metrics/what_does_fmri_measure/. Accessed May 2019.
Stone, D., *Breeding Superman: Nietzsche, Race and Eugenics in Edwardian and Interwar Britain* (Liverpool: Liverpool University Press, 2002).
Sumner, J., and Gooday, G., 'Introduction: Does Standardization Make Things Standard?', *History of Technology*, 28 (2008), 1–13.
Szanton, S. L., Gill, J. M., and Allen, J. K., 'Allostatic Load: A Mechanism of Socioeconomic Health Disparities?', *Biological Research for Nursing*, 7:1 (2010), 7–15.

Thaczyk, V., 'Archival Traces of Applied Research: Language Planning and Psychotechnics in Interwar Germany', *Technology and Culture*, 60:2 (2019), 564–595.
Thompson, E., *The Soundscape of Modernity* (Cambridge, MA: MIT Press, 2002).
Timmermans, C., and Berg, M., *The Gold Standard: The Challenge of Evidence-Based Medicine and Standardization in Health Care* (Philadelphia: Temple University Press, 2003).
Turner, D., and Blackie, D., *Disability in the Industrial Revolution: Physical Impairment in British Coalmining, 1780–1880* (Manchester: Manchester University Press, 2018).
Ueyama, T., *Health in the Marketplace: Professionalism, Therapeutic Desires, and Medical Commodification in Late Victorian London* (Palo Alto, CA: Society for the Promotion of Science and Scholarship, 2010).
Valier, H., and Timmermans, C., 'Clinical Trials and the Reorganization of Medical Research in Post-Second World War Britain', *Medical History*, 52 (2008), 493–510.
Van den Bergh, O., Witthoft, M., Petersen, S., and Brown, R. J., 'Symptoms and the Body: Taking the Inferential Leap', *Neuroscience and Behavioral Reviews*, 74 (2017), 1–79.
Van der Kloot, W., 'Lawrence Bragg's Role in the Development of Sound-Ranging in World War I', *Notes and Records of the Royal Society*, 59:3 (2005), 273–284.
Vargha, D., *Polio across the Iron Curtain: Hungary's Cold War with an Epidemic* (Cambridge: Cambridge University Press, 2018).
Virdi [Virdi-Dhesi], J., 'Curtis's Cephaloscope: Deafness and the Making of Surgical Authority in London, 1816–1845', *Bulletin of the History of Medicine*, 87:3 (2013), 347–377.
Virdi [Virdi-Dhesi], J., 'From the Hands of Quacks: Aural Surgery, Deafness, and the Making of a Surgical Speciality in 19th-Century London' (PhD dissertation, University of Toronto, 2014).
Virdi, J., 'Between Cure and Prosthetic: "Good Fit" in Artificial Eardrums', in C. Jones (ed.), *Rethinking Modern Prostheses in Anglo-American Commodity Cultures, 1820–1939* (Manchester: Manchester University Press, 2017), pp. 48–69.
Virdi, J., 'Prevention and Conservation: Historicizing the Stigma of Hearing Loss, 1910–1940', *Journal of Law, Medicine and Ethics*, 45:4 (2017), 531–344.
Virdi, J., *Hearing Happiness: Fakes, Frauds, and Fads in Deafness Cures* (Chicago: University of Chicago Press, forthcoming).
Virdi, J., and McGuire, C., 'Phyllis M. Tookey Kerridge and the Science of Audiometric Standardisation in Britain', *British Journal for the History of Science*, 51:1 (2018), 123–146.
Wakefield, J. C., 'The Biostatistical Theory versus the Harmful Dysfunction Analysis, Part 1: Is Part-Dysfunction a Sufficient Condition for Medical Disorder?', *Journal of Medicine and Philosophy*, 39:6 (2014), 648–682.
Wallis, J., 'A Machine in the Garden: The Compressed Air Bath and the Nineteenth-Century Health Resort', in J. Agar and J. Ward (eds), *Histories of Technology, the Environment and Modern Britain* (London: UCL Press, 2018), pp. 76–100.
Waring, M., *If Women Counted: A New Feminist Economics* (London: Macmillan, 1989).

Warman, C., 'From Pre-Normal to Abnormal: The Emergence of a Concept in Late Eighteenth-Century France', *Psychology & Sexuality*, 1:3 (2010), 200–213.

Wasserman, D., and Asch, A., 'Understanding the Relationship between Disability and Well-Being', in J. E. Bickenback, F. Felder and B. Schmitz (eds), *Disability and the Good Human Life* (Cambridge: Cambridge University Press, 2014), pp. 139–167.

Weber, R. N., 'Manufacturing Gender in Commercial and Military Cockpit Design', *Science, Technology, and Human Values*, 22:2 (1997), 235–253.

Williams, T., and Carel, H., 'Breathlessness: From Bodily Symptom to Existential Experience', in K. Aho (ed.), *Existential Medicine: Essays on Health and Illness* (London: Rowman & Littlefield, 2018), pp. 145–159.

Williamson, B., 'Electric Moms and Quad Drivers: People with Disabilities Buying, Making, and Using Technology in Postwar America', *American Studies*, 52:1 (2012), 5–30.

Wilson, D., 'Calculable People? Standardising Assessment Guidelines for Alzheimer's Disease in 1980s Britain', *Medical History*, 61:4 (2017), 500–525.

Wilson, D. J., *Living with Polio: The Epidemic and Its Survivors* (Chicago: University of Chicago Press, 2005).

Woods, B., and Watson, N., 'In Pursuit of Standardization: The British Ministry of Health's Model 8F Wheelchair, 1948–1962', *Technology and Culture*, 45:3 (2003), 540–568.

Worboys, M., 'The Hamilton Rating Scale for Depression: The Making of a "Gold Standard" and the Unmaking of a Chronic Illness, 1960–1980', *Chronic Illness*, 9:3 (2012), 202–219.

Wyatt, S., 'Non-Users Also Matter: The Construction of Users and Non-Users of the Internet', in T. Pinch and N. Oudshoorn (eds), *How Users Matter: The Co-Construction of Users and Technology* (Cambridge, MA: MIT Press, 2005), pp. 67–79.

Young, I. M., *On Female Body Experience: 'Throwing Like a Girl' and Other Essays* (Oxford: Oxford University Press, 2005).

Index

Page numbers in **bold** refer to figures.

accent 6, 70, 100n52
advertisements 117–118, 120–124
advertising 82, **84**, 106, 119–120, 122, 124
age 4, 24, 43–44, 52, 70, 75, 120, 144–145, 164
allostatic load theory 44–45, 142
ambulatory oxygen *see* oxygen
American–English 113
American Telephone and Telegraph company *see* AT&T
Amplivox 88, 111, 119
Amundson, Ron 41–42, 46, 55, 59, 205
Anderson, Julie 19
army 70, 72–73, 113, 117, 145
 see also military
artificial respiration 178, 180–181, 183–184
AT&T (American Telephone and Telegraph company) 94–95
audiogram 109, 112, 202
 see also zero line
audiology 108, 114
average 3, 15–16, 36, 66, 78–79, 95, 114, 147, 193–194, 205–206, 208

Barnes, Elizabeth 38, 41, 51–52, 53, 56, 208
Baynton, Douglas 8, 9
BBC 36, 113, 182
Behnke, Emil 149
Bell, Alexander Graham 5, 9, 66, 112
bell curve 21–22, 39
Bell Laboratories 77, 95, 107, 112, 114
biomedicine 24, 206–207
biopower 24, 25, 60, 204
bio-statistical theory *see* BST
blended measurement *see* measurement
blind 75–76, 110
Bloor, Michael 153
BMI (Body Mass Index) 1, 13–14, 44

Body Mass Index *see* BMI
bone conduction 79, 86, 111, 114, 125
Boorse, Christopher 39, 40, 49, 58
Bouk, Dan 23
Bourke, Joanna 15
Bowker and Star 144
Bragg–Paul pulsator 175, 179, 181–185, 188, **189**, 190, 207
Braun, Lundy 24, 47–48, 58, 80, 141, 157, 160, 163
breathlessness 7, 18, 19, 20, 146, 153–155, 157, 159, 163, 175, 191, 206
 measurement of 2, 20, 140
 see also dyspnoea
Bridgeman Report *see* reports
British Medical Journal see publications
Brompton Hospital 174, 194
Browne, Lennox 149
BST (bio-statistical theory) 39–43, 48, 61n16
Buckley H. C. 83–84

Canguilhem, Georges 15
Carel, Havi 18, 38, 56–57, 131, 154, 176, 180
children 4, 9, 11, 22, 74, 77, 79, 112, 113–115, 119, 132, 191
chronic fatigue 58, 206
complex obstructive pulmonary disease *see* COPD
 see also pneumoconiosis
class *see* social, class
classification 4, 8, 11, 23–24, 28, 43, 46–49, 53, 60, 95, 97, 109, 117, 141, 144, 159, 160, 164, 203, 208
classified 1, 49, 59, 74, 111, 122, 142, 207
clinic *see* hearing, clinic
Committee on Physical Deterioration 7

compensation 4, 18, 26–28, 47–48, 59, 66, 105, 108, 113–114, 140, 154–160, 162–163, 202–203, 207–8
  see also welfare
Cooper, Rachel 41, 43, 49
COPD (complex obstructive pulmonary disease) 47, 164
corsetry 147, 148–149, 150
costal breathing 148–149, 150
Cotes, John E. 150–153
Cryle and Stephens 15
curse of Kelvin 12, 114

Darwin, Charles 21
Davis, Lennard 4, 5, 8
deafened 18, 66–67, 74–76, 96, 98n17, 106, 114–117, 121
  see also noise–induced hearing loss
Deafened Ex-Service Men's Fund 75, 115, 123
Deaf history 18
Deaf Subscribers 66–67, 82, **84**, 85, 87–89, 106, 124, 127, 130
decibel 14, 106, 107, 112, 118, 120, 144, 206
degeneration 7, 11, 25, 202
  see also eugenic
Disabilities Act 50
disability
  data gap 26, 42, 66–67, 146, 163, 205
  history 1, 5, 8, 17–18
  invisible 2, 25, 28, 37, 58, 85, 175, 194
  measurement of 17, 39, 207
  paradox 54, 193
  studies 17, 18, 49, 97
doctor 109, 120, 122, 157–158, 162, 183, 188, 190, 192
  see also physician
Doll, Richard 12, 151, 168n71
dresses 131, 147–148
Dreyer, Georges 144–146
Drinker device 181–183, 185, **186**, 188, 190–191
  see also iron lung
Drinker, Philip 181
dust 155, 159, 162

dyspnoea 19, 163–164, 191
  see also breathlessness

Ellis, Havelock 148–149
embodied knowledge 27, 58, 86–88, 175, 194–195, 204, 207
  see also subjective, experience
England 184
  see also parentage, English
Enke, Julia 111
epistemic injustice 17, 37, 57–59, 91
  see also mechanical epistemic injustice
Epstein, Steven 3, 43–46, 207
eugenic 4, 7–8, 69, 25, 74, 202
  see also degeneration; eugenicists
eugenicists 25, 117
European Coal and Steel Community 153

Faulkner, Joan 151–152, 168n71
Final Report of the Anthropometric Committee of the British Association for the Advancement of Science see reports
First World War 66, 68–70, 72, 74–76, 109, 110, 124, 144–145, 150, 178–179, 202
fMRI see MRI
Foucault, Michel 24
Fremantle, Sir Francis Edward 123

Galton, Francis 7, 21, 22, 147
GDP (Gross Domestic Product) 14
gender, 9, 25, 44, 48, 141–142, 208
  see also sex
gendered imperative 118
  see also sex differences
Gilson, John C. 152–153, 160, 162
Goldberg, Daniel 6
Gooday, Graeme 12–13, 75, 117–118
Gotzsche, Peter 16–17
Gould, Stephen Jay 8, 21–22, 52
Gross Domestic Product see GDP

Hacking, Ian 8, 23, 24, 46
Haldane, John Scott 155, 178
Harris, Raymond 86–89, 90
Hart, Phillip D'arcy 158, 160, 162

Health and Safety Executive *see* HSE
hearing
    aid 67, 70, 72, 74, 79, 88, 91, 94, 106,
        111, 115–119, 120, 122–126,
        127, 128–129, 130, 131–132
    clinic 115
    loss 5–6, 10–11, 17–18, 26–27,
        37, 65–97 *passim*, 105–132
        passim, 144, 175, 206–207
    measurement of 2, 6, 67, 109
    norms of 67, 205
        see also norms
    pass as 85, 97, 111
heart disease 4, 23–24, 44, 141–142, 206
hedonic
    adaptation 55
    psychology 38, 54–55
Heggie, Vanessa 25, 178
height 3–4, 8, 13, 21, 41, 43–44,
    143–145, 148, 162, 164
hospital 14, 146, 155, 174, 178,
    181–182, 190–191, 194
HSE (Health and Safety
    Executive) 150–52
Hutchinson, John 142–145, 147–148
hysteria 49, 111
hysterical 17, 59, 76, 110, 111, 191, 206

intersectional 48, 204, 208
intersectionality 131
invisible disability *see* disability,
    invisible
IQ 13, 22, 23
iron lung 180, 181, 185, 192
    see also Drinker device

Jewson, Nicolas 6

Kay, Michael 67, 108
Kerridge, Phyllis Margaret Tookey 4, 85,
    91, 114–115, 118, 194
Kingma, Elselijn 40, 47, 49
Kudlick, Catherine 9

Lancet, The see publications
life insurance 8, 13, 23, 143

Life of Breath Project 19, 140
lip–reading 111, 113, 116
    see also oralism
lung
    capacity 7, 16, 27, 141, 143–144,
        149, 162
        see also vital capacity
    function 25, 44, 47, 144, 150–151,
        153, 160, 162–164
    volume 141, 158, 162

Macnaughton, Jane 14, 154–155
malingerers 17, 59, 76, 111, 146, 206
malingering 105, 110, 111, 146
mean *see* average
measurement
    blended 14
    ease of 3, 12–13, 17
    indirect 13–14
        see also proxy measures
    instruments 3, 37, 154
    objective 2, 20, 67, 107, 153
    quantitative 6, 23, 109
    technologies 2, 5, 13, 19
mechanical epistemic injustice 17, 28,
    37–38, 110, 124, 194, 206
    see also epistemic injustice
mechanical objectivity 5–7, 26
Medical Research Council *see* MRC
Medresco 79, 106, 124–126, 128, **130**
Melling, Joseph 155–157, 160
men 3, 16, 22–24, 26, 52–53, 66,
    75–78, 129, 130–131, 141, 144,
    146–147, 148–149, 150, 153,
    158–160, 162, 164
Milan Conference (1880) 9
military 71–73, 111, 114, 116,
    145–146, 179
    assessment 11
    hospitals 11
    industrial complex 17, 108, 113,
        202, 207
    see also army
Mills, Mara 88, 94–95, 99n30, 112, 118
miners 7, 141–142, 146, 155–159,
    160, 162

INDEX

miners' lung 150, 154
  see also pneumoconiosis
mining 150, 154, 155–156, 158, 162
Ministry of Health, 69, 106, 124–129, 132, 182
Ministry of Pensions 69, 106, 110, 116, 128
Mousley, Mr 90–91
MRC (Medical Research Council) 8, 11, 12, 27, 58, 106, 113–114, 125, 144–145, 150–154, 156–159 160, **161**, 162–163, 175, 184–185, 187–188, 190, 194, 202, 205
MRI 14, 163
music 106, 125, 131

National Benevolent Society 75, 115, 117
National Bureau for the Promotion of the General Welfare of the Deaf (the Bureau) 74, 75, 79
National Health Act 129
National Health Service see NHS
National Institute for the Deaf see NID
National Insurance Act 11, 69, 74–75
nationalised 5, 26, 68, 70, 94
National Telephone Company see NTC
naturalist account 36–37, 39, 42, 49, 59, 206
  see also bio-statistical theory
natural kinds 46, 144
NHS (National Health Service) 116, 124, 126–128, 132, 203
NID (National Institute for the Deaf) 79, 106, 109, 113, 119, 120–123
noise 18, 106–107, 120, 144, 182, 187
noise-induced hearing loss 66, 69, 109, 114
  see also deafened
Norma and Normman 15–16
normality 16, 20, 36, 43, 59, 115, 145
normativism 38–39, 49
norms 2, 15, 22, 28, 38, 53, 57, 67, 97, 117, 205
  see also hearing, norms of
NTC (National Telephone Company) 5, 10, 68–69, 77, 81

NTC report see reports

oralism 9, 113, 29n3
  see also lip-reading
oxygen 174, 176–179
  ambulatory 176

parentage
  English 162
  Welsh 160
patent medicines 122, 138n121
  Act 122
  Report of the Select Committee on
    see reports
Perez, Caroline Criado 2–3
physician 43, 52, 80, 174, 190–191
  see also doctor
pneumoconiosis 27, 58, 156, 159, 160, 162
  see also COPD; miners' lung; silicosis
Pneumoconiosis Research Unit
  see PRU
polio 175, 184, 188, 190–192
Porter, Ted 8, 23
Postmaster General 68, 83, 90, 121–123
Post Office
  Engineering Department 68, 73, 81, 83, 92, 107, 124–127
  engineers 5, 76, 78, 87–88, 106, 108, 125, 129
  Post Office Electrical Engineer's Journal
    see publications
  signal services 72
  Telecommunications Department 10, 11, 68–69, 81, 88, 90, 124, 127
Prescott, Heather 16
Priestley, Joseph 176–177
prosthetic 42, 83, 85, 97, 128, 176, 191, 193, 175–176, 191, 193, 207
proxy measures 13–14, 44, 106, 205
  see also measurement, indirect
PRU (Pneumoconiosis Research Unit) 150–152, 163
psychological 55, 76, 111, 146, 154, 187

publications
- *British Medical Journal* 85, 91, 109–110, 123, 146, 163, 179
- *Lancet, The* 110–111, 113–114, 119, 145, 192
- *Post Office Electrical Engineer's Journal* 73–74
- *Times, The* 121, 123

quacks 118–119, 123
Quetelet, Adolphe 13, 21

race 4, 21, 25, 38, 43, 44, 47, 77, 142, 144–145, 148, 162–163
   differences 47, 162
   groupings 23, 25, 45
   Welsh 162
randomised control trial 12
reference classes 4, 26, 37, 38, 42–46, 48, 52, 60, 204
rejection 28, 67, 188, 194–195
Repeater 9A 82, 86–87
   see also telephone service for the deaf
Repeater 17A 76, 84, 89, 129
   see also telephone service for the deaf
Repeater 17B 89, 90
   see also telephone service for the deaf
reports
   Bridgeman 10, 68
   NTC 77
   of the Anthropometric Committee of the British Association for the Advancement of Science 147
   of the Select Committee on Patent Medicines 121–122
Respirators (Poliomyelitis) Committee 184

scales 13–15, 144
Scotland 21, 162
Scottish accent 100n52
Second World War 12, 25, 66, 108, 113–114, 124, 190
self-tracking 203–204
sex 4, 25, 38, 43, 44, 77, 144–145, 147
   see also gender

sex differences 3, 23, 147, 164
   see also gendered imperative
sexuality 148
Shakespeare, Tom 50, 51, 56
shell shock 76, 109, 110, 146
Shim, Janet 4, 44, 141
silicosis 146, 154–156, 158, 162
   see also pneumoconiosis; Various Industries (Silicosis) Scheme
Smith Brothers 80–81
smokers 43, 164
smoking 153
social
   class 4, 9, 25, 38, 44, 66, 120, 143, 145
   groups 3, 4, 7, 27, 45, 48, 58–59, 144
   kinds *see* natural kinds
   model of disability 18–19, 50–53, 208
somatic conditions 37, 110, 206
stamp books 120–121, 124
statistics 1, 3–5, 11–12, 14, 22, 154
stigma 85, 96, 117–118, 131
subjective
   experience 2, 20, 28
   see also embodied knowledge
   individuality 20, 140

Telegraph Act (1869) 5, 68, 98n12
telephone service for the deaf 66–67, 74, 77, 79, **89**
   see also Repeater 9A; Repeater 17A; Repeater 17B
telephone system 5–6, 26, 69, 90, 94–96, 106–107
   see also trench, telephony
Thackray Museum 143
Thompson, Emily 107, 114
Times, The see publications
Treasury 10, 68, 82, 124
trench
   telephony 70, 73–74
   warfare 72, 76
tuberculosis 11, 155–156
tuning forks 3, 66, 108, 110
Turner, William Alden 110

US 1, 17, 22, 23, 25, 68, 82, 107, 113, 185, 192–193

users 7, 19, 26, 28, 67, 80, 86–88, 94, 96–97, 124, 126, 128, 131, 176, 187, 192, 194–195, 207

valves 73–74, 81, 82, 84, 87, 91–92, 113, 119
Various Industries (Silicosis) Scheme 156, 158
see also silicosis
Victorian 7, 147, 155, 159
Virdi, Jaipreet 108, 113
vital capacity 141, 143, 145, 175
see also lung, capacity

Wales 150, 156, 158, **160**, 163, 184
see also parentage, Welsh; race, Welsh
Waring, Marilyn 14
Weber, Rachel 16, 80
weight 3–4, 8, 13, 21, 43–44, 144–145, 148, 162, 179, 186

welfare 10, 37, 69, 83, 117, 202
see also compensation
well-being 51, 53–56, 57, 58, 128–129, 193
WHO (World Health Organization) 1, 16, 48
women 3–4, 44, 77, 118, 129, 130–131, 140–141, 147–149, 150, 152–153, 164
Workmen's Compensation Act 156
World Health Organization *see* WHO
World War One *see* First World War
World War Two *see* Second World War

X-ray 155, 157–159, 160, 162

zero line 95, 115
see also audiogram

EU authorised representative for GPSR:
Easy Access System Europe, Mustamäe tee 50,
10621 Tallinn, Estonia
gpsr.requests@easproject.com